T0155868

The Psychiatric Report

Principles and Practice of Forensic Writing

The Psychiatric Report

Principles and Practice of Forensic Writing

Edited by

Alec Buchanan

Associate Professor, Law and Psychiatry Division, Department of Psychiatry, Yale University School of Medicine, New Haven, CT, USA

Michael A. Norko

Associate Professor, Law and Psychiatry Division, Department of Psychiatry, Yale University School of Medicine, New Haven, CT, USA

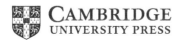

CAMBRIDGE
UNIVERSITY PRESS

CAMBRIDGE
UNIVERSITY PRESS

University Printing House, Cambridge CB2 8BS, United Kingdom

One Liberty Plaza, 20th Floor, New York, NY 10006, USA

477 Williamstown Road, Port Melbourne, VIC 3207, Australia

314-321, 3rd Floor, Plot 3, Splendor Forum, Jasola District Centre, New Delhi - 110025, India

103 Penang Road, #05-06/07, Visioncrest Commercial, Singapore 238467

Cambridge University Press is part of the University of Cambridge.

It furthers the University's mission by disseminating knowledge in the pursuit of
education, learning and research at the highest international levels of excellence.

www.cambridge.org
Information on this title: www.cambridge.org/9780521131841

© Cambridge University Press 2011

First published 2011

A catalogue record for this publication is available from the British Library

Library of Congress Cataloging in Publication data
The psychiatric report : principles and practice of forensic writing / [edited by] Alec Buchanan,
Michael A. Norko.
    p.   cm.
Includes bibliographical references and index.
ISBN 978-0-521-13184-1 (pbk.)
1. Evidence, Expert.   2. Forensic psychiatry.   3. Report writing.   4. Medical writing.
I. Buchanan, Alec.   II. Norko, Michael A.   III. Title.
RA1056.P79 2011
808′.066614–dc22
2011011261

ISBN 978-0-521-13184-1 Paperback

To Aidan (A. B.) and Albert and Anne Norko (M. N.)

Contents

Contributors

Paul S. Appelbaum, MD

Elizabeth K. Dollard Professor of Psychiatry, Medicine & Law; Director, Division of Law, Ethics, and Psychiatry, Department of Psychiatry, Columbia University, New York, NY, USA

Peter Ash, MD

Chief, Division of Child and Adolescent Psychiatry; Director, Psychiatry and Law Service; Associate Professor, Department of Psychiatry and Behavioral Sciences, Emory University, Atlanta, GA, USA

Madelon V. Baranoski, PhD

Associate Professor, Law and Psychiatry Division, Department of Psychiatry, Yale University School of Medicine, New Haven, CT, USA

Alec Buchanan, MD

Associate Professor, Law and Psychiatry Division, Department of Psychiatry, Yale University School of Medicine, New Haven, CT, USA

Philip J. Candilis, MD

Associate Professor, Department of Psychiatry, University of Massachusetts Medical School, Worcester, MA, USA

J. Richard Ciccone, MD

Professor of Psychiatry and Director, Psychiatry and Law Program, Department of Psychiatry, University of Rochester Medical Center, Rochester, NY, USA

Eric Elbogen PhD, ABPP

Associate Professor, Department of Psychiatry, University of North Carolina at Chapel Hill, Chapel Hill, NC, USA

Graham D. Glancy, MB, ChB, FRCPsych, FRCP(C)

Forensic Psychiatrist, Assistant Professor, Department of Psychiatry, University of Toronto, Ontario, Canada

Robert P. Granacher, Jr., MD, MBA

Lexington Forensic Neuropsychiatry, Clinical Professor of Psychiatry, University of Kentucky, College of Medicine, Lexington, KY, USA

Ezra E. H. Griffith, MD

Professor of Psychiatry and African-American Studies, Department of Psychiatry, Yale University School of Medicine, New Haven, CT, USA

Jeffrey S. Janofsky, MD

Associate Professor and Director, Psychiatry and Law Program, Department of Psychiatry and Behavioral Science, Johns Hopkins University, Baltimore, MD, USA

Sally Johnson, MD

Professor, Department of Psychiatry, University of North Carolina at Chapel Hill, Chapel Hill, NC, USA

Joshua Jones, MD

Clinical Assistant Professor of Psychiatry, University of Rochester Medical Center, Rochester, NY, USA

Alyson Kuroski-Mazzei, DO

Clinical Assistant Professor, Department of Psychiatry, University of North Carolina at Chapell Hill, Chapel Hill, NC, USA

Li-Wen Grace Lee, MD
Assistant Clinical Professor, Department of
Psychiatry, Columbia University, New York,
NY, USA

Gregory B. Leong, MD
Clinical Professor of Psychiatry and
Behavioral Sciences, University of
Washington School of Medicine, Seattle,
WA, and Staff Psychiatrist, Center for
Forensic Services, Western State Hospital,
Tacoma, WA, USA

Barbara McDermott, PhD
Professor, Division of Psychiatry and
the Law, Department of Psychiatry
and Behavioral Sciences, University
of California, Davis Medical Center,
Sacramento, CA, USA

Richard Martinez, MD, MH
Robert D. Miller Professor of Psychiatry
and Law, University of Colorado at Denver
Medical Center and Director of Forensic
Programs, Denver Health Medical Center,
Denver, CO, USA

Michael A. Norko, MD
Associate Professor, Law and Psychiatry
Division, Department of Psychiatry, Yale
University School of Medicine,
New Haven, CT, USA

John O'Grady, MB, ChB
Formerly, Consultant Forensic Psychiatrist,
Ravenswood House MSU, Fareham,
Hampshire, UK

Debra A. Pinals, MD
Associate Professor of Psychiatry, Director
of Forensic Education, University of
Massachusetts Medical School, Worcester,
MA, USA

Marilyn Price, MD
Clinical Instructor, Harvard Medical
School, Law and Psychiatry Service,
Massachusetts General Hospital, Boston,
MA, USA

Patricia Ryan Recupero, JD, MD
Clinical Professor of Psychiatry,
Warren Alpert Medical School of
Brown University, President and CEO,
Butler Hospital, Providence,
RI, USA

Phillip J. Resnick, MD
Professor of Psychiatry, Case Western
Reserve University School of Medicine,
Cleveland, OH, USA

Robert L. Sadoff, MD
Clinical Professor of Forensic Psychiatry,
and Director, Forensic Psychiatry
Fellowship Program, University of
Pennsylvania, Philadelphia, PA, USA

Charles Scott, MD
Chief, Division of Psychiatry and the
Law; Clinical Professor of Psychiatry and
Director, Forensic Psychiatry Residency
Program, Department of Psychiatry
and Behavioral Sciences, University
of California, Davis Medical Center,
Sacramento, CA, USA

J. Arturo Silva, MD
Private Practice, Forensic Psychiatry,
San Jose, CA, USA

Sherif Soliman, MD
Senior Clinical Instructor, Case Western
Reserve University, School of Medicine,
Associate Director, Forensic Services,
Northcoast Behavioral Healthcare,
Cleveland Campus, Cleveland,
OH, USA

Aleksandra Stankovic, MA
Research Assistant, Department of
Psychiatry, Yale University School of
Medicine, New Haven, CT, USA

Robert Weinstock, MD
Clinical Professor of Psychiatry,
Department of Psychiatry,
University of California Los Angeles,
CA, USA

Kenneth J. Weiss, MD

Clinical Associate Professor of Psychiatry and Associate Director, Forensic Psychiatry Fellowship Program, University of Pennsylvania School of Medicine, Pennsylvania, PA, USA

Robert M. Wettstein, MD

Clinical Professor of Psychiatry, University of Pittsburgh, Pittsburgh, PA, USA

Cheryl Wills, MD

Assistant Professor of Psychiatry, Case Western Reserve University, Cleveland, OH, USA

Howard Zonana, MD

Professor, Law and Psychiatry Division, Department of Psychiatry, Yale University School of Medicine, New Haven, CT, USA

Foreword

Paul S. Appelbaum

Asked what forensic psychiatrists do, laypeople – and indeed, most psychiatrists – are likely to respond, "Testify in court." The prototypical image of the forensic psychiatrist is the expert in the witness box, and little wonder given the attention to this role by print and broadcast journalists, in cases involving the insanity defense, will contests, and other contentious disputes. Complementing this nearly exclusive focus in the popular media has been a similar concentration of the scholarly and professional literature on expert testimony and its vicissitudes, including debates on what psychiatric experts have to contribute in different types of cases, the legal rules that govern their testimony, and the ethical considerations guiding their behavior.

Forensic psychiatrists are well aware, however, that only a small percentage of cases, whether civil or criminal, ever get to trial, and many "expert witnesses" stay quite busy while only occasionally setting foot in a courtroom. That is because a written report of a psychiatric evaluation of a party to the case or of relevant documentation serves as the basis for settlement, plea bargaining, or other disposition far more frequently than testimony is required. Indeed, one might fairly claim that, despite its near absence from the popular media and its neglect in the professional literature, the *sine qua non* of the function of a forensic expert is the production of a written report embodying his or her findings. And formulating and writing reports turns out to be every bit as challenging a task as ultimately taking the stand.

As the reader prepares to explore this volume with its unique, in-depth look at the forensic psychiatric report, it might be helpful to reflect on some of the ethical principles and their practical consequences that should shape that product. This is not the place for an exhaustive discussion of forensic ethics, and fortunately my views on that topic are well known and available elsewhere. Nor is it an attempt to preempt the more rigorous ethical explorations of the chapters that follow. Rather, I offer some reflections on the overarching ethical considerations that often do and I believe should guide the work of the forensic psychiatrist as he or she crafts the expert's report.

The role of any witness – expert or lay – begins with the presumption that the witness will be truthful, hence the solemn oaths that uniformly precede testimony and the affirmations frequently required on affidavits and other written submissions. Thus, the Ethics Guidelines of the American Academy of Psychiatry and the Law (AAPL), the leading organization of forensic psychiatrists in the United States, suggest that "honesty and striving for objectivity" is one of the hallmarks of an ethical forensic psychiatrist. When examined closely, however, the assertion that an expert should be honest, a seemingly uncontroversial proposition, turns out to contain unexpected complexities. Telling the truth is not as simple a task as it may seem.

We might, to begin with, think about two classes of truth-telling, subjective and objective. *Subjective truth-telling* resembles the common view of honesty, i.e., saying what one believes. A subjectively truthful person does not hold one opinion but express another because doing so will bring financial gain, avoid embarrassment, or win admiration. But truth-telling has another component as well that is captured by the witness's oath "to tell the truth, the whole truth ..." I call this *objective truth-telling* and by that I mean placing the conclusions of a report in a sufficient context that the reader is not misled into believing something that is likely untrue. Objective truth-telling might be thought of as a proactive duty to avoid a sin of omission by volunteering information that allows one's data and conclusions to be more accurately interpreted. This includes noting the limitations of one's evaluation (e.g., lack of sufficient time, absence of important records, uncooperativeness of the evaluee, one's own inexperience) and their consequences for the certainty with which one can state one's opinion. It also encompasses limitations on scientific knowledge that may preclude definitive answers to a question or make even the best assessments inherently tentative. When an expert draws a conclusion that stands in opposition to the weight of the existing literature, that circumstance and its justification ought to be made clear as well.

All this may seem unobjectionable in the abstract, but in formulating a report the forensic psychiatrist faces a variety of temptations and pressures, if not to lie, then at least to "fudge" on both objective and subjective truthfulness. Attorneys are the source of much of this pressure, but some may derive from the people being evaluated and many temptations are endogenous, i.e., their source is forensic psychiatrists themselves.

Attorneys' interests in an expert's report are generally self-evident: they want a document that will provide the maximum assistance possible in winning the case. Hence, attorneys will often ask to see a draft of a report or to discuss the psychiatrist's conclusions prior to the report being written. Typically what follows is an extended negotiation over content and tone. As supportive as a report may seem to a psychiatric expert who genuinely believes that the attorney has a strong case, few legal advocates fail to spot ways in which it could be even better. They may ask for an adjective to be replaced, an inconvenient fact to be omitted, or qualifiers that appear to weaken the conclusion to be dropped. If the expert indicates an intention to write an unfavorable report, the attorney may ask what evidence it would take to change the psychiatrist's mind and then try to persuade the expert that such evidence exists but may have been overlooked.

Sometimes, of course, attorneys are right. Information in a report may be factually incorrect, adjectives can be freighted with unintended meanings, and much information that would ordinarily go into a clinical anamnesis is simply irrelevant to a forensic report. Thus, it is only the overly rigid (and maybe a bit self-righteous) expert, as opposed to the wise one, who says, "I never change my drafts, regardless of what the attorney says." Complicating the assessment of when to respond positively to attorneys' requests are some of the other pressures at play on the forensic psychiatrist. Good attorneys woo their experts, making them feel like valued members of a team that is working together toward a common purpose: a legal victory for the client. The intrinsically human tendency to identify with the group of which one is a part may, in all but imperceptible ways, make it difficult for the expert to judge when to resist an attorney's blandishments. Here is where it may help to recall that the experts' duty of truth-telling is not homologous with the attorney's commitment to zealous advocacy. The "team" metaphor goes just so far in the forensic setting.

The person being evaluated can also be the source of pressure on the forensic psychiatrist to compromise, maybe just a bit, on the truthfulness of the written evaluation. An evaluee may plead for assistance from the psychiatrist or confide that all of his or her hopes for a better life rest on the outcome of the examination. Whether deliberately or not, evaluees can evoke powerful feelings of empathy and pity – perhaps even fantasies of rescue – in the forensic expert. These feelings may be especially potent when the person being evaluated is also the psychiatrist's patient and thus someone to whose well-being the psychiatrist is committed. There are many reasons why it is best to avoid combining forensic and thera-peutic roles (though sometimes – as with Social Security Disability evaluations – that may be impossible, since the Social Security Administration insists on a report from the treating psychiatrist), but this is one of the strongest. It is difficult to put aside loyalties that have become firmly embedded in a relationship with another person, and indeed, in that context, are praiseworthy. Yet, that is precisely what the therapist turned forensic expert must do to produce a truthful report. Certain temptations are best avoided.

Not all threats to the truthfulness of a forensic report are external. A variety of practical and emotional considerations can play on the mind of a forensic expert and influence the shape of the report. At the most basic level, forensic psychiatrists make (or supplement) their livings by working for attorneys, who like any other kind of customer, may well turn elsewhere if not satisfied with the product they receive. Thus, failure to deliver a report that the attorney thinks is maximally useful may not only truncate the expert's engagement in the case at hand, but may – or so the expert may fear – foreclose the possibility of future employ-ment by the attorney and his or her firm. It takes a certain degree of courage to resist the temptation to change a problematic word, shade a conclusion, or drop an offending passage. An old adage, but a true one, suggests that the expert who cannot afford to walk away from any case is the one at greatest risk of having his or her integrity compromised. At a time like that, it is worth recalling that every experienced forensic psychiatrist has at least one story of having told an attorney of an unfavorable conclusion with trepidation, only to hear, "That's what I thought. But I owed it to my client to find out for sure." Indeed, I once had an attor-ney call to ask if I would be willing to do another case precisely because I had returned an unfavorable evaluation in a previous outing and thus, "I know I can trust you."

Marx notwithstanding, money is not the only motivating factor, nor necessarily the most important one, when it comes to influencing a psychiatric report. Most forensic experts covet the big case, with a high-profile defendant or plaintiff, extensive media coverage, and the prospect of impacting a significant verdict. It is immensely gratifying to think of one-self not just as a good forensic psychiatrist, but an important one. But staying in a case like that means being prepared to offer an opinion that assists the party that is employing the psychiatrist, and that is not always possible to do without shading the truth. The temptation to do so may be even more pronounced when the psychiatrist has strong views, most often political or moral, about the favored outcome of the case. Whether it is the belief that big business is always trying to take advantage of the average working person or that psychi-atric facilities should never use physical restraint to control disruptive patients, the chance to promote one's causes and support one's prejudices can be a potent influence on behavior. It may be impractical to suggest avoiding such cases, but at the least participation calls for a degree of caution.

Critical to understanding the impact of these pressures and temptations to veer from adherence to subjective and objective truth is the recognition that very few forensic psychia-trists consciously "sell-out." No one says to himself or herself any of the following: "I can't let my attorney and the defense team down"; "Gee, I feel so badly for this poor guy, the least I can do is to say that he couldn't form a criminal intent"; or "With two kids in college next year, I've got to find some way to increase my income, and if I say what they want in this case, this law firm could be a gold mine of referrals." These forces almost always act below the level of conscious awareness, making the attorney's arguments for altering a report seem just a bit more plausible and the possibility of producing a supportive conclusion well within the range of reasonable inferences from the evidence. Thus, the expert who says, "I could never be corrupted," has missed the point. Few experts can be bought – at least overtly. But we are all susceptible to more potent forces that act on us without our awareness, their surreptitious character offering us "cover" – plausible deniability, if you will – from charges that we were less than truthful.

How then does a forensic expert who wants to perform with integrity resist the effect of pressures that are often unseen? No perfect approach has yet been devised, but such experts are not without stratagems of their own. A good place to start is with awareness of one's vulnerability to these pressures and their potential impact on one's performance. During the report drafting process, a self-aware psychiatrist might ask whether the evidence warrants this favorable turn of phrase or the certainty with which a conclusion is stated, or whether the desire to please the attorney or to be of help to the client is at play. Since we are far from the best judges of our own behavior, it sometimes helps to consult an experienced colleague, who can offer an outside perspective. There are good reasons why lawyers are reluctant to permit their experts to talk about cases with others prior to offering their testimony – such discussions may be discoverable – but there often are ways of presenting issues to another forensic psychiatrist and getting useful feedback without talking about a case per se. Certainly there is usually no reason after the termination of a case why reports cannot be shared – albeit with some redaction to protect the privacy of the parties – to obtain input on one's performance. Formal peer review of forensic reports and testimony may also be available through academic departments, professional associations (such as AAPL), or groups of colleagues.

Truthfulness is a necessary but not sufficient guideline for forensic practice, including in the forensic report. Respect for the people whose cases we are evaluating – what ethicists call simply *respect for persons* – is equally important. Our respect for the humanity of the evaluee in front of us is manifest by making clear our purpose, the party for whom we are working, and the disposition of the information that we obtain in the course of the evaluation. All that, however, precedes the crafting of a report. As the forensic psychiatrist sits at the computer, respecting the evaluee means protecting his or her privacy by excluding irrelevancies from the report. Many staples of a clinical assessment have no place in a forensic evaluation. Although the scope of appropriate information will vary depending on the purpose at hand, early developmental history (e.g., "The defendant wet his bed until he was 7 years old") is unlikely to be relevant to an assessment of a defendant's competence to stand trial and a plaintiff's sexual history (e.g., "She first had intercourse with her boyfriend at age 15") will have little to add to an evaluation of work-related disability. The greater the potential that data have for embarrassing the evaluee, the higher should be the threshold of pertinence for their inclusion. We owe to all persons, wherever we encounter them, the obligation to avoid gratuitous harm, including in the forensic setting.

Once a report is written and, when called for, testimony has been given, the forensic expert's role in a case may be at an end. However, I would suggest that even then the expert has residual obligations to the evaluee that fall under the rubric of respect for their personhood. Not every forensic psychiatrist will agree on the dimensions of those obligations, but I suggest that they extend to ongoing efforts to protect evaluees' privacy, even after the conclusion of the case. As the AAPL Ethics Guidelines frame this, "The psychiatrist maintains confidentiality to the extent possible given the legal context." On its face, this obligation may seem puzzling, especially when a case has been heavily covered in the media. Why should an expert not feel free to discuss it with a reporter, share details with family members, and answer questions from inquisitive friends at social gatherings? The answer, I believe, is that implicit in the interaction with the evaluee is an agreement that he or she will disclose certain information to the examiner for a specific purpose: formulation of an opinion, writing of a report, and testimony in court. Few forensic psychiatrists have failed to be impressed by the general level of openness and the personal details revealed by many subjects of forensic evaluations. Were these evaluees anticipating the forensic psychiatrist taking what he or she learned to Court TV or the local 6 o'clock news, they might not be nearly as forthcoming. Moreover, the frequent retort that after one has testified all the information is already in the public domain is rarely true. There is much that a forensic psychiatrist learns that is not embodied in the report or revealed on the witness stand. Perhaps there is some justification for discussing just that information and no more – but in the heat of a television interview or under a reporter's probing it is not easy to remember what is already in evidence, and hence publicly available, and what is not. As flattering as the attentions of the press may be, they are more safely avoided if one is not to needlessly infringe the evaluee's privacy, even if he or she is now someone who is a very public person.

Surely, there is much more that could be said about forensic psychiatric ethics as they apply to the forensic report. And ethics, of course, are just one of the considerations for the expert as an evaluation is formulated and put on paper. But thinking through the ethics of the process may not be a bad place to start one's exploration of the report writing process, as well as a good place to return from time to time. More practical considerations have a way of forcing themselves to the front of one's mind; ethics often seem theoretical and hence remote from everyday forensic work. Psychiatrists retain their value to the justice system, however, by virtue of their integrity; allow that integrity to be undermined and the contributions of forensic psychiatry quickly unravel. The ethics of our field are central to the entire forensic process, including the writing of the forensic report. As for everything else one needs to know, the chapters that follow are an ideal place to start.

Editors' preface

Alec Buchanan and Michael A. Norko

As the list of contributors indicates, this is a largely American book. Much of the recent literature on report writing comes from the United States. An international literature informs the content of the chapters, however, and the principles underlying successful writing do not respect national boundaries. While the psychiatric report has to acknowledge local needs and conditions, therefore, we have sought to ensure that the ideas presented here are not limited in their application to any particular jurisdiction.

Introduction

Michael A. Norko and Alec Buchanan

The writing of clear, precise examination reports that are cogent and engaging is a practice that lies at the heart of the work in forensic psychiatry. There are many skills that are necessary to successful forensic practice, including the abilities to conduct a productive examination of the subject, distill the most important and relevant information from a large quantity of data, and process information in a rational manner in order to answer the legal questions posed. Yet it is the skill at report writing that largely defines forensic practice; it demarcates evaluators' abilities and demonstrates their usefulness to those who enlist their efforts. The written report illustrates the importance of expert mental health evaluation to critical questions posed by the legal system. It reveals the care and competence with which the evaluation was conducted. It represents the value of the mental health professions and the contributions they make to public life. The written forensic report is thus a highly complex body of work that signifies more than a pragmatic response to the particular questions posed to the evaluator.

The development of skill at forensic report writing requires knowledge, experience, and guidance. Yet, as Wettstein points out, there is relatively little discussion in the literature on the precise subject of report writing; what exists has mostly focused on "mechanics and organization" of reports (Wettstein 2010a, p. 46). It is, of course, necessary to discuss these dimensions of report writing, and much will be said about them in this textbook. But it is also vital to the professional development of forensic evaluators to engage in serious circumspection about the multiple dimensions of the work that are less often or less fully discussed. This, too, is part of the intention of this textbook.

A broader conceptualization of report writing is informed by dynamic and evolving reflections upon the work. Moving beyond the structure of reports, Enfield contributed several conceptual embellishments to descriptions of the forensic report. He described it as a form of expert witness testimony and an example of "applied scientific writing" (Enfield 1987, p. 386). Griffith and Baranoski have conceived of the forensic report as "performative writing" (Griffith & Baranoski 2007). They have challenged the notion that such reports are merely impersonal, objective documents but are inherently complex narratives requiring of the examiner a developed skill in crafting this performative element (Griffith & Baranoski 2007; Griffith et al. 2010). (These ideas are discussed in detail in Chapter 5.)

It has been argued persuasively that forensic report writing is a core competency in forensic practice (Griffith & Baranoski 2007; Simon 2007; Griffith et al. 2010). As one anonymous reviewer of this textbook proposal put it, mental health professionals are often taught to write forensic reports "via folklore and tradition." Proficiency at report writing is more than learning and practicing construction techniques passed down from generation to generation. The complex task of effective report writing can be understand as occupying a

The Psychiatric Report, ed. Alec Buchanan and Michael A. Norko. Published by Cambridge University Press. © Cambridge University Press 2011.

central position in the professional development of the forensic practitioner. This is one perspective on the forensic report, viewing it as a component of professional skill development for certain mental health practitioners. Fleshing out this perspective is the task of much of this textbook, which will explore ethics, narrative, and draftsmanship in addition to a study of preparatory elements, special considerations in the content of various reports, and a range of special issues.

Other perspectives are equally important. The forensic report must also be understood as part of an evolution of professional practice in recent decades. It fulfills various functions that are required by the legal marketplace, and which are integral to a set of interactions between mental health professionals and legal professionals. The forensic report is an instrument of enormous consequence for the individuals evaluated; circumspection is required in the task. Evaluators should reflect upon the nature of professional identity and the presence or absence of normative ethics relevant to a series of overlapping but distinct identities and roles. In this chapter, we will frame some of these perspectives and at least begin their exploration.

Context of the forensic report

The forensic report exists within a universe of rich, complicated, overlapping and sometimes competing connections and interactions among societal, legal, medical, psychological, and professional forces. Forensic evaluators do not simply perform a mental health evaluation and document its results (Griffith & Baranoski 2007). Understanding this work requires an appreciation not only of the subtleties and sophistications of the craft, but of the full context within which the work is conducted.

Effects upon evaluees

It is an obvious point – though rarely discussed – that forensic evaluations and the opinions and wording of written reports hold potentially enormous and irreversible consequences for the evaluee and other legal stakeholders in various disputes (Silva et al. 2003). Thus, society has a significant interest in the skills and ethical behavior of forensic evaluators. Several of the authors in this text have taken up the task of describing various aspects of the ethics of forensic practice and report writing. It is worth being circumspect, in particular, about the effects of forensic reports on the evaluees.

How should health care professionals approach tasks in which the legal questions posed are limited to concerns for the protection of the public? O'Grady asked this question about detention in the United Kingdom under the Mental Health Act (O'Grady 2002). In the United States, a similar question can be posed regarding the various Sexually Violent Predator statutes, which require no promise of treatment in exchange for the loss of liberty. Some authors have argued that forensic evaluators must demonstrate restraint in service delivered to society because of such concerns (see Allnutt & Chaplow 2000). Others argue that service to the state is not problematic if there is simultaneous assistance to the evaluee who will thereby receive beneficial interventions (Mullen 2000). There are situations in which the evaluation report will be the first step toward the evaluee receiving needed clinical services (Enfield 1987). Some forensic determinations simply will not align with the best interests of the evaluee, depending on the perspective taken. That reality, however, does not free the writer to adopt a countertherapeutic tone in the report (Enfield 1987). Whether forensic reports become the connection to countertherapeutic results depends on the outcome of the case except in the unlikely event that the forensic writer clumsily offends the evaluee unnecessarily. If a report leads to a period of incarceration or other detention, the presence or absence of appropriate care in the custody environment would determine the outcome along the countertherapeutic-nonthera-peutic-therapeutic dimension. Whether one sees the report as a nexus to such outcomes or not depends on whether one takes a view that insists upon some direct or indirect benefit to the evaluee as a part of ethical practice or adopts another ethics frame in which the consequence is irrelevant as long as other values like respect for persons and honesty have been promoted.

A related caution has to do with the use of empathy in forensic evaluations. Appelbaum describes "forensic empathy" as the quest for "awareness of the perspectives and experiences of interviewees" in an effort to give voice to their concerns in the report (Appelbaum 2010, p. 44). Shuman distinguishes between "receptive empathy" and "reflective empathy." The former he describes as "the perception and understanding of the experiences of another person." This seems to be the form of empathy that Appelbaum has in mind. Shuman agrees that this is an appropriate use of empathy in forensic evaluations. Reflective empathy, on the other hand, communicates an "interpretation or understanding to the defendant in a man-ner that implies a therapeutic alliance" (Shuman 1993, p. 298). This, of course, undermines the warnings that are given to evaluees at the initiation of the examination about the limits of confidentiality and the lack of a treatment relationship.

Candilis and colleagues describe such receptive empathy as an attitude of the "com-passionate professional" who is drawn into the multiple aspects of the subject's suffering (Candilis et al. 2001, p. 169). Griffith has described the compassionate approach to an eval-uee as part of the task of constructing narrative (Griffith 2005). Simone Weil observed that, "Every created thing is an object for compassion because it is limited" (Weil 1998, p. 143) and that the use of power must be entrusted only to those who understand this obligation toward all human beings (Weil 1998, pp. 137–138). Norko has argued that the use of power in forensic evaluations calls for an ethics construct in which compassion plays a central role (Norko 2005). However one parses these concerns, they are certainly manifest as context for the forensic report that is worth contemplating.

Professional identity and its implications

Wettstein (2010a, 2010b) has provided a listing of ways in which forensic report writers see themselves (see Table 1). How report writers see their role in this context is likely to have at least some effect upon how the role is performed. This has many pragmatic dimensions of style, attitude, quality of interactions, objectives, etc., but also includes an obvious ethics dimension. What rules would simultaneously and adequately cover the scientist and the artist? Or the business person and the policy advocate? Does it matter what the role of self-identity is, as long as the behavior conforms to necessary and appropriate guidelines that apply broadly? This might be part of the consideration in O'Grady's call for a "robust ethical framework" (O'Grady 2002, p. 179) or the notion of "robust professionalism" as developed by Candilis, Martinez, and Dording (Candilis et al. 2001; Martinez & Candilis 2005). (See Chapters 4 and 19 for further discussions.)

Pellegrino has offered a similar list of the various roles which physicians in general have come to play: clinical scientist, body mechanic, businessperson, social servant, and helper/healer (Pellegrino 2003). Pellegrino argues that the role of healer is primary to all the others, and forms the true foundation of medical ethics. He would not look, for example, to a businessperson's ethics and work backward to an ethic of the physician as

Table 1 Possible self-identities of forensic report writers*

Scientist

Clinician

Investigator

Journalist-reporter

Quasi-attorney

Judicial decision-maker

Court educator

Businessperson

Health care administrator

Artist-writer

Policy advocate

* See Wettstein 2010a and 2010b

businessperson. Given that forensic practitioners deliberately eschew the role of healer in conducting forensic evaluations, Pellegrino's alternate theory of virtue ethics may be more workable in relation to role identity. He offers examples of the following virtues for physicians: fidelity to trust, benevolence, effacement of self-interest, compassion and caring, objectivity, courage, intellectual honesty, humility, and prudence (Pellegrino 2003, pp. 14–15). Forensic practice might more easily apply these virtues to the various role identities listed by Wettstein.

Expectations from the legal system

Rix has provided an account of expectations that the court system in the United Kingdom has of its experts as part of the so-called "Woolf Reforms" of 1996 (Rix 1999). Lord Woolf undertook an inquiry to examine needed changes in the civil justice system. The expectations that the courts should have of experts' written reports are listed in Table 2. What the legal system in the UK anticipates from its experts confirms the need for appropriate knowledge, skill, and experience in writing forensic reports. Many of these expectations have face validity. Some have been expressed quite directly in professional guidelines. For example, in conformity to the third item in Table 2, the American Academy of Psychiatry and the Law (AAPL) guidelines for competency to stand trial evaluation reports make the explicit recommendation that the writer "should also state clearly any limitations or qualifications of which the psychiatrist is aware" (Mossman et al. 2007, p. S48). It is one of our objectives in this textbook to articulate the principles of practice in the forensic report that would fulfill expectations such as those proposed by the legal system in the UK.

There are some items here that are worthy of additional comment. The issue of the expert forming an "independent view" of suggestions made to the expert by outside sources is not often discussed explicitly. This might include comments from counsel, hoping to influence the expert's thinking. It might also include the "voices" of evaluees or collateral informants hoping to have their viewpoints validated. Evaluators should consider all sources of

Table 2 Courts' expectations of experts' written reports from the "Woolf Reforms"*

The overriding duty is to help the court on matters of the report writer's expertise

The writer believes that the facts of the report are true and opinions expressed are correct and within the writer's field of expertise

Any matters which may affect the validity of the opinions are represented in the report

When there exists a range of opinions about the legal questions posed, the writer summarizes the range of opinion and gives reasons for the writer's chosen opinion

All material instructions given to the writer, and all sources of information, are detailed in the report

Nothing suggested by another party is included or excluded from the report without the writer forming an independent view of it

The writer believes the report to be complete and accurate, and that it describes all matters believed relevant to the expressed opinion

If at any time, the existing report requires correction or qualification, the writer will give written notice of that fact to the appropriate instructing authority

The report is understood to form the evidence that will be given under oath or affirmation

The writer may expect the public adverse criticism of the court if the writer has not taken reasonable care in meeting these standards

The writer confirms that no contingency fees have been arranged for the writer's work in the case

The report is for the sole purpose of assisting those authorities requesting the report, and may not be used for any other purpose

* Adapted from Rix (1999)

information, and represent them in a final report in an authentic manner. Clearly, though, such authentic representation does not presume or prevent the report writer from coming to an independent opinion about the relevant legal matters.

The issue of expressing a range of possible opinions is a point on which there might be a reasonable difference of opinion among forensic report writers. Describing the range of possible opinions and the data supporting each might increase the transparency of the report. It could also lead to greater confusion than clarity. Some report writers might adopt this approach in some cases, but avoid it in others when it would render the report unclear or confusing.

Few experts in the United States would expect public criticism by the court for failing to attend to the expectations for effective report writing. They might expect embarrassment at mistakes revealed under cross-examination, or private criticism for failing to assist retaining counsel appropriately (although the latter is more likely to be manifested by a lack of repeat invitation to participate in forensic work with the attorney). The possibility of public criticism by the court itself for less than satisfactory work would have an interesting effect upon the practice of forensic report writing; perhaps not necessarily an adverse effect on quality, but likely an adverse effect upon the anxiety experienced by many report writers anticipating oral testimony.

Table 3 Academy of Experts' four principal hallmarks of a good report*

A stand-alone, concise, user-friendly format, expressed in the first person singular by the person whose opinion has been given or who adopts as his own the opinion of others

Text which is arranged in short sentences and paragraphs

Judicious use of appendices

Matters of fact being kept separate from matters of opinion

* Reproduced with permission from Rix (1999), p. 157.

Principles, guidelines, and standards

Many clinical practice guidelines are unsuitable as practice standards in that they do not define standards of care or practice. Guidelines should not be developed to articulate a single, acceptable approach, but rather should allow flexibility and a range of potential approaches to the task (see Zonana 2008). Rix has conveyed a similar approach taken by the Academy of Experts in the UK, which is a professional society and an accrediting body concerned with promoting the use of independent experts (Rix 1999). The Academy of Experts has described four principal hallmarks of a good report, which it intends as a model rather than a standard, acknowledging the same concerns as noted by Zonana above (see Table 3).

We stand in agreement with these approaches. We offer a caution that the act of "adopting" the opinions of others (see Table 3) might more readily be described as the notion of coming to agree with an opinion that is shared by another, after thorough and careful review of all relevant data. Rix affirms that "slavish adherence" to the model principles is not required (Rix 1999, p. 159). As an example of adherence to these model principles, Mossman and colleagues make explicit their recommendation for a stand-alone format in the guidelines for competency to stand trial evaluation reports (Mossman et al. 2007, p. S48).

Each of the guidelines for forensic evaluations promulgated by the American Academy of Psychiatry and the Law has made a statement reflecting that there are multiple formats that might be adopted by a writer in a given case (Giorgi-Guarnieri et al. 2002, pp. S24–S25; Mossman et al. 2007, p. S52; Gold et al. 2008, pp. S20–S21). For example, AAPL's practice guideline on insanity defense evaluations includes this statement: "There is no one correct style or format for writing a report" (Giorgi-Guarnieri et al. 2002).

In our planning for this textbook we have adopted that same strategy, including the contributions of colleagues who differ on some issues of report writing. For example, some of our authors are adherents of the strategy of short, concise reports, which are user friendly, and focus attention to the most relevant matters, while others prefer lengthy reports with the belief that they will be more persuasive, more demonstrative of the professional practice involved in the evaluation, and will assist in anticipated oral testimony. There are similar differences of opinion about offering ultimate issue testimony in written or oral form. Some of those differences are derived from jurisdictional proscriptions, but others are matters of preference in professional practice. Differences also exist in the matter of inquiring into a defendant's version of the alleged criminal act during an evaluation of competency to stand trial, again with some jurisdictional constrictions, as specifically described in the AAPL guidelines on competency to stand trial evaluations (Mossman et al. 2007, pp. S35–S36).

It has been our explicit desire to avoid setting standards of practice. We have attempted to develop a rich and far-reaching discussion of principles of practice, acknowledging fair variations within acceptable or even exemplary parameters. Professional efforts in report writing serve many functions and are produced within contexts both internal and external to particular disciplines. Given those realities, no other approach seems reasonable.

Purpose of textbook

Our goal in designing this textbook was to express a comprehensive set of principles of writing the forensic report, taking into account the complexity and variability of report writing tasks. Recent work has begun to address the conceptual issues that frame and instill aspects of forensic writing (Griffith & Baranoski 2007; Appelbaum 2010; Griffith et al. 2010; Wettstein 2010a). This textbook attempts to broaden the inquiry toward a more comprehensive set of tasks, and to formulate the principles that underlie and inform those tasks.

We have decided to sketch the major elements and challenges of effective report writing through a series of 19 chapters organized in 3 conceptual sections. Section 1 ("Principles of writing") explores general principles that apply to the work of any type of forensic report, including processes that prepare the writer to engage the work and conceptual approaches that ought to infuse the writing itself. Section 2 ("Structure and content") examines the essence of principles and practice in various types of forensic report-writing endeavors. In Section 3, several chapters explore a range of topics that we have included under the heading of "Special issues." In the Conclusion, we attempt to identify a number of themes that have emerged in the chapters which precede it, including narrative, respect for persons, ethics, the role of clinical guidelines, and the opportunities for further empirical research related to report writing.

Professionals looking for guidance about aspects of types of reports in which they are not yet fully practiced will find Section 2 of particular interest. We hope that all forensic report writers will consider the ideas presented in Section 1. The special issues raised in Section 3 will apply variously to both particular and common circumstances in report writing.

We have attempted to distill the experience of forensic report writing into a guide meant to both transmit knowledge and insights and to stimulate internal reflection and serious self-examination of one's tangible work and its broader implications. There exists significant variation in styles of practice within generally acceptable professional guidelines. We have asked our authors to focus on abstracting the most important principles of their assigned topics so that they may each be presented in a single, concise chapter. Readers may wish to augment this discussion of principles by referring to the templates and sample reports that are already available in the literature (e.g., Melton et al. 2007; Berger 2008; Greenfield & Gottschalk 2009).

Finally, we counsel readers of the importance of finding opportunities for skillful review of their work by senior colleagues who are willing to share their expertise. This may occur in formal training programs, but should also be found in peer consultation and peer review in the formative stages of forensic practice.

The ability to write effective forensic reports and to be circumspect about the processes, implications, and consequences of forensic report writing will serve mental health professionals well. Their input is continuously required by courts, attorneys, and boards. Performing this work with distinction serves not only the individual practitioner and the legal marketplace, but the mental health professions as a whole. We hope that this textbook will assist our readers in taking their necessary and appropriate places in describing the many and complex issues of mental health and mental illness in the legal arena.

References

Allnutt, S. H. & Chaplow, D. (2000) General principles of forensic report writing. *Australian and New Zealand Journal of Psychiatry* 34: 980–987.

Appelbaum, K. L. (2010) Commentary: the art of forensic report writing. *Journal of the American Academy of Psychiatry and the Law* 38: 43–45.

Berger, S. H. (2008) Template for quickly creating forensic psychiatry reports. *Journal of the American Academy of Psychiatry and the Law* 36: 388–392.

Candilis, P. J., Martinez, R., & Dording. C. (2001) Principles and narrative in forensic psychiatry: toward a robust view of professional role. *Journal of the American Academy of Psychiatry and the Law* 29: 167–173.

Enfield, R. (1987) A model for developing the written forensic report. In *Innovations in Clinical Practice: A Sourcebook*, vol. 6, ed. P. A. Keller & S. R. Heyman. Sarasota, FL: Professional Resource Exchange, Inc., pp. 379–394.

Giorgi-Guarnieri, D., Janofsky, J., Keram, E., et al. (2002) AAPL practice guideline for forensic psychiatric evaluation of defendants raising the insanity defense. *Journal of the American Academy of Psychiatry and the Law* 30 (suppl): S1–S40.

Gold, L. H., Anfang, S. A. S., Drukteinis, A. M., et al. (2008) AAPL practice guideline for the forensic evaluation of psychiatric disability. *Journal of the American Academy of Psychiatry and the Law* 36 (suppl): S1–S50.

Greenfield, D. P. & Gottschalk, J. A. (2009) *Writing Forensic Reports: A Guide for Mental Health Professionals.* New York: Springer Publishing.

Griffith, E. E. H. (2005) Personal narrative and an African-American perspective on ethics. *Journal of the American Academy of Psychiatry and the Law* 33: 371–381.

Griffith, E. E. H. & Baranoski, M. V. (2007) Commentary: the place of performative writing in forensic psychiatry. *Journal of the American Academy of Psychiatry and the Law* 35: 27–31.

Griffith, E. E. H., Stankovic, A., & Baranoski, M. V. (2010) Conceptualizing the forensic psychiatry report as performative narrative. *Journal of the American Academy of Psychiatry and the Law* 38: 32–42.

Martinez, R. & Candilis, P. J. (2005) Commentary: toward a unified theory of personal and professional ethics. *Journal of the American Academy of Psychiatry and the Law* 33: 382–385.

Melton, G. B., Petrila, J., Poythress, N. G., et al. (2007) *Psychological Evaluations for the Courts: A Handbook for Mental Health Professionals and Lawyers*, 3rd edn. New York: Guilford, pp. 606–691.

Mossman, D., Noffsinger, S. G., Ash, P., et al. (2007) AAPL practice guideline for the forensic psychiatric evaluation of competence to stand trial. *Journal of the American Academy of Psychiatry and the Law* 35 (suppl): S1–S72.

Mullen, P. E. (2000) Forensic mental health. *British Journal of Psychiatry* 176: 307–311.

Norko, M. A. (2005) Commentary: compassion at the core of forensic ethics. *Journal of the American Academy of Psychiatry and the Law* 33: 386–389.

O'Grady, J. C. (2002) Psychiatric evidence and sentencing: ethical dilemmas. *Criminal Behaviour and Mental Health* 12: 179–184.

Pellegrino, E. D. (2003) The moral foundations of the patient-physician relationship: the essence of medical ethics. In *Military Medical Ethics*, vol. 1, ed. T. F. Beam & L. R. Sparacino. Washington, DC: The Borden Institute, pp. 5–21.

Rix, K. J. B. (1999) Expert evidence and the courts 2. Proposals for reform, expert witness bodies and 'the model report.' *Advances in Psychiatric Treatment* 5: 154–160.

Shuman, D. W. (1993) The use of empathy in forensic examinations. *Ethics and Behavior* 3: 289–302.

Silva, J. A., Weinstock, R., & Leong, G. B. (2003) Forensic psychiatric report writing. In *Principles and Practice of Forensic Psychiatry*, 2nd edn., ed. R. Rosner. London: Arnold, pp. 31–36.

Simon, R. I. (2007) Authorship in forensic psychiatry: a perspective. *Journal of the*

American Academy of Psychiatry and the Law
35: 18–26.

Weil, S. (1998) *Writings Selected*, with an
Introduction by Eric O. Springsted.
Maryknoll, NY: Orbis Books.

Wettstein, R. M. (2010a)
Commentary: conceptualizing the forensic
psychiatry report. *Journal of the American
Academy of Psychiatry and the Law* **38**:
46–48.

Wettstein, R. M. (2010b) The forensic
psychiatric examination and report. In *The
American Psychiatric Publishing Textbook of
Forensic Psychiatry*, ed. R. I. Simon & L. H.
Gold. Washington, DC: American
Psychiatric Publishing, Inc.,
pp. 175–203.

Zonana, H. (2008) Commentary: When is a
practice guideline only a guideline? *Journal of
the American Academy of Psychiatry and the
Law* **36**: 302–305.

Chapter

History and function of the psychiatric report

Kenneth J. Weiss, Robert M. Wettstein, Robert L. Sadoff,
J. Arturo Silva, and Michael A. Norko

The psychiatric report made a relatively late appearance in psychiatric jurisprudence. This has not prevented it from becoming the primary mechanism by which psychiatric opinions are communicated to courts. Today, the written report informs legal decisions in the absence of oral testimony (Silva et al. 2003). This chapter first explores the history of those developments. Changes in the form and function of the report have been driven by statute, by regulation, and by the activities of professional organizations representing forensic psychiatrists. As a result of those changes, today's psychiatric reports have come to fulfill a range of functions beyond the simple communication of a psychiatric opinion. Those functions are reviewed later in the chapter.

1.1 Origins

We take for granted the present requirement of producing written expert psychiatric reports, but this was not always the situation even in recent American jurisprudence. In the historical literature relating to the use of experts in court reference to the written expert report is uncommon. References to expert psychiatric reports are less common still. The first instances of physicians assisting fact finders are in Roman cases (Lewis 1894) such as that following the death of Julius Caesar (Gutheil 2005). In medieval Europe physicians were called upon to interpret wounds (Overholser 1953) and to testify in cases of violent death (Ciccone 1992).

In America, medical experts seem first to have appeared in courtrooms in the nineteenth century. By 1900 their use was commonplace (Mohr 1993). After the appearance of T. R. Beck's *Elements of Medical Jurisprudence* in 1823, courtrooms seem to have admitted evidence from an increasing number of medical experts, often with dubious credentials. Mohr (1993) observes that Beck cautioned physicians about obscure language, verbal pyrotechnics, and becoming courtroom bullies. Beck was dismayed by the increasing use of experts, who he thought often made fools of themselves on the stand. The possibility of using written reports to tone down the rhetoric is not mentioned: there was no incentive for attorneys to have their experts prepare written reports, as the important action took place in the form of verbal debates. Accounts of nineteenth-century trials note that experts adopted an adversarial stance, confusing juries as to where the truth lay. The problem was compounded by the experts being paid by their respective sides. The first widespread use of psychiatric reports seems to have come in civil cases, and especially in will contests. The pattern, it appears, was that the experts were asked to read transcripts of fact witnesses and then to prepare narrative reports addressing the question of insanity at the time the will was written or amended.

The Psychiatric Report, ed. Alec Buchanan and Michael A. Norko. Published by Cambridge University Press. © Cambridge University Press 2011.

The reports seem to have included much of what one might expect today: reviews of records, critiques of other experts' opinions, and scholarly discussions of the manner in which disease affects sanity. The experts' written opinions were sometimes published after the trial.

In his last book, *Contributions to Mental Pathology* (1873), an anthology of selected publications, Isaac Ray included his commentary on five criminal trials (Abner Rogers, Abner Baker, C.A., Bernard Cangley, and George Winnemore) and one civil case (Morgan Hinchman), as well as his expert opinions in two will contests (Henry Parish and Eliza Angell). There is no evidence from these accounts, with the exception of the Parish Will Case, that written reports played a role in assisting the parties or the court in adjudicating the criminal cases. There were instances of psychiatrists examining prisoners and listening to testimony before testifying on the question of insanity, but the entire focus of Ray's reporting is on the live testimony. In an account of the Rogers trial by attorneys Bigelow and Bemis (1844), the material was gathered from their own notes, those of the Chief Justice, and the opening and closing remarks of the State's Attorney "so far as he could write them out from memory after the trial" (p. 1). There were written medical reports from a pathologist, Dr. Gay, whose opinions were not admissible because he died before the trial (barring cross-examination) and from a group of pathologists commenting on the autopsy findings. There is no indication that the psychiatric experts had prepared written reports.

Among the best examples of the early use of expert reports is the 1856 Parish Will Case in New York City. Records of the evidence and testimony are preserved in three volumes and over 2300 pages. In addition to Ray's publishing his opinion in 1873, the opinions of all the psychiatric experts were published in a volume collected by one of the experts, Dr. John Watson of the New York Hospital (Watson et al. 1857). The other experts included prominent asylum doctors or medical superintendents: Dr. D. Tilden Brown of the Bloomingdale Asylum, Dr. M. H. Ranney of the New York City Lunatic Asylum at Blackwell's Island, Dr. Pliny Earle of the Bloomingdale Asylum, Dr. Luther V. Bell of the Massachusetts Medical Society (late of the McLean Asylum near Boston), Dr. Isaac Ray of the Butler Hospital for the Insane, and Sir Henry Holland, a London physician.

Dr. Watson's opinion occupied about 350 pages; others ranged from 4 to 64. There were references to the evidence by way of volume and page, and the reports were generally logical and carefully written. There is nevertheless evidence of hostility among these experts, suggesting overreaching opinions and partisanship. Other examples of expert witnesses publishing their opinions in will contests are readily available (Hammond 1866; Lee 1870), though it is not obvious, aside perhaps from self-aggrandizement, why they did so.

The book comprising the collected opinions of the psychiatric experts in the Parish Will Case may be the most spectacular example of nineteenth-century forensic reportage. The reports followed a pattern that could be used as a template today – statement of the issues, review of available data, integration of the data with the legal question, and the expert opinion. Watson's massive report, replete with a detailed table of contents, is prefaced by a modest statement: "For the facts of the case I have, throughout, relied exclusively upon the evidence taken before the Surrogate; referring directly to the folios in the printed evidence for every statement I have had occasion to borrow, and, in part third, referring, for the opinions advanced, to the most reliable medical and medico legal authorities" (Watson et al. 1857, p. 4).

Earle, in a self-effacing introduction to his report in Parish, cites the difficulty in judging insanity. He notes that:

> no accurate definition of insanity has ever been devised. It follows that there is no test for it,
> no *experimentum crusis* which, in equivocal cases, may be applied with certainty of a positively

accurate result, or demonstration, such as in the results of the exact sciences divests of all doubt the solution of a problem or a proposition (Watson et al., 1857, p. 413).

Bell, by contrast, is less modest, leading with his credentials:

> I have entered upon the consideration of the questions involved in this case, under the best lights afforded me in a professional experience of nearly thirty years; two-thirds or more of which time has been passed in the care and treatment of those mentally disordered, while at the head of the oldest and one of the largest of the curative institutions for the insane in the country. During this period I have been very frequently called upon to appear before the courts of justice, and afford the aids of my experience in the solution of medico-juridical questions touching the condition of the mind. (Watson et al., 1857, p. 461).

1.2 Uses and abuses

The testimony of paid expert witnesses raised considerable consternation among nineteenth-century legal authorities. In *The Law of Wills* Redfield (1866) noted:

> [W]hen we consider the conflicting character of testimony coming from experts; and often its one-sided and partisan character; and above all, the tendency of most mature and well-balanced minds, to run into the most incomprehensible theorizing and unfounded dogmatism, from the exclusive devotion of study to one subject, and that of a mysterious and occult character, we cannot much wonder that some of the wisest and most prudent men of the age are beginning to feel, that the testimony of experts is too often becoming, in practice, but an ingenious device in the hands of unscrupulous men, to stifle justice, and vindicate the most high-handed crime. (Redfield 1866, p. 132, notes omitted)

Redfield quotes US Supreme Court Justice Grier, who characterized conflicting expert testimony as "perplexing, instead of elucidating, the questions involved in the issue" (Redfield 1866, p. 133).

The view from London was no less blunt, as physician Forbes Winslow warned:

> The position of the medical witness, even under the most favourable circumstances, is perplexing, anxious, and embarrassing. The character of his education, the peculiarity of his habits of thought, the philosophic cast of his mind, his constant and earnest search after truth, the nature of his daily professional occupation, ill adapt him for contending in the forensic arena with the knowledge, ability, and subtle acumen which are so often brought to bear (in courts of justice) against those little skilled in the art of legal fence. (Winslow 1854, p. 82)

Given this level of criticism, the modern observer might wonder why the experts could not simply be reined in, relegating their roles to advisors providing written opinions. It may be that attorneys were loath to give up the adversarial process in favor of cool deliberation.

The pressure for change seems to have become increasingly compelling, however. Isaac Ray's speech to the 1870 meeting of the American Social Science Association in Philadelphia (Ray 1873) saw him comment twice on the use of written reports as a solution to corruption brought about by the adversarial system. First:

> It is not very obvious how this course could be followed under our present mode of procedure. Not being called by either party, their evidence could not be elicited like that of other witnesses, by examination in chief and cross examination [sic]. It would have to be given to the court or jury in the shape of a report, which might or might not be received with the binding force of evidence (p. 424).

Then, commenting on the power of cross-examination to diminish the potency of witnesses, Ray writes:

> This evil would be entirely avoided if the testimony of experts could be given in writing and read to the jury without any oral examination. It would thus be deliberately prepared, its explanations well considered, and its full force and bearings clearly discerned. It would go to the jury on its own merits, no advantage being gained by either party by the superior adroitness of counsel in embarrassing the witness, and pushing his statements to a false or ridiculous conclusion … It would work no injustice to either party, and it could be managed without additional inconvenience. There certainly can be no difficulty in civil cases, where both parties consent to the arrangement (pp. 429–430).

Here is an example of one of Ray's lead-balloon ideas of how to reform the law (others are having judges take a back seat in civil commitment and abolishing the cognitive test for insanity in criminal cases).

Ray extended his advice about the use of reports in the 1873 introduction to his 1857 opinion in the Parish Will Case. Here one can infer that the practice of submitting written reports was still relatively unusual and, at times, controversial:

> It is a noteworthy fact, in the trial of this case, that the Surrogate wisely determined that the medical opinions should be given in writing, with the understanding that, though not clothed with the authority of legal evidence, they would be carefully considered and credited with all the weight to which they were really entitled. Such a remarkable disregard of technicalities was at once significant of his own breadth of mind, and conducive to the most exact and complete expression of belief. It enabled the expert to utter – what is impossible in the usual method of examination and cross-examination – his opinions and the reasons for opinions, with that coherence and logical relation absolutely necessary to show their full force and significance. This was a movement in the right direction, and is well worthy of imitation wherever the mode of procedure admits of it. (Ray 1873: 1973 edition, p. 316)

Shorn here of his earlier suggestion that oral examination be dispensed with entirely, Ray's suggestion seems forward thinking and likely to make the experts of the time more helpful to courts. Is his comment definitive evidence that there were no psychiatric expert reports prior to 1857 and that even by 1873 they were unusual? It appears so. If there were narrative reports by expert witnesses before that time these were probably private documents that were not discoverable in court. They would have served simply to inform the parties of what the witness was likely to say at trial.

Ray died in 1881. Shortly following his death, President Garfield was assassinated by Charles Guiteau. Guiteau's highly public trial included a significant amount of expert testimony. Rosenberg's (1968) review includes a variety of source materials, relying principally on published trial transcripts (Report 1882) and newspaper accounts. It is clear that court procedure continued to permit witnesses, some of whom (Drs. John P. Gray and Edward C. Spitzka, for example) were known for their theatricality, to exercise their verbal skills. By contrast, there is little evidence that reports played a role, although Rosenberg makes fleeting reference to Gray's "formal report to the District Attorney." Guiteau's trial was followed by vitriolic attacks between professionals. Gray and others published their views of the case and trial excerpts in the *American Journal of Insanity* (Anonymous 1882a, 1882b, 1882c; Bucknill 1882).

1.3 Statutory regulation and academic input

In the early twentieth century, more attention was paid to the shape and form of expert testimony. Wigmore (1910) comments on the expert's exemption from answering hypothetical questions if the data underlying the testimony were from personal observation. Still, there was no specific recommendation that the expert supply a written narrative that would be open to scrutiny.

In the late 1930s the Uniform Expert Testimony Act, a legislative proposal made by the National Conference of Commissioners on Uniform State Laws, attempted to correct the perceived polarization of experts in civil cases (see Anonymous 1938; Harno 1938; Overholser 1953). The Act, if adopted by a jurisdiction, empowered the trial court to appoint experts in any criminal or civil proceeding when any party or the court itself deemed such evidence desirable. It did not go so far as to eliminate partisan experts by replacing them with court appointments in all circumstances. Second, the Act stated, in Section 1, "An expert witness may be required, on direct or cross-examination, to specify the data on which his inferences are based." This is significant, because it speaks to the questions of how experts' evidence is derived and the problem of testimonial privilege of the litigants. Finally, the Act granted:

> Power in the court to require its own experts to file a written report, to be open for inspection by the parties, and to be read by the witness at the trial upon request of court or of any party, subject to "lawful objections" as to its admissibility; [and] power in the court to require a conference before trial among any of the experts, two or more of whom may thereupon prepare a joint report which may be introduced at the trial by party or court, subject to "lawful objections" as to its admissibility.

Other features of the Act addressed uniform compensation of experts. The overall tone of the document suggests that expert testimony generally had become a blight on the legal system.

In 1942 the American Law Institute, drafters of the Model Code of Evidence, sought to make expert reports lucid by having them read into evidence (Rule 408) (Overholser 1953). By the early 1950s the states had done little to adopt the substance of either this part of the Model Code or the Uniform Expert Testimony Act (Overholser 1953; Ordover 1974). The consequent reliance on oral testimony thus seems an artifact of an adversarial legal system that relies on argumentation. As one commentator put it: "In order to preserve the opportunity to object, we have foregone the lucidity of the direct narrative presentation … Resistance to the introduction of written evidence is largely based upon traditional adversary concepts of jury trials and the hypertechnical forms of objections which have evolved to 'protect' the jury within this framework" (Ordover 1974, pp. 68–69, footnote omitted).

Ordover (1974) pointed out also that resistance to the written report was much less evident in other areas of legal practice, for instance in arguments before government agencies. In a direct attack on the misuse of expert witnesses, he proposed a set of procedures that would help jurors cope with technical or complex expert testimony, consistent with Uniform Rules of Evidence (Model Code Rule 401[2]): "The trial judge shall have the discretion to permit or require expert, skilled, or other complicated testimony to be prepared in written form prior to the trial and to be presented in narrative form before the court and/or jury in any case where such a presentation will serve the interests of justice" (Ordover 1974, p. 69, footnote omitted). The written report in these cases is to be accompanied by a sworn affidavit. Ordover suggests different provisions to improve *voir dire* and discovery. The application would be in the hands of the trial judge, who is empowered to take an active, directorial role in the trial – not simply one of a referee or umpire.

In Ordover's model, the jury gets to hear the expert's opinions on direct examination in the narrative form, unhampered by the awkwardness of objections, questions of form, or the need to refresh memory. A variant would be to have the direct testimony delivered to the jury in video format. Beyond that, they experience a live cross-examination, which will attenuate attempts at advocacy on the part of the expert. Questions arise as to whether the expert actually presents the direct testimony, since it can be colored by demeanor. In this model, there is always an opportunity for the jury to assess the expert's demeanor on cross-examination.

1.4 The rise of the guilds and professional self-regulation

The contemporary view of written forensic reports is closely related to the development and contributions of professional organizations. The American Academy of Psychiatry and the Law (AAPL) was founded in 1969. A founder, Seymour Pollack, argued in 1974 that forensic reports should present, as briefly as possible, only the most probative data that support the reasoning behind the relevant legal opinion offered (Silva et al. 2003). He thought this should not take more than three pages (Simon 2007). Pollack urged that only material relevant to the psychiatric-legal inquiry be included in the forensic report, which should be free of psychiatric jargon and idiosyncratic terminology, and that the reader be able to clearly distinguish data, inferences, and conclusions (Pollack 1971). In this advice, one sees the desire for quick and effective communication to the legal audience. Pollack produced a suggested format for reports to attorneys or the courts. The heart of the format consisted of an outline of psychiatric-legal issues, the psychiatrist's opinions about those issues, and the data and reasoning relevant to the opinions (Pollack 1974).

Other authors at that time provided cautions about requirements to share the written report with opposing counsel (Danto 1973; Watson 1978). Danto extolled the virtue of effective communication to the legal system, but also suggested the possibility that the "more experienced forensic psychiatrist may prefer not to commit his opinion in writing in order not to give the 'other side' the advantage of knowing the report in advance of the trial and thus being able to prepare the cross-examination more carefully" (Danto 1973, p. 123). This represents an early acknowledgement that report writing must anticipate testimony, as well as a strategy that we have seen among forensic experts, but which finds few adherents today.

The American Board of Forensic Psychiatry (ABFP), founded in 1976, generated a report format, by which it judged candidates' submitted work products in its certification examination processes through 1993 (see Silva et al. 2003, p. 34, for the full ABFP format). This was an early construct of the mechanics of report writing, which has survived to contemporary practice. AAPL practice guidelines on insanity defense, competence to stand trial, and psychiatric disability evaluations have produced expansions and minor variations of the basic theme of the ABFP format (Giorgi-Guarnieri et al. 2002, pp. S24–S25; Mossman et al. 2007, p. S52; Gold et al. 2008, pp. S20–S21). Hoffman advanced a structure for forensic reports in civil litigation related to personal injury, elaborating principles of the evaluation and report (Hoffman 1986). With these significant portrayals of appropriate content for forensic reports, it is not surprising that Nicholson and Norwood observed from a review of recent studies of forensic report content that practice had improved compared with the anecdotal characterizations of these reports from the 1970s and 1980s (Nicholson & Norwood 2000).

1.5 Contemporary views on the function of the psychiatric report

In modern forensic practice, the written report is the centerpiece of psychiatric evidence and the expert's major work product; it is not merely the documentation of how the actual work was performed (Griffith et al. 2010) (see Chapter 5 for further discussion of these ideas.). In most cases, the report is the only work product placed on display following many hours of

Table 1.1 Roles of the forensic report

1. Communicating information
2. Preparing the ground for testimony
3. Facilitating treatment
4. Demonstrating proper conduct of the evaluation
5. Aiding the measurement of clinical and forensic practice

labors and interactions (Silva et al. 2003; Mossman et al. 2007). Forensic reports serve many functions, which can be summarized into five conceptual roles (see Table 1.1)

Recent authors usually describe the primary function of the psychiatric report as the effective communication of information (Svendsen 1971; Danto 1973; Appelbaum 2010). The literature emphasizes the problems inherent in speaking to an audience of a different discipline, one with its own peculiar education, culture, and language (Silva et al. 2003; Hecker & Scoular 2004; Griffith & Baranoski 2007). The literature emphasizes also the layers of narrative complexity present in many reports, and the added challenges this can present to effective communication (Griffith et al. 2010).

The forensic evaluator, in preparing the report, narrates the evaluee's story, providing the evaluee's particular perspective about his or her life experience regarding the events which gave rise to the litigation or legal situation (Griffith & Baranoski 2007; Griffith et al. 2010). Presenting the evaluee's narrative is an essential component of the forensic evaluation; therefore, using the evaluee's own words and language is generally recommended when possible. Skill at describing important dimensions of the lives of real people provides to the legal audience a portrait of the evaluee that may not be fully visualized by non-clinicians. The expert forensic writer uses such "portraiture" (Griffith et al. 2010) to help the legal audience understand how the evaluee's legal history fits into a larger psychological understanding of the evaluee, and conversely to see how the fuller portrait informs the relevant legal considerations at hand.

The evaluator, in the report, also tells the stories of the other individuals involved in the litigation, either as opposing parties, witnesses, or others (Griffith et al. 2010). These other narratives emerge through the presentation of documents such as police reports, victim statements, or the evaluator's interviews. The evaluee may well have a different account of the underlying events than those provided by the opposing parties, witnesses, or others.

A report communicates the results of the evaluation to the retaining attorney or agency. They not only need to know that an evaluation was conducted, and that it was conducted appropriately, but that the evaluator was able to reach, or not reach, specific expert opinions based on data developed according to the methodologies of the evaluator's profession. In addition, the report must communicate to the retaining party the expert's reasoning in reaching specific opinions and in not reaching or rejecting others. The effective report serves as a vehicle through which the retaining party persuades others about the desired legal result. Of course, the retaining attorney may instruct the evaluator not to prepare a report when the forensic opinion is adverse to the client's legal interests to protect the attorney from having to provide the adverse opinion to the opposing side.

Similarly, the report communicates the results of the evaluation to the opposing parties. The retaining attorney can thus utilize the evaluation, as evidenced through the report, to negotiate with the opposing side to further the legal interests of the evaluee. Attorneys may, for instance, request that the evaluator conduct an unusually thorough evaluation, and prepare a lengthy report documenting the evaluee's mental disorder to then persuade the opposing side of the significance of the evaluee's disorder and legal incapacity. In some situations, the report communicates the results of the evaluation to the responsible court or agency. Reports will necessarily differ when the retaining party is the responsible judge, rather than an attorney or agency. Given that the court-retained expert serves as a nonpartisan court consultant, such court-retained reports can flesh out more fully the strengths and weaknesses of forensic opinions on all sides of a given case.

At times, the report may communicate the results of the evaluation to the evaluee/litigant. Retaining attorneys sometimes encounter an uncooperative or challenging client and use the evaluator as an intermediary. The report can persuade the evaluee to proceed to trial, settle the litigation, dismiss the litigation, or accept a higher or lower settlement amount. An adverse report, in the face of an obstreperous evaluee, may prompt the retaining attorney to resign his or her representation of the client. At the outset of the evaluation, some retaining agencies query the evaluator regarding the advisability of disclosing the report to the evaluee; many experts operate under the assumption that all evaluees will have access to the report.

The second role for the psychiatric report emphasized by contemporary literature is to prepare the stage for oral testimony and cross-examination. For the expert, the written report is important to preparation for trial testimony, which may take place long after the evaluation is complete (Wettstein 2010a, 2010b). In such cases and in especially complex ones, a carefully prepared report may be essential to effective testimony (Enfield 1987).

Because the opinions expressed in reports may well need to be defended in court (Hecker & Scoular 2004; Wettstein 2010a, 2010b), the care with which the report is generated is critical to the ultimate success of the expert's efforts. As Weiner observed, "Unlike clinical reports, which are typically either praised or ignored but are rarely demeaned, at least not publicly, forensic reports are fair game to opposing counsels whose proper task and duty to their client calls for them to challenge and poke holes in what the psychologist has written, as publicly and embarrassingly as they can" (Weiner 1999, p. 517). Thus, forensic writers are advised to choose their words carefully and construct the report in a way that allows it to be defended successfully upon cross-examination (Appelbaum 2010). The evaluator can repeatedly refer to the report during the testimony rather than having to search through the entire file on the witness stand for particular quotations from the evaluee, clinical data, or other information.

A third role for psychiatric reports emphasized by some authors is facilitating subsequent mental health treatment for the evaluee. (Mullen 2000; Lindqvist & Skipworth 2000) Reports do this by communicating relevant history, clinical findings, diagnosis, and conclusions. The report of mental status examination findings can assist the legal audience in appreciating the evaluee's strengths and deficits, which may be important to issues of disposition. A well-written report of these findings helps the legal audience to understand psychiatric methodology and the conclusions that may be drawn from mental status findings. Experts may be asked to offer treatment or disposition recommendations in conjunction with their psycho-legal opinions.

Fourth, some have noted the "insurance" or "defensive" value to the author of the psychiatric report. Forensic evaluators, as licensed health care professionals, are subject to professional negligence litigation, professional association ethics complaints, licensing board complaints, and criminal prosecution in their forensic work (Gold & Davidson 2007). A report allows the evaluator to document the database for the evaluation, evaluation methods, and legal decision-making process in defending against claims of negligence or intentional misconduct, even if the interview with the evaluee is documented on audio- or videotape. Forensic reports which, for instance, document the informed consent process for the evaluation may later be useful to the evaluator if questions arise regarding release to others of information contained in the report.

Finally, a group of related claims concern the possibility that the psychiatric report offers a means by which psychiatric practice, including the practice of the author, can be evaluated and credentialed (Fein et al. 1991; Farkas et al. 1997). The forensic report opens windows to the evaluator's professionalism and skill (Enfield 1987). It can illustrate the methodologies and utility of the evaluator's profession (Allnutt & Chaplow 2000; Griffith & Baranoski 2007; Wettstein 2010b). Forensic reports can serve as a quality assessment tool in health services research (Skeem et al. 1998; Wettstein 2005; Robinson & Acklin 2010). Forensic reports, it has been argued, can serve as the database for empirical research by the evaluator and others regarding case type, psychopathology, and forensic opinion. They can be compiled and examined by researchers to study forensic methods and expert opinions, and help establish relevant standards of conduct for forensic evaluators themselves (Wettstein 2005; Grisso 2010; Robinson & Acklin 2010).

1.6 Conclusion

Psychiatry in America achieved acknowledgement and identity in the nineteenth century, the same era in which medical expert testimony flourished amid wide criticism. The evils of partisan, paid experts were understood to confuse the jurors. In criminal cases, with little guidance on mutual discovery of evidence, there seems to be little in the way of extant examples of written reports by expert witnesses before the twentieth century. In civil cases, such as the Parish Will Case, the court's decision to require written expert reports appears to have been an innovation.

This was to the delight of Isaac Ray, who, as usual, was a voice in the wilderness calling for reform. By the time of the 1881 Guiteau trial, however, it was business as usual, with battling experts providing verbal testimony and only publishing their opinions and commentary later. There were reasons enough to look to reform as a solution to the problems caused by experts' disparate opinions, but none sufficient in the nineteenth century to cause the legal establishment to change to a system of written documents, subject to live cross-examination.

The widespread introduction of the written psychiatric report in the twentieth century has been followed by professional, judicial, and academic input as to what structure the report should have and what its function should be. That function has come to be seen as both broader and deeper than the simple communication of an opinion. Broader, because the report serves other functions too, including preparing the ground for oral testimony. Deeper, because it is now clear that the provision of even the most basic elements of a report, including a narrative account of events, requires more rigorous description and analysis than it has so far received.

References

Allnutt, S. H. & Chaplow, D. (2000) General principles of forensic report writing. *Australian and New Zealand Journal of Psychiatry* **34**: 980–987.

Anonymous (1882a) The Guiteau trial. *American Journal of Insanity* **38**: 303–448.

Anonymous (1882b) Guiteaumania. *American Journal of Insanity* **39**: 62–68 (reprinted from *British Medical Journal*, June 24, 1882).

Anonymous (1882c) Case of Guiteau. *American Journal of Insanity* **39**: 199–207 (reprinted from the *Journal of Medical Science*, July 1882).

Anonymous (1938) The Uniform Expert Testimony Act. *Columbia Law Review* **38**: 369–375.

Appelbaum, K. L. (2010) Commentary: the art of forensic report writing. *Journal of the*

American Academy of Psychiatry and the Law **38**: 43–45.

Bigelow, G. T. & Bemis, G. (1844) *Report of the Trial of Abner Rogers, Jr.* Boston: Charles C. Little and James Brown.

Bucknill, J. C. (1882) The plea of insanity in the case of Charles Julius Guiteau. *American Journal of Insanity* **39**: 181–198.

Ciccone, J. R. (1992) Murder, insanity, and expert witnesses. *Archives of Neurology* **49**: 608–611.

Danto, B. L. (1973) Writing psychiatric reports for the court. *International Journal of Offender Therapy and Comparative Criminology* **17**: 123–128.

Enfield, R. (1987) A model for developing the written forensic report. In *Innovations in Clinical Practice: A Sourcebook*, vol. 6, ed. P. A. Keller & S. R. Heyman SR. Sarasota, FL: Professional Resource Exchange, Inc., pp. 379–394.

Farkas, G. M., DeLeon, P. H., & Newman, R. (1997) Sanity examiner certification: an evolving national agenda. *Professional Psychology* **28**: 73–76.

Fein, R. A., Appelbaum, K. L., Barnum, R., et al. (1991) The designated forensic professional program: a state government-university partnership to improve forensic mental health services. *Journal of Mental Health Administration* **18**: 223–230.

Giorgi-Guarnieri, D., Janofsky, J., Keram, E., et al. (2002) AAPL practice guideline for forensic psychiatric evaluation of defendants raising the insanity defense. *Journal of the American Academy of Psychiatry and the Law* **30** (suppl): S1–S40.

Gold, L. H. & Davidson, J. E. (2007) Do you understand your risk? Liability and third-party evaluations in civil litigation. *Journal of the American Academy of Psychiatry and the Law* **35**: 200–210.

Gold, L. H., Anfang, S. A. S., Drukteinis. A. M., et al. (2008) AAPL practice guideline for the forensic evaluation of psychiatric disability. *Journal of the American Academy of Psychiatry and the Law* **36** (suppl): S1–S50.

Griffith, E. E. H. & Baranoski, M. V. (2007) Commentary: the place of performative writing in forensic psychiatry. *Journal of the American Academy of Psychiatry and the Law* **35**: 27–31.

Griffith, E. E. H., Stankovic, A., & Baranoski, M. V. (2010) Conceptualizing the forensic psychiatry report as performative narrative. *Journal of the American Academy of Psychiatry and the Law* **38**: 32–42.

Grisso, T. (2010) Guidance for improving forensic reports: a review of common errors. *Open Access Journal of Forensic Psychology* **2**: 102–115.

Gutheil, T. G. (2005) The history of forensic psychiatry. *Journal of the American Academy of Psychiatry and the Law* **33**: 259–262.

Hammond, W. A. (1866) Opinion Relative to the Testamentary Capacity of the Late James C. Johnston, of Chowan County, North Carolina. New York: Baker, Voorhis & Co.

Harno, A. J. (1938) Uniform Expert Testimony Act. *Journal of the American Judicature Society* **21**: 156–159.

Hecker, J. E. & Scoular, R. J. (2004) Forensic report writing. In *Handbook of Forensic Psychology: Resource for Mental Health and Legal Professionals*, ed. W. T. O'Donohue & E. R. Levensky. New York: Elsevier Science, pp. 63–81.

Hoffman, B. F. (1986) How to write a psychiatric report for litigation following a personal injury. *American Journal of Psychiatry* **143**: 164–169.

Lee, C. A. (1870) Medical Opinion of Charles A. Lee, M.D., in the Matter of Carlton Gates, Deceased. New York: William J. Read.

Lewis, E. B. (1894) *The Law of Expert Testimony.* Philadelphia: Rees Welsh & Co.

Lindqvist, P. & Skipworth, J. (2000) Evidence-based rehabilitation in forensic psychiatry. *British Journal of Psychiatry* **176**: 320–323.

Mohr, J. C. (1993) *Doctors and the Law: Medical Jurisprudence in Nineteenth-Century America.* Baltimore: The Johns Hopkins University Press.

Mossman, D., Noffsinger, S. G., Ash, P., et al. (2007) AAPL practice guideline for the forensic psychiatric evaluation of competence to stand trial. *Journal of the American Academy of Psychiatry and the Law* **35** (suppl): S1–S72.

Mullen, P. E. (2000) Forensic mental health. *British Journal of Psychiatry* **176** 307–311.

Nicholson, R. A. & Norwood, S. (2000) The quality of forensic psychological assessments, reports, and testimony: acknowledging the gap between promise and practice. *Law and Human Behavior* 24: 9–44.

Ordover, A. P. (1974) The use of written direct testimony in jury trials: a proposal. *Hofstra Law Review* 2: 67–95.

Overholser, W. (1953) The psychiatrist as expert witness. In *The Psychiatrist and the Law*. New York: Harcourt, Brace and Co., pp. 103–134.

Pollack, S. (1971) Psychiatric consultation for the court. In Offender Therapies Series APTO Monograph #3: The Court and the Expert: Writing Reports, vol. 1, Essays in Comparative Psychiatry, ed. F. Ferracuti. Published by The International Journal of Offender Therapy, July.

Pollack, S. (1974) Suggested format for psychiatric report to attorney or court. In *Forensic Psychiatry in Criminal Law*. Los Angeles: University of Southern California, pp. 171–173

Ray, I. (1873) *Contributions to Mental Pathology*. Boston: Little, Brown and Co. Facsimile edition (1973) with an introduction by J. M. Quen. Delmar, NY: Scholars' Facsimiles & Reprints.

Redfield, I. F. (1866) *The Law of Wills*, 2nd edn. Boston: Little, Brown, and Co., Part I.

Report of the Proceedings in the Case of the United States vs. Charles J. Guiteau, tried in the Supreme Court of the District of Columbia, holding a Criminal Term, and beginning November 14, 1881, 3 vols. (1882). Washington, DC.

Robinson, R. & Acklin, M. W. (2010) Fitness in paradise: quality of forensic reports submitted to the Hawaii judiciary. *International Journal of Law and Psychiatry* 33: 131–137.

Rosenberg, C. E. (1968) *The Trial of the Assassin Guiteau*. Chicago: University of Chicago Press.

Silva, J. A., Weinstock, R., & Leong, G. B. (2003) Forensic psychiatric report writing. In *Principles and Practice of Forensic Psychiatry*, 2nd edn., ed. R. Rosner. London: Arnold, pp. 31–36.

Simon, R. I. (2007) Authorship in forensic psychiatry: a perspective. *Journal of the American Academy of Psychiatry and the Law* 35: 18–26.

Skeem, J. L., Golding, S. L., Cohn, N. B., et al. (1998) Logic and reliability of evaluations of competence to stand trial. *Law and Human Behavior* 22: 519–547.

Svendsen, B. B. (1971) Denmark: Psychiatrists, the medico-legal council and the courts. In *Offender Therapies Series APTO Monograph #3: The Court and the Expert: Writing Reports, vol. 1, Essays in Comparative Psychiatry*, ed. F. Ferracuti. Published by The International Journal of Offender Therapy, July, 1971.

Watson, A. S. (1978) On the preparation and use of psychiatric expert testimony: some suggestions in an ongoing controversy. *Bulletin of the American Academy of Psychiatry and the Law* 6: 226–246.

Watson, J., Brown, D. T., Ranney, M. H. G., et al. (1857) *The Parish Will Case Before the Surrogate of the City of New York*. New York: John F. Trow.

Weiner, I. B. (1999) Writing forensic reports. In *The Handbook of Forensic Psychology*, 2nd edn., ed. A. K. Hess & I. B. Weiner. New York: John Wiley & Sons, Inc., pp. 501–520.

Wettstein, R. M. (2005) Quality and quality improvement in forensic mental health evaluations. *Journal of the American Academy of Psychiatry and the Law* 33: 158–175.

Wettstein, R. M. (2010a) The forensic psychiatric examination and report. In *The American Psychiatric Publishing Textbook of Forensic Psychiatry*, 2nd edn., ed. R. I. Simon & L. H. Gold. Washington, DC: American Psychiatric Publishing, Inc., pp. 175–203.

Wettstein, R. M. (2010b) Commentary: conceptualizing the forensic psychiatry report. *Journal of the American Academy of Psychiatry and the Law* 38: 46–48.

Wigmore, J. H. (1910) *A Pocket Code of the Rules of Evidence in Trials at Law*. Boston: Little, Brown and Co.

Winslow, F. (1854) *Lettsomian Lectures on Insanity*. London: John Churchill.

Section 1 Principles of writing

Chapter

2

Preparation

Cheryl Wills

Report writing is an essential skill which involves accessing, examining, analyzing, interpreting, prioritizing, and communicating clinical and other data that the psychiatrist will use to formulate opinions about legal questions posed by attorneys. Formulating a forensic psychiatric report is an activity which must be taken seriously, because a report can affect the freedom, safety, assets, occupation, and emotional well-being of litigants. It is therefore important to give thoughtful consideration to how an expert prepares to write a forensic report.

Prior to writing a report, the forensic psychiatrist must be cognizant of the fundamental concepts of forensic practice. The expert must meet legal, ethical, and professional obligations, including ensuring that there is sufficient time in one's schedule to research and produce a quality report. Failure to fulfill these obligations may result in unpleasant outcomes for the attorney and the client, especially if a judge rules that a psychiatric report is not admissible in court. In such cases, there also may be adverse professional consequences for the psychiatrist.

The expert must accomplish several tasks of various levels of complexity when preparing to write a report. A forensic psychiatrist who is well prepared to write a report has effectively set the stage for an accurate, objective, and effective response to the question(s) posed by the attorney. As with the clinical psychiatric interview, a consistent approach to preparing to write psychiatric reports for courts will help the expert concentrate on key information and produce a quality product.

A purposeful approach to report preparation should not confine the expert to a rigid set of rules. Rather, the report preparation outline, like the clinical interview, should serve as flexible scaffolding which permits fluid progression of required evaluative and determinative activities. A framework for report preparation will streamline the referral process from legal professionals, aid with organizing large amounts of data, enhance the consistency of the report, and help the psychiatrist marshal and clarify compelling data that will be used to formulate opinions.

This chapter describes the process by which the forensic psychiatrist prepares the report in three stages: deciding whether or not to accept the case; procuring, examining, and categorizing forensic data that will serve as the body of the psychiatric report; and formulating forensic opinions for the report.

2.1 The initial contact

The initial contact between a forensic psychiatrist and an attorney or judge sets the tone for the working relationship. During this encounter, the psychiatrist must determine whether

The Psychiatric Report, ed. Alec Buchanan and Michael A. Norko. Published by Cambridge University Press. © Cambridge University Press 2011.

the requested service is within the parameters of sound forensic psychiatric practice. A psychiatrist who does not complete this analysis may encounter challenging situations, including: being overwhelmed by having too many cases, accepting cases outside of one's area of expertise, and/or becoming involved in cases that may compromise one's objectivity. These situations can be avoided when the psychiatrist uses a consistent approach to reduce the likelihood of accepting unsuitable referrals.

The psychiatrist who is considering accepting a case should determine whether there are barriers to serving as an expert witness in the identified jurisdiction. State medical boards and physician professional organizations have begun to regulate medical expert witness testimony. In July 2008, the Federation of State Medical Boards identified 31 states with minimum standards for physician expert testimony. Most of these states either require the expert to hold an active medical license or to be actively involved in clinical practice. In Ohio, for example, at least 75% of an expert witness's professional time must be spent teaching or providing patient care. In Connecticut, a medical expert witness in malpractice litigation must demonstrate active involvement in teaching or practicing medicine in the 5-year period prior to the alleged offense which resulted in the claim.

According to the Federation of State Medical Boards, which stresses the importance of physicians providing ethical expert witness testimony, a physician who proffers false expert testimony may be subject to disciplinary action for unprofessional conduct. The American Medical Association (AMA) has also taken this position (AMA 2005). Additionally, AMA policy states that physician expert witness testimony "should be subject to peer review" (AMA 2005). In view of these policies, the psychiatric expert should ask the attorney to research expert qualifications in the identified venue, to avoid the uncomfortable situation of having the expert's report rejected by the court due to jurisdictional barriers.

If the psychiatrist has sufficient time to consult on the case and there are no judicial or licensure obstacles, the expert should determine whether the case is within his or her scope of practice. For example, a psychiatrist whose clinical practice is limited to evaluation and treatment of college students may be ill suited to provide expert consultation in a case involving an elderly person with head trauma and multiple medical problems. Also, if a psychiatrist is asked to formulate an opinion regarding whether or not a particular medical intervention, with which the psychiatrist is not familiar, is the definitive test in a particular area, the expert should decline to participate and advise the attorney to retain a different expert to address that particular concern.

A psychiatrist who is comfortable with the general aspects of the case should ascertain the primary legal question(s) the attorney wants the expert to address, as well as any secondary concerns. For example, an attorney representing the plaintiff in a malpractice case seeks expert consultation. In Case "A," the attorney requests an opinion about causation and damages. In Case "B," the attorney also is seeking to reform a system of care. In Case "C," the attorney wants to sue the hospital, which is trying to shift all responsibility for damages to a physician who is indemnified by a third party. Although the expert will likely examine the same documents in each situation, Case "A" requires the expert to formulate opinions related to the standard of care, causation, and damages. In Case "B," the expert is expected to proffer the opinions in Case "A" along with opinions about why and how the system of psychiatric care needs to improve. The expert in Case "C" will describe the damages that can be attributed to the facility and to the physician. The expert who is able to provide the consultation proposed by the attorney should ask the attorney to describe the requested service(s), in writing, to avoid confusion.

Next, the psychiatrist's role in the case should be clarified. The psychiatrist may be asked to work as an expert for plaintiff's counsel, defense counsel, or the court. An expert preparing a report for a defense attorney will be asked to describe exculpatory findings. A plaintiff's attorney will ask the expert to formulate opinions that support the plaintiff's complaint.

After these tasks have been completed, the forensic psychiatrist should identify and address any perceived barriers to objectivity, such as compensation arrangements. The psychiatrist should present the rate of compensation and retainer agreement to the attorney. The American Academy of Psychiatry and the Law (AAPL), has provided a useful criterion for professional compensation agreements in the "AAPL Ethics Guidelines for the Practice of Forensic Psychiatry" (AAPL Ethics Guidelines), which says that contingency fees "should not be accepted" from attorneys because they "undermine honesty and efforts to attain objectivity" in forensic psychiatric practice (AAPL 2005). Also, a forensic psychiatrist should not have a personal interest in the outcome of a case. Additionally, the agreed upon services and compensation should be documented in a signed agreement contract or letter, to reduce the likelihood of future misunderstandings between the attorney and the expert.

The psychiatrist, also, should address other potential barriers to objectivity before agreeing to serve as a psychiatric consultant. Several professional organizations, including the AAPL, have addressed the need for professionals to strive to reduce bias during expert witness consultation. The AAPL Ethics Guidelines offer direction to forensic psychiatrists seeking to engage in objective consultation. During forensic examinations, psychiatrists can reduce internal bias by differentiating between verified and unverified data and by distinguishing between facts and conclusions (AAPL 2005). The Guidelines also dissuade practices that may increase external bias, including offering opinions before evaluating examinees and performing forensic evaluations on one's own patients (AAPL 2005).

Although the AAPL Guidelines help a forensic psychiatrist diminish bias, the challenge of maintaining neutrality during forensic consultation, while satisfying the requirements of the retaining attorney, requires thoughtful navigation of medico-legal terrain and constant self-examination. Struggling to maintain objectivity is conducive to dispassionate forensic psychiatric practice. However, when the expert finds that there is not sufficient evidence to support the retaining attorney's position, the expert should decline or withdraw from the case (Diamond 1959; Katz 1992; Gutheil et al. 2004; Goldyne 2007).

Narcissism can influence an expert's capacity to render unbiased forensic opinions. Stable narcissism, such as a realistic appraisal of one's professional abilities and a healthy conscience, generally promotes objective expert consultation; skewing data to curry favor with an attorney is not a viable option. Fragile narcissism, on the other hand, is perpetuated when one's sense of importance depends on external reinforcement and validation by others. Fragile narcissism, consequently, may lead an expert to develop a "win-at-all-costs" mindset which favors conscious distortion of data and opinions (Gutheil & Simon 2004). Practices that enhance a psychiatrist's neutrality include: describing limitations of provisional opinions proffered before the expert has analyzed all the data; identifying additional information that may help the expert formulate a more comprehensive opinion; and communicating with attorneys in an effort to increase the likelihood that the expert's findings will be fairly represented (Gutheil & Simon 2004).

The last step in determining whether or not to accept a case involves special arrangements. The expert who expects special consideration, such as having resident physicians

Table 2.1 SLED-SOS referral checklist

Schedule	Check schedule for availability
Licensure	Jurisdictional requirement for expert testimony
Expertise	Experience in the specific area of litigation
Duty	Identify the required task
Stance	Expert's role in the case
Objectivity	Identify barriers to neutrality
Supplemental information	

present during an examination, should discuss this with the attorney, before accepting the case, so that additional accommodations may be anticipated, and to allow the attorney to decline the arrangement if it is not suitable.

The process of determining whether or not to accept a forensic case is a complex series of steps that may be simplified by using the acronym "SLED-SOS" to help the expert recall the information needed during the initial contact with an attorney. The SLED-SOS referral checklist contains six items: S, checking one's schedule to determine availability to provide the requested service; L, verifying that the expert meets licensure requirements for expert testimony in the identified jurisdiction; E, determining whether the requested service is within the scope of the psychiatrist's expertise; D, learning the duty of the consultant; that is, the specific legal question(s) the attorney wants the psychiatrist to address; S, identifying the expected stance or position the psychiatrist will be taking in the case (plaintiff's perspective, defense perspective, court-appointed consultant, trial preparation, policy analysis, etc.); O, identifying potential barriers to the expert's objectivity; and S, supplemental information, including special arrangements (Table 2.1).

2.1.1 Case example

Psychiatrist I. M. Skilled is contacted by Attorney X to proffer an opinion about the role of a mental health crisis worker in the sexual assault of a hospital volunteer by a patient. The attorney, who represents the crisis worker, wants Dr. Skilled to examine records, to interview the plaintiff, and to prepare a report. Attorney X says he hopes the case will not go to trial.

Although Attorney X anticipates an early settlement in the case, Dr. Skilled ponders the referral as if the case will go to trial; the attorney's aspirations should not alter the quality of the services provided by the expert. Dr. Skilled determines that she has sufficient time to perform the examination, to prepare a quality report, and, if needed, to provide expert witness testimony.

Attorney X asks Dr. Skilled if she is comfortable providing expert consultation in cases that involve sex offenses. Dr. Skilled, who has provided compassionate psychiatric care to victims of sexual assault and to insanity acquittees who have engaged in violent behavior, including sex offenses, believes that she will be able to be objective in this case. Dr. Skilled also determines that she has no interest in the outcome of the case.

Attorney X asks the psychiatrist about her professional background. Dr. Skilled reviews her credentials and the limits of her practice and licensure with Attorney X, who asks Dr. Skilled about her professional arrangements. The psychiatrist reviews compensation arrangements, including the retainer agreement with Attorney X. He agrees to these conditions and requests a copy of Dr. Skilled's curriculum vitae.

The psychiatrist agrees to send the document, along with compensation and retainer agreements, to Attorney X. Dr. Skilled also requests a letter from the attorney which describes the requested services; mentions the compensation agreement and retainer; lists the legal complaint; and cites the applicable legal standard(s). Attorney X asks whether the case file should be sent along with the other documents. Dr. Skilled tells Attorney X that the case file may be sent at any time; however, work will not commence on the case until the other documents and the retainer have been received and examined by the psychiatrist.

The documents arrive in Dr. Skilled's office. If there is confusion about the consultation agreement, Dr. Skilled will contact Attorney X. Otherwise, Dr. Skilled will accept the referral.

2.2 Obtaining and examining the data

The precision of a forensic report depends on the quality of the data and how they are analyzed by the expert. Bias can be introduced into the forensic report when a psychiatrist does not effectively coordinate the tasks of examining and summarizing large volumes of data. For example, an expert who randomly interprets data may fail to prioritize information that favors the position of the retaining attorney. The expert may also fail to concede data that weaken the position of the retaining attorney. Ultimately, this carelessness may subject the expert to increased scrutiny during cross-examination.

A more consistent approach to data categorization and analysis will permit the expert to elucidate favorable data, acknowledge weak data, and consider alternate perspectives. Of course, if the expert, who is preparing to write the report, determines there are not sufficient data to support the attorney's position, the expert should contact the attorney to discuss the situation and consider whether the attorney wishes the expert to continue with any aspect of the consultation. Prior to reaching this conclusion, however, the expert must evaluate the data.

The first stage of data analysis is the paper review, which involves gathering, examining, and tabulating data that will be used by the expert to prepare the report. Data are studied early during the consultation process, so that the expert can identify and request missing documents. The expert recognizes weak data that require additional corroboration to support the claim. Also, the expert will note gray zones of information that cannot be remedied by reviewing additional data.

Although the types of documents examined will vary from case to case, there are certain materials that should be examined during each consultation project. These include: a signed contractual agreement, a letter from the attorney describing the requested services and deadlines, a copy of the legal complaint, and a copy of the applicable legal standard (Table 2.2). These essential resources help the psychiatrist construct a medico-legal scaffold that will be filled as the expert examines records, conducts interviews, analyzes the case, and formulates opinion(s).

Technology has increased the variety and, at times, the quality of resources that may be scrutinized during the paper review stage. The psychiatrist may examine electronic records including digital recordings, websites, electronic presentations, and digital images. Regardless of the format, the psychiatrist lists and describes each information source. The expert will also attempt to create an accurate timeline of events by citing dates listed on each resource. (Authentication of dates falls outside the scope of the psychiatrist's reasonably expected duty.)

Table 2.2 Documents examined in each case

Signed contractual agreement

Letter from the attorney describing the requested services and deadlines

Copy of the legal complaint

Copy of the legal standard to be applied in the case

The expert who is preparing to write a psychiatric report should catalog data so that they will be more accessible when the expert begins to marshal the evidence and formulate opinions. The data also should fit into the timeline described above. The source of each item, including the author, date(s), and organization, if applicable, should be described along with the content. The importance of distinguishing factual data from opinions is critical, as are the relevance and accuracy of each datum. These details, along with the clarity of the information, may affect the opinions that will be crafted by the expert.

The expert should maintain a record of documents requested but not received so that this information can be included in a report, if appropriate. This practice illuminates the psychiatrist's efforts to conduct a comprehensive examination. Also, the expert who has access to this information will be in a better position to dispel efforts, by opposing counsel, to show that the expert intentionally ignored contrary data in an effort to render a favorable opinion for the retaining attorney.

If substantial records are missing, then the psychiatrist can only prepare to generate a preliminary report for the attorney. At times, requested records may become available after the psychiatrist's final report has been submitted to the retaining attorney. For this reason, the expert preparing to write a report should include a reminder, in the notes, to reserve the right to revise the opinion(s) and to submit an addendum to the report, if critical information that substantially alters the opinion becomes available.

The forensic psychiatrist who has completed the paper review stage has produced a preliminary psycho-legal blueprint of the case, including the allegations, legal standards, identified parties (persons, organizations, and property), quality and types of evidence, etc. The psychiatrist uses these data to determine how best to acquire additional information to augment the database during the second stage – the psychiatrist's real-time view of the case. This stage is controlled by the psychiatrist, using applicable clinical and forensic skill sets to formulate questions designed to clarify details of the case. The information gathered by the psychiatrist will fill in the scaffolding created during the paper review. The expert may interview the retaining attorney, plaintiffs, defendants, and other witnesses. At times, the expert may also conduct a tour or site visit to glean information about the case from a specific vantage point.

In forensic psychiatry, the process of preparing for interviews can be cumbersome. Of course, the expert should attempt to review the records before conducting the interview, but there are several potentially rate-limiting steps between deciding to interview a person and conducting the actual interview.

The expert requests interviews during a collaborative consultation with the retaining attorney. Experts and evaluees may be stationed in different towns, states, or countries, so travel may be involved for one or both parties. Also, the expert should state, up front, whether special adaptations should be made for physical disabilities, trainees, etc.

The expert should ask the retaining attorney about special needs of interviewees, so that reasonable accommodations may be arranged for the interview. When the attorney has confirmed the interview time and location, the expert should request a letter from the attorney which details these adaptations.

Special arrangements must be made for the psychiatrist to conduct an examination when an interviewee is remanded to a secure facility, such as a locked psychiatric unit or a prison. The retaining attorney should assist the expert by contacting the appropriate authorities and obtaining a security clearance, an appointment time, and a confidential area where the interview may take place. Although some facilities do not require written documentation from the hospital administrator, warden, etc. for the expert to be admitted to the facility, a letter of introduction from the facility administrator, or designee, may facilitate access to the institution in case there are bureaucratic barriers to entry.

Experts who must travel to evaluations should plan to arrive early because security protocols may preclude changing the time of the interview on a particular day. Also, the psychiatrist should be familiar with general security rules at an institution before entering the campus. For example, an expert who enters a prison will be subject to inspection and contraband protocols, and risks being held hostage if a riot occurs during the visit.

In the free world, regardless of where the evaluation occurs, the expert should be familiar with resources in the vicinity of the interview room, including restrooms and refreshments, in order to review the resources with the interviewee(s). Also, people who accompany the evaluee should feel comfortable in the waiting area.

During a forensic interview, the psychiatric expert obtains information from the evaluee, at the request of a third party. Although the expert may use clinical interviewing skills to gather data, the evaluation is not clinical, but forensic. The evaluee will not receive a diagnosis or treatment recommendations; there is no actual or implied therapeutic relationship between the psychiatrist and the evaluee. Also, any report generated as a result of the interview will be the property of the retaining attorney. The evaluee who requests a copy of the report should be advised to consult with the retaining attorney regarding that matter.

The evaluator must explain the unique nature of the interview to each interviewee. Also, the interviewer must determine how well each interviewee understands this information before the forensic interview begins. Additionally, the expert should verify the identity of the interviewee. Unless the examination is ordered by a court, Health Insurance Portability and Accountability Act (HIPAA) confidentiality rules will likely apply, and the interviewer will need to obtain releases of information from the interviewee in order to share the information with retaining counsel. (For examples of such releases, see Gutheil 2009, pp. 121–123; Chapter 3.)

The forensic psychiatrist adapts the structure of each interview to obtain specific information which may corroborate, clarify, or contradict existing evidence. During an evaluation of criminal culpability, for example, the expert seeks to understand the defendant's psychiatric history in addition to details about the defendant's mental state and behavior about the time of the alleged offense.

Data gathered during the interviews will be used to fill gaps in the paper review database. Pertinent data will be used to form a coherent narrative which approximates the alleged incident and its aftermath. Also, in some cases, the psychiatrist may tour key venues to develop additional insight into the case.

The psychiatrist combines, prioritizes, and organizes data from the paper review and real-time view before moving to the next stage – identifying data that do not support the position the psychiatrist intends to take – which can be thought of as "aggravating circumstances." Each aggravating circumstance will be accompanied by supporting evidence. During this

Table 2.3 PRAMS system for data organization

Paper review

Real-time view (psychiatrist)

Aggravating circumstances

Mitigating circumstances

Supplemental information

stage, the psychiatrist also should note limitations of the case analysis, including the absence of critical records, failure to interview key witnesses, etc.

In the next stage, the psychiatric expert identifies mitigating circumstances – evidence which supports the expert's position. Mitigating circumstances corroborated by interviews, records, and other data provide a framework for opinions which will be proffered in the psychiatric report.

During the final stage, the psychiatrist considers supplemental information that was not examined during the paper view or real-time view. Resources may include literature searches, records that were not previously available, and other salient data. The forensic psychiatrist should determine if there are restrictions associated with the information that is being examined. For example, if a case involves medical malpractice, the expert should limit the review to policies, laws, literature, etc. that were available or enforceable when the alleged incident occurred. Also, the expert should distinguish between anecdotal information and evidence-based research when cataloging and prioritizing data. Supplemental information should be categorized as aggravating or mitigating circumstances for the case analysis.

The psychiatric expert should examine the relevance and strength of each aggravating and mitigating circumstance. If the strength of the aggravating circumstances substantially outweighs that of the mitigating evidence, the expert may not be able to say much in support of the attorney's position. However, if the reverse is true, the expert will be in a position to proffer an accurate, objective, and effective response to the question(s) posed by the attorney(s).

The data analysis exercise, described above, helps the expert categorize large volumes of data and facilitates describing the evaluation method to others. The five steps outlined in the activity are represented by the acronym PRAMS, which may serve as an aide-memoire for this stage of report preparation: Paper review, psychiatrist's Real-time view, Aggravating circumstances, Mitigating circumstances, and Supplemental information (Table 2.3) (Wills 2007).

2.2.1 Case example

Dr. Skilled uses the methodology outlined above to examine the case submitted by Attorney X. The following information is gathered during the paper review stage: Jake is a 20-year-old man, with mild mental retardation and psychosis, who is escorted to Stabler Hospital by police officers, after Jake threatened to harm his mother. While there, Jake lunges at an emergency room nurse and is given injectable medication. Don, a mental health crisis worker, takes a history and tells Jake's mother, who has legal guardianship of Jake, that Jake likely will be admitted to the psychiatric unit. Jake's mother completes the required paperwork and goes home.

Don presents Jake's history to Dr. Learner, the attending psychiatrist, who says that Jake "seems calm and rational right now." There are no vacant hospital beds, so Dr. Learner decides to send Jake home over Don's objection. Don phones Jake's mother/guardian so she may return to the hospital to bring Jake home. She is upset about the disposition; Don advises her to speak directly with Dr. Learner and with a patient advocacy administrator.

While Don is speaking to Jake's mother, Dr. Learner instructs Trina, a hospital volunteer, to escort Jake to the bus stop, so that he can go home. Trina complies and Jake breaks her arm when he attempts to rape her in the hospital lobby. Don sees Trina when she returns to the emergency room on a gurney. Trina sues Don and Stabler Hospital.

Dr. Skilled requests Trina's medical records from Attorney X. Trina received emergency and surgical care after she was attacked by Jake. Also, Trina had several subsequent emergency room visits for chest pain and fainting due to panic attacks.

During the psychiatrist interview stage, Dr. Skilled interviews Don, whose statements corroborate the medical record. Don advises Dr. Skilled to speak with Jake's mother. Her report is consistent with Don's report and the medical record. Dr. Learner, who no longer works at Stabler Hospital, declined to be interviewed by Dr. Skilled. Attorney X will forward Dr. Learner's deposition to Dr. Skilled as soon as it becomes available.

Dr. Skilled interviews Trina, who has stopped attending college, has been unable to work, and isolates herself at home. She alleviates her anxiety with medication she receives from a family physician. Trina has not met with a psychiatrist; she has intrusive recollections of the attack whenever she thinks about mental health, emergency care, physical intimacy, or bus stops. She stopped watching her favorite medical and law enforcement television shows because they remind her of the trauma. Also, Trina ended her engagement to her fiancé because physical intimacy triggers flashbacks of the attack.

Trina and Don were friends and colleagues before the incident. He always looked out for her. Trina believes that Don's failure to warn her about Jake's history is what ultimately caused Jake to harm her. During separate interviews, Trina's roommate and ex-fiancé each corroborate Trina's report.

Dr. Skilled decides that Dr. Learner's and Stabler Hospital's decision to release Jake and to instruct Trina to escort him to the bus stop contributed substantially to Trina's injuries and subsequent decline. Dr. Skilled must now determine how, if at all, Don's actions contributed to Trina's injuries.

Aggravating circumstances which are directly related to Don's behavior include several facts: Don did not attempt to protect Trina by sharing Jake's history with her. Also, Don did not insist that Jake remain in the hospital until his mother could be notified about Dr. Learner's decision. The fact that Dr. Learner discharged Jake from the emergency room is not an aggravating circumstance for Don, because he did not have the authority to overrule Dr. Learner's decision.

Mitigating circumstances include the following facts: Don did not have authority to overrule Dr. Learner. Also, Don did not have authority to review Jake's history with Trina; he did not know she was involved with Jake's care.

Supplemental information, in this case, would include job descriptions for mental health crisis workers, psychiatrists, and volunteer workers at Stabler Hospital which may clarify lines of authority and the scope of Don's professional responsibilities. Although policies regarding involuntary hospitalization and transferring patients to outlying facilities may be useful for psychiatric malpractice litigation, the documents do not specifically relate to Don's behavior or his professional obligations in the case.

2.3 Marshaling the evidence

The forensic psychiatrist who has gathered and prioritized the evidence must complete one additional task before writing a thoughtful and concise report. The expert must scrutinize the data and craft opinions which address the question(s) posed by the attorney.

When formulating an expert opinion, the expert should be cognizant of how attorneys interview witnesses under oath. During direct examination of an expert, a skilled attorney strives to illuminate favorable evidence that the expert has documented in the psychiatric report. The cross-examining attorney poses questions to the expert that are designed to reduce the impact of the initial testimony to deliberating judges and jurors. Although attorneys are expected to provide zealous representation to those who retain them, forensic psychiatrists are supposed to conduct dispassionate examinations of cases and to filter bias from their opinions. The psychiatric expert, therefore, should anticipate vigorous cross-examination of proffered testimony and be prepared to concede to well-founded conclusions which do not support the retaining attorney's position.

A skilled expert knows that dispassionate opinion formulation facilitates one's ability to serve as an advocate for those opinions. Psychiatrists should not advocate for an attorney or a specific outcome. The observant expert uses the principles of direct and cross-examination to inform the opinion crafting exercise when preparing to write the psychiatric report.

The following method for formulating final opinions is recommended. The psychiatrist composes a preliminary opinion or claim. The expert assures that the claim is logical, relevant, and valid. Mitigating data are used to support the claim. The hierarchy is key; the strongest evidence is presented first. Next, the expert examines the preliminary opinion and supporting evidence for areas of potential vulnerability or exposure in anticipation of what the expert may be asked during cross-examination. Aggravating evidence marshaled above will be used to facilitate this process. The expert will study the data and determine how best to respond to these weaknesses. Weaker supporting evidence should be omitted or reformulated to produce a more cogent opinion. Also, concessions may be incorporated into the opinion. After completing these four steps, the expert synthesizes a revised opinion that should be examined for potential vulnerability as if it were a preliminary opinion. The process should be repeated until the expert crafts a cogent work product with logical opinions, strong supporting arguments, and appropriate concessions.

This method of forensic opinion formulation strengthens report preparation by compelling the expert to anticipate and to incorporate concessions into each crafted opinion. The acronym CHESS (Wills 2008) will help the reader recall the steps used to produce opinions. The exercise contains five steps: C, formulating the claim or preliminary opinion; H, establishing a hierarchy of supporting evidence; E, examining the evidence for exposure; S, studying the evidence; and S, synthesizing a revised opinion (Table 2.4).

2.3.1 Case example

Dr. Skilled is ready to craft an opinion in support of Don's behavior.

Claim

The preliminary opinion is that Don's involvement in Jake's care was not a cause of Trina's injuries.

Table 2.4 The CHESS method of forensic opinion formulation

C	Claim (state a preliminary opinion)
H	Hierarchy (of supporting evidence)
E	Exposure (examine for)
S	Study (and revise)
S	Synthesize (a revised opinion)

Hierarchy of supporting evidence

Don evaluated Jake and recommended psychiatric hospitalization to Dr. Learner. Don did not have authority to override Dr. Learner's decision to release Jake from the hospital. Don did not violate Jake's confidentiality by telling Trina about Jake's behavior because she was not initially involved in Jake's care. Don reasonably believed that Dr. Learner would not release Jake from the hospital until his mother/guardian arrived to escort him home. Don was not present when Dr. Learner instructed Trina to escort Jake to the bus stop. Don did not learn of Trina's involvement in Don's care until after she was attacked by Jake.

Examine for exposure

Don could have alerted his superiors to Dr. Learner's ill-informed decision before Don contacted Jake's mother. Don could have insisted Dr. Learner not release Jake until his mother arrived, since she had legal guardianship of Jake.

Study and revise

Because Don was obligated to follow the chain of command at Stabler Hospital, he did not have authority to overrule Dr. Learner's decision to release Jake to the community. Don reasonably believed Dr. Learner would not release Jake from the hospital until his mother/guardian returned to complete the requisite paperwork. Don advised Jake's mother to review her concerns with Dr. Learner and with a patient advocate because she feared bringing him home.

Privacy rules precluded Don from reviewing Jake's case with Trina. Don did not learn that Trina had escorted Jake from the emergency room until after Trina had been injured by Jake.

State the reformulated opinion

Although Don was involved in Jake's emergency room care, his actions were not a cause of Trina's injuries. Don believed Jake needed to be hospitalized, but Don did not have authority to override Dr. Learner's decision to send Jake home. Don informed Jake's mother/guardian of Dr. Learner's decision. When she objected to the plan, Don suggested she speak with Dr. Learner and with the patients' rights coordinator.

Don reasonably assumed that Jake would not be released from the hospital until his mother signed the requisite paperwork. He did not review Jake's case with Trina, because she initially was not involved with Jake's care; Don was obligated to adhere to hospital privacy rules. He did not learn that Trina had escorted Jake from the emergency room until after Jake attacked her.

2.4 Communicating the opinion

Preparation for writing the psychiatric report requires hours of hard work and reflection. The expert who has crafted the opinion(s) should review the findings with the retaining attorney. During this discussion, the attorney(s) may provide feedback about the findings to the expert. Requests for changes should be given due consideration. For example, an expert should be willing to clarify technical matters that may be confusing to laypersons. Also, an expert may decide to abridge the report preparation database in anticipation of preparing a concise report which will allow the jury to examine key information without being over-whelmed by voluminous details. Changes to the opinions should reflect only what the expert is comfortable explaining in court in terms of the content and the rationale for change.

The skilled expert knows that, when possible, changes to opinions should occur before the report has been written. Opposing counsel can use findings documented in a draft, preliminary, or final report, to unsettle and discredit the psychiatric expert. If the cross-examining attorney can show that changes between the draft and final reports alter the sub-stance of the report, then the expert's credibility will be diminished, along with the strength of the retaining attorney's case. If opposing counsel can show that the retaining attorney has influenced the substantive content of the psychiatric report, the judge may decide to exclude the psychiatric report from the evidence database. This can have adverse professional conse-quences for the psychiatrist, who should avoid preparing unnecessary drafts of reports and should not be bullied into altering the psychiatric report. A psychiatric report should not be written unless the attorney requests one.

At times, a psychiatrist has not acquired all the data before an attorney asks for a report. When this occurs, the expert should prepare to write a "Preliminary Report" and should list the limitations of the information database during the preliminary report preparation exercise. If a "Final Report" is required, the expert will identify changes, in the report prep-aration database, that alter the substance of the preliminary opinions. The expert also will anticipate explaining the rationale for such revisions in the final report and under cross-examination.

2.5 Summary

A forensic psychiatric report is designed to answer specific questions posed by the retaining attorney(s). The document may impact the outcome of a case and may alter the lives and livelihoods of others. As such, preparing to write a psychiatric report is a critical component of forensic psychiatric practice, which should not be delayed until the last minute.

Preparing to write a report begins when the expert receives a consultation request from an attorney. The steps involved in report development, including accepting the case, ana-lyzing the evidence, and formulating expert opinions, are critical to the success of the final product, the written report. The quality of the report is enhanced when the expert anticipates and plans for each of these activities, rather than adopting a more spontaneous approach. The preparation work should drive the writing of the report, not a spontaneous creative-writing process. Preparation for writing a forensic report is an essential skill that will affect the quality of the forensic report and, ultimately, the career of the expert.

References

American Academy of Psychiatry and the Law (AAPL). (2005) *Ethical Guidelines for the Practice of Forensic Psychiatry*. Adopted May 2005. Available at: http://www.aapl.org/pdf/ethicsgdlns.pdf [Accessed May 23, 2009].

American Medical Association (2005) Peer Review of Medical Expert Witness Testimony. H-265.993. Chicago, IL: American Medical Association, Available at: http://www.ama-assn.org/ama/no-index/advocacy/11760.shtml [Accessed September 30, 2009].

Diamond, B. (1959) The fallacy of the impartial expert. *Archives of Criminal Psychodynamics* **3**: 221–230.

Federation of State Medical Boards. *Expert Witness Qualifications by State* (Updated July 1, 2008). Available at: http://www.fsmb.org/pdf/grpol_expertwitness.pdf [Accessed October 15, 2009].

Goldyne, A. J. (2007) Minimizing the influence of unconscious bias in evaluations: a practical guide. *Journal of the American Academy of Psychiatry and the Law* **35**: 60–66.

Gutheil, T. G. (2009) *The Psychiatrist as Expert Witness*, 2nd edn. Washington DC: American Psychiatric Publishing, Inc.

Gutheil, T. G. & Simon, R. I. (2004) Narcissistic dimensions of expert witness practice. *Journal of the American Academy of Psychiatry and the Law* **33**: 55–58.

Gutheil, T. G., Bursztajn H, Hilliard J. T., et al. (2004) "Just say no": experts' late withdrawal from cases to preserve independence and objectivity. *Journal of the American Academy of Psychiatry and the Law* **32**: 390–394.

Katz, J. (1992) "The fallacy of the impartial expert" revisited. *Bulletin of the American Academy of Psychiatry and the Law* **11**: 379–382.

Wills, C. (2007) PRAMS: a systematic method for evaluating penal institutions under litigation. *Journal of the American Academy of Psychiatry and the Law* **35**: 103–108.

Wills, C. (2008) The CHESS method of forensic opinion formulation: striving to checkmate bias. *Journal of the American Academy of Psychiatry and the Law* **36**: 535–540.

Chapter

Confidentiality and record keeping

3

Howard Zonana

Confidentiality questions are much more varied and complicated in a forensic setting than they are in treatment settings as legal jurisdictions and judges vary in their rules and interpretations of statutes, regulations, legal precedents, and relevance. Inevitably, there are situations when legal rules conflict with ethical guidelines for psychiatrists. The ability to successfully negotiate through this maze is aided by familiarity with the ethical guidelines that have been developed by the American Psychiatric Association (APA 2009), the American Medical Association (AMA 2009), and the American Academy of Psychiatry and the Law (AAPL 2008). In difficult cases, consultation with these groups or members of ethics committees of these groups may also be helpful. This chapter will review some of the major principles relating to confidentiality and record keeping as they apply to the preparation of psychiatric reports.

3.1 Confidentiality

3.1.1 General principles

Psychiatrists conducting forensic evaluations or consultations for attorneys and courts have confidentiality obligations that relate to the agency commissioning the report (prosecution, defense, court, insurance company, corporation) as well as their own role in the legal proceedings (fact witness, expert witness or consultant to the attorney, court or employer). In criminal cases psychiatrists are typically approached by prosecution or defense attorneys, but they may also be asked by judges, parole or probation officials to provide evaluations or other relevant information. In civil cases, plaintiffs and defense counsel seek expert opinions, but also schools, employers, insurance companies, or administrative bodies such as licensure boards may request psychiatric evaluations to address specific issues such as custody of children, psychic harm or damages, malpractice, and fitness for work or duty.

The obligations of the expert with respect to confidentiality vary with the nature of his or her involvement in the case. Experts generally fit into three groups:

1. Treating psychiatrists who are asked to provide expert opinion or information relating to diagnosis or treatment. This group is most frequently called in personal injury litigation to testify about the impact of an injury to the plaintiff. Although AAPL ethical and practice guidelines for forensic psychiatry advise against using the treating psychiatrist as an expert witness for many reasons (Strasburger et al. 1997), attorneys often seek out treatment providers as fact witnesses as well as expert witnesses.

The Psychiatric Report, ed. Alec Buchanan and Michael A. Norko. Published by Cambridge University Press. © Cambridge University Press 2011.

2. Forensic psychiatrists specifically hired for the evaluation that have no prior treatment relationship with the evaluee, but have knowledge and experience in the issue related to the legal proceeding.
3. Consulting experts who review records, reports, and other data and consult to the attorney but provide only reports or other material that are usually protected as attorney work product.

The US Supreme Court in *Ake* v. *Oklahoma*, in recognizing a constitutional right to an expert in criminal cases and in defining the scope of the right, wrote that the expert would "conduct a professional examination on issues relevant to the … defense, to help determine whether the insanity defense is viable, to present testimony, and to assist in preparing the cross-examination of a State's psychiatric witnesses" (*Ake* v. *Oklahoma*, at 82, 1985). Thus, *Ake* encompassed more than a testifying defense expert; it also required a consulting expert.[1] Sometimes the roles of the consulting and testifying expert are combined, but it is not uncommon for an attorney to use a different psychiatrist as a consultant to aid in cross-examination of opposing experts, overall strategy, or as an aid in jury selection.

Since psychiatric evaluations gather health care information for diagnostic and evaluation purposes, the subsequent release of that information requires either a signed release by the evaluee or prior notification to the evaluee that the information that is being gathered is not confidential. The main sources of law and guidance in the United States are state statutes, APA ethical guidelines governing psychiatric records (APA 2009, Section 4), and the Health Insurance Portability and Accountability Act of 1996 (HIPAA 1996).

When working for the prosecution or court

Typically, when working for the court or the prosecution, the initial disclosure prior to beginning the evaluation will be something similar to:

> Since I have been asked by the court or prosecutor to perform this psychiatric evaluation what we discuss is not confidential, as I have to prepare a report and might be called to testify. My understanding of the purpose of the evaluation is to …

Clear notification of the lack of confidentiality is given. If the examination is for competency to stand trial or other court-ordered assessment, the evaluation can then proceed, as it is only notification that is required, not informed consent. Some ethical complications may arise if the individual is thought to be incompetent to stand trial and has also been ordered to have their state of mind at the time of the crime assessed, as is the practice in some states. In those circumstances, ethical issues may arise for the prosecution or court-retained evaluator if the defendant begins revealing information that may be incriminating. The American Academy of Psychiatry and the Law (AAPL) practice guidelines recommend that the evaluator stop the state of mind assessment and inform the retaining party of the defendant's incompetence (Giorgi-Guarnieri et al. 2002). Thus ethical considerations may override a rote following of the original court order.

---

[1] See, e.g., *Taylor* v. *State*, 939 S.W.2d 148, 153 (Tex. Crim. App. 1996) ("Due process, at a minimum, requires expert aid in an evaluation of a defendant's case in an effort to present it in the best possible light to the jury.").

When working for the defense

The nature of confidentiality status of the information differs when working for the defense. The "warnings" or notifications given to evaluees are different also. A typical disclosure might begin with:

> Since I have been asked by your attorney to perform this psychiatric evaluation what we discuss is initially covered under the attorney client privilege/work product rules and remains confidential. Should you and your attorney conclude that I have something useful to contribute to your case and would like a report and/or testimony, what we have talked about will cease to be confidential.[2]

When working for defense counsel, performing a state of mind evaluation on an incompetent defendant would not present an ethical conflict as any material received by the evaluating psychiatrist is protected and, even if not helpful, does not have to be revealed.

HIPAA

The Health Insurance Portability and Accountability Act and its accompanying regulations (HHS, 45 CFR 160, 164, 2010) have had a significant impact on rules concerning disclosure of health care information in the United States. The Act established a set of basic national privacy standards and fair information practices governing "protected health information" (PHI).[3] The law attempts to balance the individual's need for privacy with society's need for disclosure. Many questions remain open regarding the applicability of HIPAA to forensic work, but HIPAA does provide some guidance for court-related evaluations. For example, court-ordered evaluations do not have to be shown to the evaluee prior to submission of the report.[4]

---

[2] Although even this level of detail may not cover all of the possibilities, some states and federal courts require that an attorney who has obtained more than one opinion submit a list of the other evaluators who have examined the defendant. These other evaluators may be called by the state in rebuttal. See *US ex rel. Edney* v. *Smith* (1976) 425 F. Supp. 1038.

[3] Protected Health Information is the term used in the Health Insurance Portability and Accountability Act and the federal regulations relating to that Act (45 CFR § 160.103). It refers to "Individually identifiable health information" held or transmitted by a covered entity or its business associate, in any form or media, whether electronic, paper, or oral. "Individually identifiable health information", in turn, is information, including demographic data, that relates to:
- the individual's past, present or future physical or mental health or condition,
- the provision of health care to the individual, or
- the past, present, or future payment for the provision of health care to the individual,
and that identifies the individual or for which there is a reasonable basis to believe it can be used to identify the individual. Individually identifiable health information includes many common identifiers (e.g., name, address, birth date, Social Security Number).

[4] In particular, although the Privacy Rule generally provides significant rights with respect to health information, an individual does not have a right of access to information "compiled in reasonable anticipation of, or for use in, a civil, criminal, or administrative action or proceeding" (45 C.F.R. § 164.524(a)). For example, disclosure without authorization is permitted "[i]n response to an order of a court or administrative tribunal" (§ 164.512(e) (1) (i)), or "as authorized by and to the extent necessary to comply with laws relating to workers' compensation or other similar programs" (§ 164.512(l)). To the extent that one or more of these provisions applies (and no applicable state law provides "more stringent" protection), no authorization may be necessary. Thus, for example, if a court has requested an examination, this exception would arguably apply. A forensic psychiatrist should consult state law, however, to see whether broader access rights are applicable under HIPAA's "more stringent" state law analysis.

While HIPAA refers primarily to patients and physicians in treatment relationships, the definitions of treatment relationships are sufficiently broad that they likely include forensic evaluations. If so, forensic evaluators should provide a statement outlining their privacy practices to all evaluees and obtain signed releases when not performing court-ordered or otherwise excluded evaluations.

The American Psychiatric Association has recommended that release forms and notice of privacy practices be given to evaluees who are undergoing a forensic evaluation. The forensic program at Yale University developed a packet of such documents that has been reviewed and approved by the university's attorneys. With the caveat that these releases may not be necessary, apply only to "covered entities," and should be considered as works in progress, copies are provided in Figures 3.1 and 3.2 that can be modified to fit other university or private practice settings. Attorneys who represent the facility or organization should review any institutional use.

3.1.2 Confidentiality problems arising in practice

While notices and releases are essential starting points, they do not resolve the myriad of day-to-day situations that pose difficult problems in conducting evaluations.

Evaluee requests

One of our first "HIPAA type confidentiality problems" arose when an evaluation for a paranoid individual charged with impersonating a federal officer was requested by a defense attorney. The attorney thought the charges would be dropped if the government believed the man was mentally ill. He was seen by a psychiatrist and then, as part of the evaluation, was sent for psychological testing after signing the release forms permitting us to talk with his attorney. The psychiatrist concluded that the man understood the issues related to release of information forms but might not be competent to stand trial. During the psychological testing he told the psychologist that he did not want the psychology test results sent to his attorney as he was thinking of firing his attorney. He did not immediately fire the attorney and the attorney wanted the psychiatric report completed quickly in the hope of resolving the case expeditiously, hoping to avoid filing for a competence to stand trial evaluation, since he did not want to see the defendant hospitalized for an extended period if it could be avoided. We had to decide whether we could send the psychological testing as part of the report.

This would have been no problem if the evaluation had been court ordered but defense attorneys frequently request many evaluations without a court order. We ultimately decided to send a report but not include any data from the psychological testing after concluding that the test results were not essential for the report. If the results were critical to the evaluation then further discussion with the client would be necessary by the psychiatrist and if he still refused, a discussion with the attorney so that he could directly deal with the client about his representation agreement.

Reporting statutes

Two other cases illustrate conflicts that can arise in relation to child abuse reporting laws. In the first case a psychiatrist, hired by a defense attorney of a minor child retained by his parents, was asked to perform an evaluation in an attempt to understand why the minor brought a gun to school. During the evaluation the parents of one of his friends (collateral sources of information) revealed that the minor had revealed evidence of child abuse by his father to them.

Yale University School of Medicine
Law and Psychiatry Division

Authorization for Use or Disclosure of Protected Health Information

Name of Evaluee _____

Date of Birth _____ _____ _____

Daytime Phone # _____ Evening Phone # _____

Address _____

City _____ State _____ Zip Code _____

I hereby authorize the Law and Psychiatry Division of Yale School of Medicine to use or disclose my protected health information as indicated below to:

Name _____

Daytime Phone # _____ Fax # _____

Address _____

City _____ State _____ Zip Code _____

Information to be released:
☐ Consultation report _____
☐ Other _____

Purpose of Disclosure:
☐ Legal
☐ Insurance
☐ Workers' Compensation
☐ Other _____

I understand that this health information may include HIV-related information and/or information relating to diagnosis or treatment of psychiatric disabilities and/or substance abuse and that by signing this form, I am specifically authorizing the release of information relating to:

☐ Substance Abuse (including alcohol/drug abuse)
☐ Mental Health
☐ Psychotherapy Notes
☐ HIV related information (including AIDS related testing)

The confidentiality of this record is required under Chapter 899 of the Connecticut General Statutes, as well as, Title 42 of the United States code. This material shall not be transmitted to anyone without written consent or authorization as provided in these statutes.

X _____
Signature of Evaluee, Patient or Legal Guardian   Date

1. I understand that this authorization will expire two years from my last date of service visit. A photocopy of this form will be considered as valid as the original.

2. I understand that I may revoke this authorization at any time by notifying The YSM Deputy Privacy Officer at the address indicated below, in writing, and this authorization will cease to be effective on the date notified except to the extent action has already been taken in reliance upon it.

YSM Deputy Privacy Officer
Yale School of Medicine
300 George Street, 6th Floor
P.O. Box 9805
New Haven, CT 06535-9805

3. I understand that information used or disclosed pursuant to this authorization may be subject to re-disclosure by the recipient and no longer be protected by Federal privacy regulations. However, other state or federal law may prohibit the recipient from disclosing specially protected information, such as substance abuse treatment information, HIV/AIDS-related information, and psychiatric/mental health information.

4. My health care and payment for my health care will not be affected if I do not sign this form.

5. I understand that my refusal to sign this Authorization will not jeopardize my right to obtain present or future treatment for psychiatric disabilities except where disclosure of the information is necessary for the treatment.

6. I understand that I will get a copy of this form after I sign it.

7. Unlike medical treatment records the federal privacy rule does not give you the right of access to our reports that are prepared for use in a civil, criminal, or administrative action prior to their submission.

8. Our Division usually functions, unless otherwise contracted, as a team with individual evaluators consulting with other professionals (psychiatrists, psychologists, social workers and nurses) to be sure that comprehensive and complete evaluations are being performed. All the members of the Division (including students, as we are part of a medical school) are bound by the same confidentiality as the primary evaluator.

By signing below, I acknowledge that I have read and understand this Authorization.

X _____ _____ OR _____ _____
Signature of Evaluee   Date   Parent/Legal Guardian/Authorized person   Date

_____
Relationship to Evaluee

Form #: YSM HIP11-L&P Division
Original Date of Form: Effective Date: April 14, 2003
Revised Date: August 20, 2004

Figure 3.1 Example of a release form.

Yale University

School of Medicine
Department of Psychiatry
Connecticut Mental Health Center
Law and Psychiatry Division

Connecticut Mental Health Center (CMHC)   *34 Park Street*
Yale Department of Psychiatry   *New Haven, Connecticut 06519-1187*
NOTICE OF PRIVACY PRACTICES   *Howard Zonana, M. D.,Director*
Law & Psychiatry Division   *Telephone: 203974-7158*
                                                 Fax: 203 974-7177

THIS NOTICE DESCRIBES HOW MEDICAL INFORMATION ABOUT YOU MAY BE USED AND DISCLOSED, AND HOW YOU CAN HAVE ACCESS TO THIS INFORMATION. PLEASE REVIEW IT CAREFULLY.

The Law & Psychiatry Division is federally mandated to maintain the privacy of your medical information and wants you to know about our practices for protecting your health information.

The Law & Psychiatry Division is required to abide by the terms of this notice. The medical information we maintain may come from you or treatment providers and other medical records that have been legally authorized for release to us. The medical information we record and maintain is known as Protected Health Information, or PHI. We will not use or disclose your PHI without your permission, except as described in this notice.

Although we are not engaged in a treatment relationship with you, we do collect medical information for diagnostic assessments that are part of legal proceedings. Evaluations are most frequently requested in civil or criminal cases by:

1. Courts
2. Prosecutors or States Attorneys
3. Defense attorneys
4. Parole or probation departments
5. Administrative bodies; e.g., licensure boards, workers compensation, social security
6. Insurance companies
7. Employers

Court, prosecutor, and opposing counsel requested evaluations are not confidential, as reports have to be submitted and testimony may be required. You will be notified at the outset of the interview if the interview is confidential and to whom a report will be sent. Reports that are court ordered are usually sent to the Clerk of the court and then are distributed to both defense and prosecution attorneys (and both sides in a civil case). Such reports/testimony may become part of the public record if they are entered into evidence. Reports requested by your attorney are initially protected under the attorney–client privilege and only if you and your attorney agree that the report will be useful will a report be prepared and submitted to your attorney. If you and your attorney agree that the report should be used in the case it will be made available to the judge and opposing counsel. The report/testimony may then be entered as evidence and may become part of the public record.

USES AND DISCLOSURES:

In general, it is our policy to obtain written authorization for release of information prior to making a disclosure. However, your written authorization is not required to submit reports prepared in response to a court order. You may revoke an authorization at any time, except to the extent that we have already acted on it. Unlike medical treatment records the federal privacy rule does not give you the right of access to our reports that are prepared for use in a civil, criminal, or administrative action prior to their submission.

Our Division functions usually as a team with individual evaluators consulting with other professionals (psychiatrists, psychologists, social workers and nurses) to be sure that comprehensive and complete evaluations are being performed. All the members of the Division (including students, as we are part of a medical school) are bound by the same confidentiality as the primary evaluator.

Figure 3.2 Example of a privacy notice.

We may use your Protected Health Information (PHI) without authorization for:

- Payment, e.g., to the state Department of Administrative Services to bill for your healthcare services
- Healthcare operations, e.g., to internal staff for evaluation of the quality of services provided
- Reminding you of appointments

Other permitted disclosures of your Protected Health Information (PHI) without authorization might include the following:

- Disclosures required by law, e.g., to the Department of Children and Families when a law requires that we report suspected abuse or neglect
- Preparation of a Medical Research protocol or plan, e.g. to look at records to determine if the research project should proceed
- Public Health, e.g., mandated reporting of disease, injury or vital statistics
- To avert a serious threat to the health or safety of you or others
- As a response to a court order, e.g. a judge orders specific portions of your record as a result of a legal matter
- If deceased, limited information to coroners, medical examiners or funeral directors

HOW YOU CAN REPORT A PROBLEM?

If you feel your privacy rights have been violated, you may file a complaint with the CMHC Health Information Specialist, Beverly Clark, RHIT, (203) 974–7321, or the CMHC Privacy Officer Michael Levine, CIO, (203) 974–7570, or the State of Connecticut, Department of Mental Health and Addiction Services (DMHAS), Office of HealthCare Information (OHI) at (860) 418–6901, or the Secretary of the United States Department of Health and Human Services (DHHS), Office for Civil Rights (OCR) at: U.S. DHHS, OCR, J.F. Kennedy Federal Building – Room 1875, Boston, Massachusetts 02203. Voice phone: (617) 565–1340. TDD: (617) 565–1343. FAX: (617) 565–3809.

There will be no retaliation for filing a complaint.

WOULD YOU LIKE MORE INFORMATION?

If you have questions and would like more information, you may contact the CMHC Health Information Specialist at (203) 974–7321 or the DMHAS Office of Healthcare Information (OHI) at (860) 418–6901.

We reserve the right to change our practices and to make the new provisions effective for all medical information we maintain. Should our medical information practices change, we will amend this notice and post a notice of the changes, which will be made available to anyone upon request. This notice is effective as of November 15, 2003.

Figure 3.2 (cont.)

In the second case a man charged with pedophilic offenses revealed some additional offenses against another identifiable minor.

These cases raise the question of reporting obligations under the child abuse reporting statutes, and whether the same obligations exist when doing a forensic evaluation. The consequences can be significant: possible disruption of the child's defense and, in the second case, additional sexual charges could be added to the existing ones. Our research has revealed that attorneys are not mandated reporters for child abuse in most states, and most states have not created exceptions for reporting abuse when the information arises during an evaluation requested by an attorney or court. Maryland has a short attorney general's opinion that protects evaluations done at an attorney's request (75 Md. Op. Atty. Gen.

76, 1990, see also *State* v. *Pratt*, 1979), and Oregon has a statute that limits disclosures for professionals treating sex offenders (ORS § 419B.010 (2007)). At the beginning of a psychiatric evaluation, it is useful for both the attorney and psychiatrist to inform an evaluee, in states that mandate child abuse reporting with no exceptions for forensically related examinations, of the reporting obligations if identifiable information of possible or additional child abuse is revealed.

3.1.3 Confidentiality issues other than to the evaluee

During the course of a forensic evaluation it is likely that interviews with collateral sources will be part of the evaluation. There is some debate as to whether respect for the defendant requires specific consent to speak with collateral sources of information that do not have privileged material, such as family, employers, friends, or acquaintances. Some experts will not make such contacts and note in their reports that consent was asked for but not given. Others feel that as long as they explain their role and goals to the collateral source before the interview is agreed to, it is ethical and appropriate to conduct the interview. Collateral data enhance the report and allow for a rebuttal to the typical cross-examination question, "You mean to tell the court that you relied only upon what the defendant told you?" Any interviews of collateral sources should be cleared with the retaining attorney prior to initiating contact so as to be clear if there are any restrictions or other reasons that would preclude an interview with that person.

3.1.4 Duty to third parties – the *Tarasoff* question

There are several types of *Tarasoff* situations that can occur during forensic evaluations. For example, during a competency to stand trial evaluation, the defendant makes several references to attacking or killing the judge in his case as he feels the judge is treating him unfairly. If you consider the threat to be significant and/or the defendant's control of his behavior is impaired, what are the ethical and legal obligations for the expert?

Can one rely on the fact that all courtrooms are considered places of risk and that is why marshals and security personnel are always present in a court setting? Should the judge or Clerk's Office be notified directly? Is it less intrusive and equally effective to notify the defense attorney and have him take the necessary steps to be sure his client does not get into additional difficulties while in the courtroom?

In a California case *(People* v. *Clark*, 1990), a defendant was charged with first-degree murder, arson, and attempted second-degree murder after burning down the house of his former therapist and killing her husband in the fire. At the request of his defense attorney, a forensic psychiatrist examined the defendant. Clark told that psychiatrist about plans to kill two additional people. The psychiatrist made a *Tarasoff* warning to those individuals. The psychiatrist later testified about these threats at the defendant's trial, and he was convicted on all counts. On appeal, the defendant argued that the psychiatrist should have been precluded from testifying at the trial, as any statements made to her were protected under both the psychotherapist–patient and attorney–client privileges.

The majority opinion in *Clark* discusses only briefly whether or not the *Tarasoff* warning made by the forensic psychiatrist was proper; it simply affirms the trial court's ruling that the warning was necessary to prevent future harm (*People* v. *Clark*, at 150, 1990). The issue of whether the psychiatrist should be allowed to testify about the threats during the murder trial was examined in more detail. The court rejected the defendant's argument that the statements to the psychiatrist were protected under the psychotherapist–patient privilege, but it agreed that the statements were protected under attorney–client privilege, taking the view that the threats were "communications made in the attorney-client relationship" (*People* v. *Clark*, at 152, 1990) and therefore should be inadmissible in any criminal proceeding.

Clark can be interpreted to mean that forensic psychiatrists who examine a defendant at the request of the defense attorney should make a *Tarasoff* warning if they deem it necessary, but their testimony about that warning may be excluded from a future criminal proceeding because of attorney–client privilege.

Subsequent cases in California have readdressed the issue of psychotherapists' testimony about *Tarasoff* warnings in criminal proceedings, first expanding and then limiting the scope of that testimony (Mosk 1993; Weinstock et al. 2001). However, it is important to note that none of these cases has suggested that a forensic psychiatrist should not issue the *Tarasoff* warning itself – the point of contention was only whether testimony about that warning is admissible in future criminal proceedings.

On June 13, 1996, the US Supreme Court established a psychotherapist–patient privilege in the federal courts in *Jaffee* v. *Redmond*. This privilege covered psychiatrists, psychologists, and social workers. Following the decision there has been some controversy between jurisdictions in several areas. The first relates to the status of the privilege following *Tarasoff* warnings (calling the police or potential victim of a patient making credible threat of harm) by a treating mental health professional. In the *Jaffee* decision, after announcing the privilege the US Supreme Court added a potential limitation in the opinion:

> [a]lthough it would be premature to speculate about most future developments in the federal psychotherapist privilege, we do not doubt that there are situations in which the privilege must give way, for example, if a serious threat of harm to the patient or to others can be averted only by means of a disclosure by the therapist. (*Jaffee* v. *Redmond*, at 18, 1996)

This has led to substantial confusion regarding whether, once a *Tarasoff* warning has been made, the psychiatrist or therapist can be forced to testify by the state against the patient about the circumstances of the warning at a subsequent criminal trial. Such testimony is used to help establish intent, premeditation, or other aggravating circumstances. The federal circuits are in disagreement in this regard. The Sixth and Ninth Circuits have held that such statements, though made without a reasonable expectation of confidentiality, are nonetheless privileged (*US* v. *Chase*, 2003 and *US* v. *Hayes*, 2000), but the Tenth Circuit and Fifth Circuit have held that, in such situations, the psychotherapist–patient privilege must give way (*US* v. *Glass*, 1998 and *US* v. *Auster*, 2008). The Supreme Court will ultimately have to resolve these differences.

Given the complexity, short of a dire emergency, it seems prudent to review the situation with the retaining attorney in forensic cases and independent consultation in treatment cases prior to making any disclosures.

3.1.5 Prosecutorial use of defense experts

Another confidentiality concern has arisen about the prosecution's ability to use defense experts if the defense declines, or is not planning to call that expert as a witness. First, the two different roles of experts must be distinguished. For the testifying expert, once on the stand, any privilege is waived. For the consulting expert who provides an adverse opinion when asked to help the attorney decide whether a scientific defense is feasible, the question may arise as to whether the prosecution can then call that expert as a government witness. Arguments to preclude the prosecution from calling such a witness have been made under the attorney–client privilege, the work product privilege, and the right to counsel (Imwinkelried 1990; Maringer 1993; Gainelli 2004).

Attorney–client privilege

The majority of courts have held that the attorney–client privilege covers communications made to an attorney by a consulting expert retained for the purpose of providing information necessary for proper representation.[5] The rationale rests on the attorney's need to obtain advice in planning a strategy for the case. As one judge commented, "Only a foolhardy lawyer would determine tactical and evidentiary strategy in a case with psychiatric issues without the guidance and interpretation of psychiatrists and others skilled in the field" (*US ex rel. Edney* v. *Smith*, 1976). Another judge remarked: "Breaching the attorney-client privilege … would have the effect of inhibiting the free exercise of a defense attorney's informed judgment by confronting him with the likelihood that, in taking a step obviously crucial to his client's defense, he is creating a potential government witness who theretofore did not exist" (*State* v. *Pratt*, 1979).

Other courts have variously rejected the extension of the privilege to consulting experts. Some have limited the privilege to attorney–client communications, excluding experts and other agents.[6] Other courts have limited the privilege to those experts who rely on

---

[5] See, e.g., *US* v. *Alvarez*, 519 F.2d 1036 at 1046–47 (1975) deciding that disclosures made by a defense-retained psychiatrist to the attorney are protected under the privilege, unless and until the psychiatrist takes the stand; *US* v. *Layton*, 90 FRD 520, 525 (N.D. Cal. 1981): "Even if the psychotherapist-patient privilege is made inapplicable by defendant's assertion of a psychiatric defense, the attorney-client privilege shields these communications."; *Houston* v. *State*, 602 P.2d 784, 791 (Ala. 1979) addressing the possibility that a claim of attorney-client privilege might be sustained vis-à-vis a psychiatrist; *People* v. *Lines*, 531 P.2d 793, 802–03 (Cal. 1975) protecting communications between a court-appointed psychiatrist and the defendant; *Miller* v. *District Court*, 737 P.2d 834, 836–38 (Colo. 1987) following "a majority of the courts" to hold that communications between a defendant and his defense-retained psychiatrist are protected; *Pouncy* v. *Florida*, 353 So. 2d at 642 (1977) applying privilege to psychiatrist; *State* v. *Pratt*, 398 A.2d 421, 423–25 (Md. 1979) concluding that communications made by the defendant to his psychiatrist are protected, even when the defendant pleads insanity as a defense; *People* v. *Hilliker*, 185 N.W.2d 831, 833 (Mich. Ct. App. 1971): "Since the privilege clearly extends to confidential communications made directly by the client to the attorney, there is nothing to dictate a different result where that communication is made to the attorney by an agent on behalf of the client, such as a doctor or psychiatrist."; *State* v. *Kociolek*, 129 A.2d 417, 423–25 (N.J. 1957) explaining that the attorney–client privilege extends to communications between the attorney and a scientific expert, such as a psychiatrist, who is aiding in the preparation of a defense; *State* v. *Hitopoulus*, 309 S.E.2d 747, 748–49 (S.C. 1983) protecting defendant-psychiatrist communications that were made to aid in the preparation of a defense. See generally Michael G. Walsh, Annotation, Applicability of Attorney-Client Privilege to Communications Made in Presence of or Solely to or by Third Person, *14 ALR 4th 594*, 2(a) (1982) summarizing court trends in the application of the attorney-client privilege when a third party is involved.

[6] See, e.g., *State* v. *Schaaf*, 819 P.2d 909, 918 (Ariz. 1991): "We find it to be within the trial court's broad discretion to determine whether an expert witness will be required to testify, even if it was the other party who initially retained the expert witness."; *State* v. *Carter*, 641 S.W.2d 54, 57 (Mo. 1982): "The privilege is limited to communications between the attorney and the client. It operates only to render the attorney incompetent to testify to confidential communications made to him by a client."; *State* v. *Hamlet*, 944 P.2d 1026, 1031 (Wash. 1997) finding that the attorney–client privilege and the Sixth Amendment are not violated when the court orders "disclosure of the name of the non-testifying

communications from the client, encompassing psychiatrists but not a ballistics expert.[7] In some jurisdictions a defendant who raises an insanity defense waives the privilege with respect to all other psychiatrists who have examined the defendant.[8] Some scholars have argued that it is not the "privilege" that should be applied here, since that overly broadens the meaning of what a privilege signifies, but rather it should be an extension of the work product rule.[9]

Work product rule

A federal district court applied the "work product rule" to prevent a ballistics expert hired by the defense from being called by the prosecution. The court acknowledged that it was entering "relatively uncharted waters and the case law is an insufficient and contradictory navigational aid," but it found that the opinions were developed at the request of the defense attorneys for strategic planning. The court noted that, "exhaustive research has disclosed no criminal case in which a federal court has permitted the government to elicit testimony from a defendant's consultative expert concerning that expert's efforts or opinions undertaken or developed at the request of a defense attorney in preparation for a criminal trial."[10] The work product rule can also be flexible if the situation is unusual. In *State* v. *Cosey*, during DNA testing, the defense exhausted the remaining crime scene specimen, which prevented the prosecution from performing more sophisticated testing similar to that performed by the defense. In that case the defendant was not planning to call the analyst or use the test results. The Louisiana Supreme Court ruled, "Fundamental fairness and the extraordinary circumstances presented by this case dictate that the prosecution be allowed to obtain copies of the test results in question" (*State* v. *Cosey*, 1995).

---

expert retained by the defense for purposes of a diminished capacity defense" or when the state calls "that expert as a State's witness to rebut evidence of a diminished capacity defense."

[7] *People* v. *Knuckles*, 650 N.E.2d 974, 978 (Ill. 1995) distinguishing the denial of the privilege to a fingerprint expert's testimony on the ground that a psychiatrist's opinion as to the defendant's sanity "will almost invariably result in large part from confidential communications with the defendant which would be directly or indirectly revealed if the psychiatrist testified on behalf of the State."

[8] See *Gray* v. *District Court*, 884 P.2d 286, 293 (Colo. 1994) holding that, when a defendant puts his mental condition at issue, he "waives the right to claim the attorney-client and physician/psychologist-patient privileges, and a prosecution's use of testimony of a defense-retained psychiatrist, who is not called by the defendant to testify at trial, is admissible at trial"; *State* v. *Carter*, 641 S.W.2d 54, 57 (Mo. 1982); *People* v. *Edney*, 350 N.E.2d 400, 402–03 (N.Y. 1976) finding no reason to protect communications made to a psychiatrist when the defendant puts his sanity in issue; *Hamlet State* v. *Hamlet*, 944 P.2d 1026, at 1030, (Wash. 1997) by asserting a defense of diminished capacity or insanity, defendant waives attorney–client privilege as to evidence concerning his mental state; *State* v. *Pawlyk*, 800 P.2d 338, 345 (Wash. 1990): "If defendant asserts an insanity defense, evidence pertaining to that defense must be available to both sides at trial."; *Trusky* v. *State*, 7 P.3d 5, 10 (Wyo. 2000): "[A defendant] may not argue a deficient mental condition and, at the same time, claim protection by privilege."

[9] See Imwinkelried (1990, pp. 21–23), surveying the recent trend in favor of extending the attorney-client privilege to expert information.

[10] See *US* v. *Walker*, 910 F. Supp. 861, at 864, 865,866 (N.D.N.Y. 1995) precluding the government from questioning defense experts on their investigation, opinions, or conclusions "unless the government first makes a showing of substantial need of that testimony and inability to obtain the substantial equivalent of that testimony without undue hardship."

The right to effective assistance of counsel

In addition to the preceding arguments, defendants have also argued that the Sixth Amendment right to effective assistance of counsel precludes the government or prosecution from using information developed by experts retained by the defense. Several courts have accepted this line of reasoning.

> A defense attorney should be completely free and unfettered in making a decision as fundamental as that concerning the retention of an expert to assist him. Reliance upon the confidentiality of an expert's advice itself is a crucial aspect of a defense attorney's ability to consult with and advise his client. If the confidentiality of that advice cannot be anticipated, the attorney might well forgo seeking such assistance, to the consequent detriment of his client's cause.[11]

Again not all courts have accepted this line of reasoning. It is also easy to lose the protection by making inappropriate disclosures. In *Taylor* v. *State*, at the request of the defense, a DNA expert was appointed only to examine semen evidence in a rape case. The expert reported that the defendant's DNA fell within a class of persons (one chance in a 12 million random match) that could have deposited the semen. The report was also sent to the prosecutor, who immediately made the expert a prosecution witness. On these grounds the court held that the expert had not been acting as a defense expert to the extent required under *Ake*. If she had, the report would never have been provided to the prosecutor (*Taylor* v. *State*, 1996). The case was remanded to see whether the expert met the threshold requirement for securing a court-appointed expert.

The ability of a defense expert to examine a victim has also been a source of controversy. The strongest cases have occurred when the prosecution has conducted an examination and intends to have an expert testify. Frequently children are the victims where experts are sought by the state (*Lickey* v. *State*, 1992 and *State* v. *Bronson*, 2001).

In sum, given some of these exceptions, any contact by a prosecutor should be reviewed with the defense counsel.

3.1.6 Psychotherapist–patient privilege

Although evaluees will typically sign releases to obtain past treatment records and permission to talk with prior therapists or treatment providers, there are many circumstances where release of prior records can be an inappropriate intrusion into a person's private life and thoughts. The balancing of legal needs and privacy rights has been an evolving process

---

[11] *State* v. *Mingo*, 392 A.2d 590, 595 (N.J. 1978); see also *Pawlyk* v. *Wood*, 248 F.3d 815, 828–29 (9th Cir. 2001) (Canby, J., dissenting): "In my view, a psychiatrist retained to assist the defense is not to be treated as a run-of-the-mill witness; due process requires recognition of his or her position as a member of the defense team. Defense counsel should be able to employ the services of such a psychiatrist in preparing an insanity defense without running the risk of involuntarily creating evidence for the prosecution."; *US* v. *Alvarez*, 519 F.2d 1036, 1047 (3d Cir. 1975): "The attorney must be free to make an informed judgment with respect to the best course for the defense without the inhibition of creating a potential government witness."; *Hutchinson* v. *People*, 742 P.2d 875, 881 (Colo. 1987): "We cannot sanction the prosecution's decision … to offer the defense's handwriting expert as a witness in its case-in-chief. Absent compelling justification or waiver, we believe that such a practice violates a defendant's right to effective assistance of counsel."; *People* v. *Knippenberg*, 362 N.E.2d 681, 684–85 (Ill. 1977) protecting statements given by the defendant to an investigator for the Illinois Defender Project that the defense attorney had contacted for assistance with the case.

that is continually being negotiated in statutes, regulations, and case law. Privileges prevent courts from obtaining information and are generally discouraged by courts. Attorney–client, priest–penitent, husband–wife as well as doctor–patient privileges are the most common and all have had substantial controversy about their limits. Since 1960, most states have developed psychiatrist-patient confidentiality and privilege statutes that codified physician ethical standards regarding confidentiality and privilege obligations along with rules denoting exceptions, e.g., civil commitment, reporting statutes, and the patient–litigant exception. The following sections discuss two additional areas that were not fully resolved by the *Jaffee* decision that affects forensic practice in military law and other waivers or exceptions to the privilege.

Military law

In forensic evaluations, the presence or absence of a psychotherapist–patient privilege can be important in preparing a case and knowing what evidence may or may not be available for review. Since the military not infrequently uses forensic psychiatric experts who are not on active duty, it is important to be aware of some of the differences in military law.

The development of the psychotherapist–patient privilege in military law has differed from that of federal law, both before and after the US Supreme Court enunciated a federal psychotherapist–patient privilege in *Jaffee* v. *Redmond* (Flippin 2003). The source of military law under Article 36 of the Uniform Code of Military Justice (UCMJ) states the President may prescribe rules of evidence "which shall, so far as he considers practicable, apply the principles of law and rules of evidence generally recognized in the trial of criminal cases in the US district courts." Under Article 36 a majority of the Military Rules of Evidence (MRE) were subsequently adopted with minor modifications from the Federal Rules of Evidence (FRE). One major difference between the FRE and the MRE relates to the rules of privilege. The analysis of MRE 501 explains that a general rule of privilege is not practical in a military setting:

> Unlike the Article III court system, which is conducted almost entirely by attorneys functioning in conjunction with permanent courts in fixed locations, the military criminal legal system is characterized by its dependence upon large numbers of laymen, temporary courts, and inherent geographical and personnel instability due to the worldwide deployment of military personnel. Consequently, military law requires far more stability than civilian law. This is particularly true because of the significant number of non-lawyers involved in the military criminal legal system. Commanders, convening authorities, non-lawyer investigating officers, summary court-martial officers, or law enforcement personnel need specific guidance as to what material is privileged and what is not.[12]

At the time of their implementation, the MRE did not recognize a psychotherapist–patient privilege, and in fact specifically rejected it. Military Rule of Evidence 501(d) provided that "notwithstanding any other provision of these rules, information not otherwise privileged does not become privileged on the basis that it was acquired by a medical officer or civilian physician in a professional capacity."[13]

---

[12] Manual for Courts-Martial, United States, Mil. R. Evid. 501 (2002) (hereinafter MCM) analysis, at A22–38 "The Committee deemed the approach taken by Congress in the Federal Rules impracticable within the armed forces."

[13] MCM, *supra* note 3, Mil. R. Evid. 501(d). See also Hayden (1987, p. 66). "The military has always been explicit and intransigent in its non-recognition of any physician-patient privilege."

Before the *Jaffee* case, military courts uniformly rejected any claim of psychotherapist–patient privilege because the rules did not explicitly recognize it, and in fact explicitly rejected a physician–patient privilege. In one case the Court of Military Appeals stated "There is no physician–patient privilege or psychotherapist–patient privilege in federal law, including military law" (*US* v. *Mansfield*, 1993).

After *Jaffee* recognized a psychotherapist–patient privilege in federal courts, military courts continued to reject it. The Navy-Marine Court of Appeals, the Air Force Court of Criminal Appeals, and the Army Court of Criminal appeals all rejected the idea that *Jaffee* applied to the military. The Court of Appeals for the Armed Forces settled the issue in *US* v. *Rodriguez* holding that the MRE 501(d) "precludes application of doctor-patient or psychotherapist privilege to the military." The privilege did not apply to the defendant's statements to an Army psychiatrist and held that:

> Prior to *Jaffee* there was no privilege. Post *Jaffee* and prior to the adoption of Mil. R. Evid. 513, there was still no psychotherapist-patient in the military because it was contrary to Mil. R. Evid. 501(d). When the President promulgated Mil. R. Evid. 513, he did not simply adopt *Jaffee*; rather, he created a limited psychotherapist privilege for the military. In the absence of a constitutional or statutory requirement to the contrary, the decision as to whether, when, and to what degree *Jaffee* should apply in the military rests with the President, not this Court." (*US* v. *Rodriguez*, 2000)

In 1999 President Clinton exercised his authority under Article 36(a) and established a psychotherapist–patient privilege for the military. Executive Order 13,140 implemented MRE 513, which protected confidential communications between a patient and psychotherapist. This rule covers any communication made after November 1, 1999 (Exec. Order, 1999).

It applies, however, only to UCMJ proceedings and does "not limit the availability of such information internally to the services, for appropriate purposes." So, in general, there is still no physician–patient privilege for members of the Armed Forces.

The rule of privilege in MRE 513(a) protects "a confidential communication made between the patient and a psychotherapist or an assistant to the psychotherapist, in a case arising under the UCMJ, if such communication was made for the purpose of facilitating diagnosis or treatment of the patient's mental or emotional condition" (Mil. R. Evid. 513(a)). The rule defines a "patient" as "a person who consults with or is examined or interviewed by a psychotherapist for the purposes of advice, diagnosis, or treatment of a mental or emotional condition" (Mil. R. Evid. 513(b)(1)). Evidence from a victim or witness can be excluded on the same basis. "Psychotherapist" includes "a psychiatrist, clinical psychologist, or clinical social worker who is licensed in any state, territory, possession, the District of Columbia or Puerto Rico to perform professional services as such, or who holds credentials to provide such services from any military health care facility"(Mil. R. Evid. 513(b)(2)).

Holder of the privilege

Under MRE 513, the privilege belongs to the patient. Military Rule of Evidence 513(a) provides that the patient has "a privilege to refuse to disclose and to prevent another person from disclosing a confidential communication" (Mil. R. Evid. 513(a)). In addition to the patient, other specified persons may claim the privilege. These specified persons include guardians, conservators, and psychotherapists or assistants to a psychotherapist acting on behalf of the patient (Mil. R. Evid. 513(c)). As a result, the patient, or the guardian or conservator of the patient may authorize the trial or defense counsel to claim the privilege on the patient's behalf.

Exceptions to the privilege

The psychotherapist–patient privilege established in MRE 513 is not an absolute privilege. There are eight exceptions where the privilege is inapplicable: (1) the patient is deceased (Mil. R. Evid. 513(d)(1)); (2) the communication evidences spouse abuse, child abuse, or neglect, or "in a proceeding where one spouse is charged with a crime against the person of the other spouse or a child of either spouse" (Mil. R. Evid. 513(d)(2)); (3) federal law, state law, or service regulation imposes a duty to report the communication (Mil. R. Evid. 513(d)(3)); (4) the patient's mental or emotional condition makes the patient a danger to himself or others (Mil. R. Evid. 513(d)(4)); (5) the communication "clearly contemplated the future commission of a fraud or crime or if the services of the psychotherapist are sought … to enable … anyone to commit or plan to commit what the patient knew or reasonably should have known to be a crime or fraud" (Mil. R. Evid. 513(d)(5)); (6) if necessary to "ensure the safety and security" of military personnel or property, military dependents, mission accomplishment, or classified information (Mil. R. Evid. 513(d)(6) and Saltzburg 2006);[14] (7) when an accused offers statements or other evidence "concerning his mental condition in defense, extenuation, or mitigation, under circumstances not covered by R.C.M. 706 or [MRE] 302" (Mil. R. Evid. 513(d)(7).); and (8) when the communication's disclosure is constitutionally required (Mil. R. Evid. 513(d)(8)).

From a defense perspective, these exceptions significantly undercut the rule. In many circumstances, a defendant's statements to treating mental health professionals may not be protected. Also, exceptions that apply to the accused may not apply to the statements that victims or witnesses make to psychotherapists. For instance, the exception in MRE 513(d)(7) concerning evidence the accused offers in defense, extenuation, or mitigation regarding a mental or emotional condition will not apply to statements of a victim or witness. Overall, MRE 513 seems to afford more protection to statements of victims and witnesses than it does to statements of an accused.

This all remains relatively new and regulations and case law by the different branches are not the same.

Waiver of the psychotherapist–patient privilege in federal courts

While *Jaffee* resolved some of the basic questions regarding whether there should be a federal psychotherapist–patient privilege, to which professions it should it apply, and whether the privilege should be absolute, the more frequent question regarding exceptions or waivers to the privilege did not arise in that case. Namely, under what circumstances should a court decline to enforce the privilege where doing so would limit a defendant's ability to access records and testimony that may be relevant to a plaintiff's claim? The courts often frame the issue as whether a plaintiff's claim has resulted in an implied "waiver" of the privilege such that psychiatric or psychotherapy records are subject to discovery. Since *Jaffee*, case law is confusing and remains unresolved.

---

[14] Mil. R. Evid. 513(d)(6). This is the broadest exception to the privilege. The privilege does not exist "if anyone believes that disclosure is necessary to protect military personnel, readiness, or the mission." See Saltzburg (2006) *Military Rule of Evidence Manual*.

The judicial approaches can be divided into two categories: broad and narrow. The "broad approach" applies to those cases where a waiver of the psychotherapist–patient privilege is found solely upon a plaintiff's assertion of a nonspecific claim for emotional distress and the plaintiff has not offered the testimony of an expert psychiatrist or psychologist to support the claim. Courts adopting a "narrow approach" will usually not find the privilege waived unless the plaintiff has listed their psychotherapist or other expert as a witness for trial or proposed to place the privileged communications as part of the case. A leading case under the narrow approach is *Vanderbilt* v. *Town of Chilmark* decided by a Massachusetts court a year after *Jaffee* (*Vanderbilt* v. *Town of Chilmark*, 1997).

A majority of courts have taken a broader direction. The court in *Doe* v. *City of Chula Vista* in 1999 analyzed the merits of both approaches and reversed the magistrate's decision on the same facts (*Doe* v. *City of Chula Vista*, 1999). In this discrimination case the defendants sought documents of "each and every mental and psychological disorder" for which the plaintiff had sought treatment in the previous 10 years. The magistrate ordered the disclosures only for the preceding year's treatment providers and allowed for inquiries into "other events and circumstances" in the plaintiff's life to look for other potential causes of emotional distress. The district court broadened the information to which the defendants could have access since they concluded the Supreme Court would adopt the broader view of waiver (*Doe* v. *City of Chula Vista*, at 568, 1999).

Three other courts of appeals have followed the approach typified by Judge Richard Posner writing for the Seventh Circuit Court of Appeals. Posner states, "If a plaintiff by seeking damages for emotional distress places his or her psychological state in issue, the defendant is entitled to discover any records of that state" (*Doe* v. *Oberweis Dairy*, 2006; *Schoffstall* v. *Henderson*, 2000; *Maday* v. *Public Libraries of Saginaw*, 2007).

More recently the Court of Appeals for the District of Columbia in *Koch* v. *Cox* adopted the narrower view. It concluded the privilege is waived only when a plaintiff has "bas[ed] his claim upon the psychotherapist's communications with him" or "selectively disclos[ing] part of a privileged communication in order to gain an advantage in litigation" (*Koch* v. *Cox*, 2007).

Several courts have used the term "garden-variety emotional distress" as a means to distinguish cases where there has not been an implied waiver of the privilege (Kent & Kent 2000). This term arose pre *Jaffee* in a Massachusetts case in 1989. In concluding there was no waiver of the privilege the magistrate judge said, "Sabree has not placed his mental condition at issue. Sabree makes a 'garden-variety' claim of emotional distress, not a claim of psychic injury or psychiatric disorder resulting from the alleged discrimination" (*Sabree* v. *United Broth. of Carpenters & Joiners of America*, 1989). In cases that employ this distinction, if a plaintiff asserts a claim for emotional distress, without alleging a specific diagnosable mental condition as a component of compensatory damages or offering the testimony of an expert witness to prove emotional distress, the courts will decline to order disclosure of psychotherapy records.

Garden-variety emotional distress is clearly a legal and not a psychiatric term. Some courts will look for a psychiatric diagnosis or ask whether the plaintiff has sought psychotherapy as a basis for distinguishing claims of garden-variety emotional distress in spite of the fact that these are poor distinguishing factors: anyone seeking treatment will have a diagnosis made for insurance purposes and whether one seeks treatment is not a good indicator of the severity of emotional distress. This approach will also lead attorneys to discourage plaintiffs from seeking treatment as well.

These balancing tests seem to eviscerate the privilege, as the rationale articulated in *Jaffee* was the broader societal interest in encouraging psychotherapy and the ability to be honest in that setting. In sum, the protection of psychiatric records in what also has been referred to as the patient–litigant exception remains quite unsettled and while the attorney's responsibility is to explore the full extent of possible damage, having some awareness of the complexity can aid in the consultative role and in being certain that the issue has been considered, especially if there is other potentially harmful material in the treatment records.

3.1.7 Confidentiality within a training program or group practice

Ethical and legal conflicts can arise in forensic training programs that need to be resolved, generally by developing additional procedures and the creation of various barriers to protect the integrity of the evaluation that is being performed. Specific disclosures with attorneys requesting evaluations should be made regarding the nature of the group and how members of the firm discuss cases within the group analogous to a law firm's discussion of cases. We begin seminars with reminders regarding the confidentiality of the discussions. Since training programs supervise the evaluations performed by the psychiatrists in the program, the question of "Whose opinion is this, the trainee's or the supervisor's?" not infrequently arises during depositions or testimony. It should be clear that the final report is the opinion of the psychiatrist signing the report and not that of supervisors or others involved in the discussion of cases. The purpose of these discussions is to insure that an appropriate evaluation has been performed and sufficient collateral data collected so that the evaluation draws appropriate and defensible conclusions from the data collected.

Sometimes placements for the trainees may pose conflicts for assigning cases or allowing trainees to participate in discussions of cases. For example, one of the placements for trainees may be in local state's attorney or public defender offices. In these placements the psychiatrists are expected to provide consultation to the attorneys in that office. These consultations often involve the review of reports submitted by other psychiatrists. Since our clinic performs competency to stand trial evaluations for the local region we exclude those psychiatrists from any discussion of cases involving evaluations that are handled by that court.

Since trainees taken from our basic residency program have had clinical assignments during their basic training, it is not unusual for them to see the name of a former patient appearing for a forensic evaluation. In these circumstances we either do not make an assignment to that resident and do not permit any discussion by that resident of the evaluation or we obtain a waiver from the attorney and client so that the evaluation can proceed with a waiver of the psychotherapist–patient privilege in cases where the prior treatment does not present a significant conflict.

3.2 Record keeping

The management and content of a forensic psychiatric file is very different from a clinical treatment record, as all or part of it usually becomes part of the legal proceedings. A forensic file is generally started upon the initial contact with a referring attorney or court, which may be by phone, letter, email, or subpoena. Copies of those phone notes or letters should be retained. This is an important date as it is the frequent opening substantive question during a deposition or testimony, "Doctor, when were you first contacted regarding this case?" A letter or court order formally requesting the evaluation with the purpose of this evaluation clearly stated and the terms of the financial arrangements will usually follow the initial phone call. A copy of the psychiatrist's response accepting the case follows. A time sheet recording the dates and hours spent for the following tracks the case and forms the basic documentation for billing:

1. Interviews with the defendant or plaintiff
2. Interviews with collateral sources
3. Consultation with the attorney
4. Review of records
5. Consultation with other professionals, e.g., psychologists, neurologists
6. Lab tests ordered, e.g., EEGs, MRIs, blood tests
7. Preparation of the report
8. Testimony/Depositions
9. Travel
10. Miscellaneous expenses, e.g., videotapes.

The case file then will consist of the notice of privacy practices given to the evaluee, appropriate signed releases of information forms for protected information, prior medical records, school records, psychological testing, depositions or statements of other experts, witnesses, plaintiffs, and defendants, police reports, and other court orders and relevant correspondence.

The record will also contain notes from the individual interviews conducted with the evaluee, collateral sources, and the final report. The file may also contain relevant articles from the scientific literature that relate to the case and were used in the formation of the final opinion. The file also contains any video- or audiotapes of interviews with the defendant or significant others. Sometimes a timeline of the important events and dates in a case can be a helpful guide.

In civil cases, trials are typically preceded by deposition testimony in an attempt to preclude "surprises" from occurring during the trial. Prior to the deposition, the expert will generally receive a subpoena asking that they bring all of the material that was generated in relation to the case. This includes all notes, documents generated, and relevant articles and treatises that were researched or used in preparation (e.g., current psychiatric diagnostic manual). Rather than having to read and explain any marginal notes made on other statements, reports, or depositions, it is often more expedient to highlight and tab areas in the chart that you may wish to be able to easily find and refer to during a deposition or testimony.

Final reports are usually generated over a period of time. The material will need to be integrated into a summary addressing the specific areas that were asked about in the referral. Not all of the material gathered will find its way into the final document. The selection, composing, and organization of the material can be extremely time-consuming, taking 10–25 hours or more to generate a complicated report.

Whether or not the expert should submit a final draft of the report to the referring attorney has been controversial in the field. In order to protect against attorney influence or the perception of influence, some experts will only send a final report, and if changes need to be made, will send an addendum letter. Other experts are willing to send a draft of a report to be certain it contains no factual or legal errors. Attorneys may ask you to consider modifications of the report if they feel material has been included that is not relevant and should not be made part of the public record. Such requests can be considered and, if the expert also agrees, may be deleted with the understanding that the expert may be questioned about draft reports and subsequent changes with inferences that the attorney influenced the expert's opinion. At times attorneys will request that material be deleted that is typically part of a psychiatric evaluation but not related to the present case and not helpful to the way the attorney wishes to present the client's case, e.g., a history of prior abortions or criminal histories of relatives. These requests present difficult judgment calls and the psychiatrist must feel comfortable explaining their absence if brought out in cross-examination. It is also prudent not to keep all the preliminary drafts of a report once the report is completed, as every editorial change may have to be explained in a subsequent deposition.

An additional difficulty for treating psychiatrists who agree to become an expert in their patient's case is that their entire psychiatric record will usually be available for review unless a court agrees to some limitations on total access.

Once a case is completed, especially ones with cartons of depositions, it is also appropriate to see whether the referring attorney would like the documents that have been made available to the expert returned or shredded.

Information disclosed and introduced as evidence during a trial becomes part of the public record and may be used in presentations at professional meetings or discussed with the press. Under other circumstances, informed consent should be obtained before making any disclosures not in the public record.

The pros and cons of video- or audiotaping interviews with the defendant or plaintiff have been discussed in an AAPL Task Force Report (AAPL Task Force 1999). Some of the advantages include being able to review the details of the interviews as part of preparation immediately prior to trial. With major crimes or protracted civil cases, trials often occur several years after the event or evaluation. Recordings also allow for more accurate quotation of statements made by the defendant. One of the cons is that the opposing side may also use them to prepare cross-examination questions. Another is that other personal information not directly relevant to the case may be more available. Such tapes in addition to verifying what was said to the expert can become part of the public record and played in the national press. The use of such aids to note taking and record keeping should be reviewed with the retaining attorney and the defendant notified in advance where feasible.

Evaluees, like patients, frequently want to see or have copies of their reports. Signed release forms are generally required, although we usually try to have them obtain copies from their attorney as the attorney requested the report and the consultation was addressed to the attorney. Most attorneys will review reports with their clients and make copies available to them. Reports are generally prepared with that fact in mind as well as the possibility the report will be entered into evidence and become more publicly available. Court-ordered competency to stand trial evaluations are maintained by our clinic and referred to when subsequent competency evaluations are requested. If we have seen a defendant or client previously and a new attorney requests an evaluation, we let the attorney know that a prior file exits and that a conflict of interest may be applicable or a waiver may need to be obtained if we are to proceed.

Although not necessarily a formal part of the forensic case record, a copy of the psychiatrist's curriculum vitae (CV) and a list of the cases in which the psychiatrist testified or gave depositions during the past 4 years is required in federal courts and should be readily available and furnished to the retaining attorney. These should be updated annually or before testimony in major cases.

3.3 Conclusion

Both confidentiality and record keeping, as the foregoing analysis has documented, are hardly fixed in stone. They seem to constantly change and require ongoing familiarity with local, national, and at times international legal and ethical rules and their evolutionary development. As with many endeavors in a field replete with shifting sands it is difficult to see all of the ramifications of the impact of the electronic medical record, as it becomes a standard of care, on forensic practice. Several of the areas discussed with different rulings from the circuit courts seem ripe for Supreme Court attention.

References

AAPL Task Force (1999) Videotaping of forensic psychiatric evaluations. Zonana, H., Bradford, J. M., Giorgi-Guarnieri, D., Dietz, P. E., Hoge, S. K., Sprehe, D. J., Teich, S. *Journal of the American Academy of Psychiatry and the Law* **27**: 345–358.

American Academy of Psychiatry and the Law (2008) *Ethical Guidelines for the Practice of Forensic Psychiatry*. Bloomfield, CT: AAPL.

American Medical Association (2009) *Code of Medical Ethics: Current Opinions With Annotations*. Chicago, IL: AMA.

American Psychiatric Association (2009) *The Principles of Medical Ethics With Annotations Especially Applicable to Psychiatry*, 2009 Edition Revised. Arlington, VA: APA.

Flippin, S. (2003) Military Rule of Evidence (MRE) 513: A shield to protect communications of victims and witnesses to psychotherapists. *Army Lawyer* 2003: 1.

Gainelli, P. (2004) Ake v. Oklahoma: The right to expert assistance in a post Daubert, post-DNA world. *Cornell Law Review* **89**: 1305.

Giorgi-Guarnieri, D., Janofsky, J., Keram, E., et al. (2002) Practice guideline – forensic psychiatric evaluation of defendants raising the insanity defense. *Journal of the American Academy of Psychiatry and the Law* **30**: S3–S40.

Hayden, D. L. (1987) Should there be a psychotherapist privilege in military courts-martial? *Military Law Review* **123**: 31.

Imwinkelried, E. J. (1990) The applicability of the attorney-client privilege to non-testifying experts: reestablishing the boundaries between the attorney-client privilege and the work product protection. *Washington Law Quarterly* **68**: 19.

Joint Service Committee on Military Justice (2008) *Manual for Courts-Martial, United States*.

Kent, M. & Kent, T. (2000) Michigan civil rights claimants: should they be required to give up their physician-patient privilege when alleging garden-variety emotional distress? *University of Detroit Mercy Law Review* **77**: 479–501.

Maringer, E. F. (1993) Witness for the prosecution: prosecutorial discovery of information generated by non-testifying defense psychiatric experts. *Fordham Law Review* **62**: 653.

Mosk, S. (1993) Psychotherapist and patient in the California Supreme Court: ground lost and ground regained. *Pepperdine Law Review* **20**: 415–424.

Saltzburg, S. A. (2006) *Military Rule of Evidence Manual*. Conklin, NY. LexisNexis Matthew Bender.

Strasburger, L. H., Gutheil, T. G., & Brodsky, A. B. (1997) On wearing two hats: Role conflict in serving as both psychotherapist and expert witness. *American Journal of Psychiatry* **154**: 448–456.

Weinstock, R., Leong, G. B., & Silva, J. A. (2001) Potential erosion of the psychotherapist-patient privilege beyond California: dangers of "criminalizing" Tarasoff. *Behavioral Sciences and the Law* **19**: 437–449.

Legal cases, statutes, and regulations

14 ALR 4th 594, 2(a) (1982) Application of the attorney-client privilege when a third party is involved.

75 Md. Op. Atty. Gen 76 (1990).

Ake v. *Oklahoma* (1985) 407 US 68.

Doe v. *City of Chula Vista* (1999) 196, FRD 562.

Doe v. *Oberweis Dairy* (2006). 456 F. 3d 704.

Exec. Order No. 13,140 (Oct. 12, 1999). 64 Fed. Reg. *55, 115.*

Gray v. *District Court* (1994) 884 P.2d 286.

Health Insurance Portability and Accountability Act (1996) (HIPAA), Public Law 104–191.

HHS (2010) Standards for Privacy of Individually Identifiable Health Information; Final Rule: 45 CFR Parts 160 and 164.

Houston v. *State* (1979) 602 P.2d 784.

Hutchinson v. *People* (1987) 742 P.2d 875.

Jaffee v. *Redmond* (1996) 518 US 1.

Koch v. *Cox* (2007) 489 F. 3d 384.

Lickey v. *State* (1992) 827 P.2d 824.

Maday v. *Public Libraries of Saginaw* (2007) 480 F.3d 815.

Miller v. *District Court* (1987) 737 P.2d 834.

ORS (2007). § 419B.010.

Pawlyk v. *Wood* (2001) 248 F.3d 815.

People v. *Clark* (1990) 789 P.2d 127.

People v. *Edney* (1976) 350 N.E.2d 400.

People v. *Hilliker* (1971) 185 N.W.2d 831.

People v. *Knippenberg* (1977) 362 N.E.2d 681.

People v. *Knuckles* (1995) 650 N.E.2d 974.

People v. *Lines* (1975) 531 P.2d 793.

Pouncy v. *Florida* (1977) 353 So.2d 640.

Sabree v. *United Broth. of Carpenters & Joiners of America*, Local No. 33, (1989) 26 FRD 422.

Schoffstall v. *Henderson* (2000) 223 F.3d 818.

State v. *Bronson* (2001) 779 A.2d 95.

State v. *Carter* (1982) 641 S.W.2d 54.

State v. *Cosey* (1995) 652 So.2d 993.

State v. *Hamlet* (1997) 944 P.2d 1026.

State v. *Hitopoulus* (1983) 309 S.E.2d 747.

State v. *Kociolek* (1957) 129 A.2d 417.

State v. *Mingo* (1978) 392 A.2d 590.

State v. *Pawlyk* (1990) 800 P.2d 338.

State v. *Pratt* (1979) 398 A.2d 421.

State v. *Schaaf* (1991) 819 P.2d 909, 918.

Taylor v. *State* (1996) 939 S.W.2d 148.

Trusky v. *State* (2000) 7 P.3d 5.

US ex rel. Edney v. *Smith* (1976) 425 F. Supp. 1038.

US v. *Alvarez* (1975) 519 F.2d 1036.

US v. *Auster* (2008) 517 F.3d 312.

US v. *Chase* (2003) 340 F.3d 978.

US v. *Glass* (1998) 133 F.3d 1356.

US v. *Hayes* (2000) 227 F.3d 578.

US v. *Layton* (1981) 90 FRD 520, 525.

US v. *Mansfield* (1993) 38 MJ 415, 418.

US v. *Rodriguez* (2000) 54 MJ 156 *cert. denied* (2001) 531 US 1151.

US v. *Walker* (1995) 910 F. Supp. 861.

Vanderbilt v. *Town of Chilmark* (1997) 174 FRD 225.

Ethics

Richard Martinez and Philip J. Candilis

4.1 Introduction

The two most important products of forensic work are expert testimony and the written reports that precede it. Experience and reflection combine to reveal certain core ethical premises.

First, forensic reports should hold to the same professional values that guide forensic practice. Dr. Robert Simon's traditional expectation that "writing with clarity and precision is a core competency in forensic psychiatry" (Simon 2007) serves as a touchstone for this discussion. For a report (or expert testimony) to be of high quality and credibility, it must be transparent, persuasive, accurate, free of jargon, consistent in its data and conclusions, useful, and non-prejudicial. However, we believe these aesthetic and technical necessities of report writing must be considered at another level. Clinical professional practice follows certain aesthetic and technical processes in order to achieve credibility, but these processes sit upon an ethical core or foundation. This foundation must be appreciated if we are to provide ethical reports.

As health care ethicists, we believe all clinical actions build on an ethical foundation that grounds professional behavior. Furthermore, certain practice habits or skills are more effective in sustaining our goals and reflecting our core values. So while we cannot completely separate the aesthetic or technical elements from the ethical elements, we can provide some reflection on the relationship between the two that may lead to more compelling and ethically sound forensic reports.

As an example, we may consider the professional habits by which informed consent is practiced before a medical procedure. Some legitimately argue that a complex discussion with the patient, where risks, benefits, and personal values are considered, is essential to achieve a practice of shared decision-making. Others may argue that it is enough to explain the procedure, present some of the more serious risks and potential benefits, and obtain the patient's signature. These are two practice habits or approaches, both sitting upon the ethical core of respect for persons and their rights to self-determination. However, most would agree that the first approach differs from the second in reflecting more accurately the core ethical values that ground the informed consent process.

Similarly in forensic practice, certain habits sustain and reflect the core ethical values of our profession. Just as with expert testimony, report writing should not only be guided by our understanding of foundational ethical values from forensic practice, but also mirror those values. A warning on the limits of confidentiality, for example, may be sketchy or

The Psychiatric Report, ed. Alec Buchanan and Michael A. Norko. Published by Cambridge University Press. © Cambridge University Press 2011.

thorough, reflecting the ethical values of informed consent. But just as with the clinical consent process, thorough habits of practice are more effective in reflecting those ethical values, whether one is testifying in a civil case or writing a forensic report. Therefore, we believe a review of what constitutes an ethical forensic practice is first necessary if we are to propose an approach to report writing that reflects and supports those values.

Second, we have argued, along with Ezra Griffith (1998) and others (Martinez & Candilis 2005; Norko 2005; Candilis et al. 2007; Candilis 2009), for a professional forensic practice that incorporates post-modern understanding of how culture and context shape claims of "objective" and "scientific" knowledge. We have argued that the modernist notion of an objective world, where the observer ("expert") is claiming truth simply by accurate and value-neutral descriptions of that world, is misleading. Post-modernism has successfully exploded the myth that one's perspective is pure, unadulterated, and unaffected by personal and contextual factors (Nagel 1986). When an evaluator makes an expert declaration, a more textured appreciation of the complexity of human experience is necessary. While acknowledging that our medical knowledge and experience provide legitimacy to our role in the legal system, we have joined Griffith and Baranoski (2007) in arguing that it is time for forensic experts to identify and acknowledge the relational and contextual subjectivities involved in forensic practice.

Specifically, culture and other aspects of context must be appreciated if we are to strive for fairness, objectivity, and honesty. At the center of this claim – as in the patient–physician relationship where dynamic subjective processes are at play – is the recognition that the subjective aspect of the forensic expert–evaluee relationship must be appreciated. This must include understanding relational complexities and dynamics in addition to culture (Gutheil et al. 1991). In the forensic evaluation and assessment process, the expert and evaluee are engaged in a complex relationship that influences perception and therefore opinions.

In turn, forensic report writing is a complex process involving the creation of a credible and persuasive narrative. Understanding the subjective dynamics inherent to the development of a narrative product must be part of the construction of that narrative. Therefore, we offer an ethical base for report writing that highlights our professional obligation to manage these subjectivities and acknowledge the complex web from which they emerge.

Third, we believe report writing, as with forensic practice and the process of evaluation, must not only consider the narrative dimension that characterizes this activity but also place it in the context of the basic professional principles that guide forensic practice. Therefore, we recommend a review of the AAPL Ethics Guidelines for the practice of forensic psychiatry (2005) as a template for evaluating reports. Guidelines based in principles of honesty and striving for objectivity are a sound foundation for recognizing the truth of complex human interactions and the limits to one's objectivity. How well does the forensic report construct a narrative that adheres to these principles? How well does the report embrace and mirror the values stated in our professional code of practice?

4.2 Ethical guidelines

In 2005, the governing council of the American Academy of Psychiatry and the Law adopted revised ethical guidelines for the practice of forensic psychiatry. In addition to defining the subspecialty and its purpose, the guidelines recognized the competing duties involved in forensic practice and the need to balance duties to the individual and to society. At the heart of the guidelines is the recognition that while certain traditional duties in medical practice may be absent, there is still the need to reconcile traditional principles with the unique conflicts of forensic practice. Respect for persons, honesty, justice, and social responsibility are therefore considered foundational to the practice.

Specifically, maintaining confidentiality, practicing a form of consent based on informed consent models, adhering to honesty, and striving for objectivity are featured elements of the guidelines. Moreover, we suspect strongly that the virtues of transparency and humility are inherently necessary for this statement of ethical practice. Therefore, all such qualities should be reflected in forensic reports.

In jail settings, for example, treating psychiatrists and psychologists are sometimes the first to hear intimate and sometimes incriminating information from recently arrested prisoners. Protecting privacy and confidentiality in this setting is directly tied to traditional patient–physician ethical obligations to avoid unnecessary harms. Here it is not appropriate to include information in the clinical chart that may be used to prosecute or harm the defendant, especially when it has no clinical purpose. In such situations, truth-seeking and honesty are balanced against primary responsibilities to avoid harms, promote benefit, and respect privacy and confidentiality.

Similarly in forensic reports, decisions to include or exclude information must be evaluated by balancing privacy with the need to include potentially harmful information that serves truth-seeking and honesty. While it is inevitable that harmful information will be included, this decision should occur with consideration of the evaluee's vulnerability in a forensic setting. A forensic evaluator's acquisition of a waiver of confidentiality at the beginning of an interview does not negate the later responsibility to assess the inclusion or exclusion of harmful information. The waiver does not mean all information is fair game in the pursuit of honesty and truth. The responsibility to minimize unnecessary harm, to respect the evaluee, to obtain information through appropriate procedures, and to examine critically the necessity and importance of the information must still be balanced, even in the context of a waiver.

4.3 Ethical forensic practice

In order to claim legitimacy as forensic experts with specialized knowledge, skills, experience, training, and education, we believe that basic professional obligations must be joined to professional aspirations that protect the integrity of our specialty. We have argued for a form of "robust professionalism" as a model for appropriate professional behavior in the forensic context (Martinez & Candilis 2005; Candilis et al. 2007; Candilis 2009). This is no minimalist professionalism that simply follows highly specialized rules set for a small group of practitioners. Robust professionalism acknowledges that our legitimacy and credibility in law is dependent on our professional background as psychiatrists and psychologists, and the ethical foundation upon which these professions are established. We return to robust professionalism in Section 4.5.

Joining this deeper, grounded view of professionalism to aspirational ethics, or what the profession should be, is a way of raising the bar – taking the discussion beyond a profession's rule-making or guidelines and setting a higher ethical standard. This joining of aspirational ethics to duties or obligations, in turn, must be reflected in the habits or practices of forensic work, including report writing. In previous publications we, along with others, proposed that forensic practice is primarily a medical practice, and as such is deeply connected to the ethical foundations and traditions in medicine (Weinstock et al. 1990; Candilis et al. 2001; Weinstock 2001).

In addition, we argue that it is not possible to define a professional ethics for forensic practice without recognizing that its foundation depends on an appreciation of how our personal and professional moralities are blended. We bring our personal virtues and vulnerabilities, along with our ethical habits and skills as professionals to each and every evaluation. Consequently, our view of professionalism recognizes duties and aspirations as health professionals linked to the unique problems and dilemmas of forensic work. Our ethical approach to forensic practice, and thus report writing, recognizes that all claims made in our role as "expert" are shaped by our limitations of perspective. Objective perspective is impossible, even in those disciplines where there is a strong presumption of objectivity (e.g., ballistics, DNA analysis).

While our expertise is rooted in elements of science, it nevertheless contains many elements of uncertainty. Our success is bound to our understanding and appreciation of how our own views of justice, retribution, and compassion may undermine our credibility to those reviewing the forensic report. It is these subjectivities that call for greater attention to forensic ethics and a more robust view of forensic work. However, this deeper, grounded, or robust view of forensic professionalism has not always been the model for forensic practice.

Previously, we traced the history of debate about professional ethics within the forensic community in the work of Seymour Pollack, Bernard Diamond, Alan Stone, and others (Candilis et al. 2007). As we shall see below, these writers did much to clarify the roles forensic psychiatrists play when they serve one side or another. Pollack, for example, generally appeared only for the prosecution, Diamond for the defense. Stone saw little psychiatry could offer the law and advised avoiding the courtroom altogether.

But we took particular interest in Appelbaum's (1997) contribution. Appelbaum stressed that forensic practitioners' primary allegiance is to justice and the legal system, not to psychiatry or the evaluee. After all, forensic practitioners may develop opinions that actually harm the evaluee – a result distinguishable from the goals of common medical ethics. Appelbaum consequently elevated truth-telling, respect for persons, and allegiance to legal questions to the status of primary values. While he recognized the importance of resisting unnecessary harms toward evaluees, he argued that values such as striving for benefit and avoiding harm must be secondary to the higher goal of seeking the truth. In concert with Diamond (1992) and Weinstock (2001), however, we propose an ethical approach that integrates our primary duties as physicians and psychiatrists with the unique duties found in the acts of forensic practice.

For example, while harms to the evaluee may be necessary in writing a competency examination (i.e., by undermining her wish to avoid trial), we have obligations to minimize this harm by the manner with which we treat information that could serve prejudicial ends – information that may unnecessarily demean the defendant. A past psychiatric history in such a defendant, depending on how this information is framed and presented, may be used to create bias in one direction or another. Descriptions of past arrests, substance abuse, or sexual history can be particularly provocative. Since the purpose of a competency examination is to answer a contemporaneous mental state question, we must take care in incorporating such information. We see this as a balancing act, recognizing the duty to strive for objectivity and present data that support one's conclusion, while avoiding gratuitous information or unnecessary passion-invoking descriptions that do not serve the goals of the legal question itself.

Consequently, we see professionalism as a process, not as a static performance of role entrenched in immutable values. We argue that our professionalism must be practiced and considered in every situation in order to hone the ideals of virtue in our practice. Virtue theorists since Aristotle stress the importance of practice in achieving excellence. In this sense, each case is an opportunity to hone one's skills and expertise, to grow in knowledge and understanding, and to achieve greater humility in the role of "expert." Likewise, each report provides a similar opportunity. Each report becomes an opportunity to reflect on how well or how poorly one is following an ethical course – a course where experts not only pursue fairness to the evaluee, but also reflect on their motives and conflicts.

A helpful and important perspective in shaping our conclusions is found in narrative ethics. This is a view of ethics that sees ethical knowledge as story-telling knowledge. Constructing the story or narrative of an event by describing the motivations and paths of the moral actors is critical to forming the complete ethical picture. Narrative is important both in the testimony of the testifying expert, and in the writing of the forensic evaluator. In the following sections, we review the importance of narrative and its connection to robust professionalism. This is where aspiration to professional ideals must join with principles of forensic practice in the act of report writing. We then argue for a set of values that should guide all forensic reports, independent of the "side" from which one entered the case. We will draw on principles of the Code of Ethics from the American Academy of Psychiatry and Law as guidance (2005). We review these principles, joined to developments in the forensic ethics literature, in order to provide direction and foundational ethical positions from which all forensic reports can be critiqued.

4.4 Narratives

Unlike the clinical report, where description and data serve the purpose of supporting diagnoses and treatment interventions (as well as creating a record for medical-legal protection), the forensic report serves other purposes at the intersection of clinic and courtroom. In order to establish an ethical orientation to forensic practice and report writing, one must appreciate that as professionals we are engaged in a process of listening and evaluating. Only then is this process followed by the act of writing.

All of these activities are elements of narrative creation. As with most forms of narrative creation, forensic report writing is a form of rhetoric and persuasion. While accurate descriptions of fact and sound demonstrations of logic are essential to reports, credibility involves additional ethical considerations. Since the forensic report is typically required to address a specific legal question involving psychiatric knowledge and experience, the report includes opinions not only of clinical observations, but also of legal questions. Therefore, the report must reflect this purpose, and do so by reflecting the values of integrity, honesty, avoiding unnecessary harms, and – always – respecting the subjects of our evaluation process.

Review of how narrative emerged in health care ethics is useful to our discussion of the ethics of report writing (Martinez 2009). In the early development of health care ethics, Thomas Beauchamp and James Childress (2001) offered a powerful principle-based approach to analyze ethical dilemmas in medicine: respect for autonomy, beneficence, non-maleficence, and justice became widely known and utilized in discussions involving health care ethical dilemmas. Recognizing that some dilemmas involve direct conflicts between specific duties (e.g., with dangerous psychiatric patients, the duty to protect third parties requires a breach of confidentiality that conflicts with the duty to respect patient confidences), other approaches emerged. Carol Gilligan (1982) and the "voice of care," and the inductive methods of casuistry (see Toulmin 1982; Toulmin & Jonsen 1988) found a foothold in health care ethics.

These approaches took different perspectives on ethical analysis: rather than principles like justice or fairness, Gilligan, for example, proposed caring as the driving force of a complete health care ethic. Richer solutions could be reached when the ethical approach was more collaborative and focused on the patient's relationships. The casuists, similarly, invoked the specifics of cases to draw broader (inductive) ethical conclusions. They emphasized context and detail to make their analyses. Legal and cultural considerations consequently became more prominent in discussions about the "correct" ethical course of action. As case law developed, certain cases created precedent; others became paradigmatic. In hospital ethics committees all over the United States, lay and professional participants could be heard stating that a case was like "the Cruzan case" or the "Debbie case" or the "Dax case," utilizing these paradigm cases as a form of argument and persuasion.

Gradually, the principle-based philosophy that helped establish health care ethics as a discipline gave ground to other disciplines – including the humanities. Literary scholars brought the tools of literary criticism to the methods and processes of health care ethics, resulting in increased appreciation for the narrative dimension of moral deliberation. Some began to critique the assumptions involved in the construction of ethics cases, recognizing that they were not reality, but "representations" told from points of view vulnerable to bias. Analysis of point of view then became essential for probing the moral dimension of ethics cases. It was no longer acceptable to assume that the narrator of an ethics case had a "view from nowhere" (Nagel 1986). As Wayne Booth (1983) noted in *The Rhetoric of Fiction*, the nature of narrative creation contains strategies by which the author "tries, consciously or unconsciously, to impose" a perspective upon the reader (p. xiii). We believe that a better appreciation of the subtleties of narrative representation is essential if we are to strive for a robust ethical approach to report writing. It is necessary to appreciate the dynamic of point of view, the relationship of stylistic choices or "framing" of the legal-medical question, and the importance of monitoring this process.

The dynamic of point of view, the position from which we listen and write, must be understood if we are earnest in our attempt to ground our effort in principles like "striving for objectivity" as outlined in the AAPL Code of Ethics. Often, trainees in the early months of specialty training exhibit significant struggles in this arena. Is one a clinician doing a clinical interview? In an insanity defense evaluation, is the psychiatrist an investigator offering a Miranda-like warning, informing the defendant that they are not for or against anything; that they want "just the facts"? Is the evaluator in the "bird's eye" position (the omniscient third-person narrative), observing from a position that is above and aloof? In each adversarial case, does the expert look for opportunities only for the side that hired them or do they remain "neutral?"

In *The Fiction of Bioethics*, Chambers (1999) argues that cases themselves are fictions or constructed literary texts and therefore subject to literary analysis. Since the 1970s, bioethicists assumed that the "case" was an objective construction, subject to moral analysis that flowed from our higher reasoning. But for Chambers and others, cases are data, packaged in the form of narrative construction that can be analyzed or deconstructed. This process of deconstruction or unpackaging leads to moral reflection and understanding that is self-reflective. By this, Chambers implies that we can achieve humility and self-criticism – values that are necessary to any moral judgment – by a fuller appreciation of the narrative dimension of all ethics cases. Chambers supports a view of cases that acknowledges context, subjectivity, ambiguity, complexity, and uncertainty thus bringing new humility to the task of ethical decision-making. Looking at cases as narratives brings new modesty to the grand claims and conclusions that too often mark expert declarations.

It is our view that this approach is useful in analyzing the ethical dimensions of forensic report writing. Chambers' approach applied to forensic report writing furthers our understanding of the many subjective elements involved. Just as there are ethical dimensions involved in all clinical encounters, we view report writing as an act entwined in ethical decisions. While this view of our reports as data to be "unpacked" lessens our hold on the comfortable myth of objectivity, we believe it is essential to reports that must stand the test of the adversarial process. In our system, this is where truth and justice are sorted.

Forensic reports, then, are a form of rhetoric, a tool for argument and persuasion. As such, they involve large and small decisions that determine what information is included or excluded, what data are stressed or minimized, what descriptions are informative or prejudicial. We believe that all forensic reports must consider this hidden element of report writing, and work earnestly toward transparency. Only then do we "strive for objectivity." The author of the report must be willing to withstand scrutiny and argument, while being guided by core values of forensic practice. This is where a robust ethic allows striving for objectivity and truth to be balanced against minimizing unnecessary harm.

4.5 Robust professionalism

In 1999, Mathew Wynia and colleagues (Wynia et al. 1999) presented a definition of professionalism as "an activity that involves both the distribution of a commodity and the fair allocation of a social good, but that is uniquely defined *according to moral relationships* [emphasis added]. Professionalism is a structurally stabilizing morally protective force in society." According to Wynia, this is a view of professionalism that "protects not only vulnerable persons but also vulnerable social values." We believe this view of professional activity – including report writing – is a good place to anchor the discussion of a forensic report consistent with the values of our profession.

With Griffith's advocacy for cultural formulation bolstering the prevailing principles of forensic ethics (1998), we recognized an advance in forensic thinking that led us directly toward Wynia's definition. It was not enough for practitioners to consider roles and principles alone; they had to consider vulnerable people and values as well. Since the writings of Bernard Diamond (1959, 1992) and Seymour Pollack (1974), forensic psychiatry had derived a vision of professionalism based on a strict view of role: experts answered either to the law or to psychiatry. But that approach was not sufficient for the complexities of forensic work. Multiple challenges to pure roles and pure objectivity had been made clear in the evolution of both bioethics and forensic ethics (recall our discussion of the post-modernists, value theorists, cultural and narrative ethicists above).

Readers may recall that Pollack practiced in a way that directed his work "primarily to the legal issues in which [the patient] is involved" (Pollack 1974). He recognized the overarching hegemony of the legal setting, its goals, and procedures. Yet, after participating in the trial of Robert Kennedy's assassin, even he developed an antipathy to capital cases – allowing his personal values to inform his work. This expansion of his role-based approach to include personal values provided an opening for the more robust kind of analysis we espouse.

Diamond, by contrast, worked in the legal setting to achieve more therapeutic ends. He worked almost exclusively for defendants. His powerful assertion that, "The psychiatrist is no mere technician to be used by the law as the law sees fit," resonates strongly for those who see beyond the minimalist requirements of the law (Diamond 1992). Diamond's defense of physicianly values in forensic work is endorsed in the more recent surveys of practitioners who identify the influence of medical ethics in their work (Weinstock 1988, 1989; Weinstock et al. 1991). Like us, today's forensic professionals consequently trace the foundational values of their work to their training first as physicians, and only then as forensic experts.

Going beyond role expectations is difficult when forensic professionalism is defined narrowly in terms of avoiding conflicts. Yet this is how early commentators defined the work. Stone (1980, 1984) noted that forensic practitioners may be limited in what they can tell the courts, leading to injustice. Or they may be tempted to offer testimony beyond their expertise, leading to ridicule. Perhaps, Stone speculated, if the results of forensic work can be injustice and ridicule, the work is best avoided. In response, Appelbaum (1997) and Strasburger et al. (1997) urged the separation of clinical and forensic roles to avoid conflicts. Indeed, this is a practice that we endorse as a starting point, but that, as we said, does not do enough to ground a complex profession. Our ethics cannot be easily splintered into opposing ethical principles, allegiances, and thus roles.

An integrated approach offers the most robust version of forensic professionalism, one that contains both traditional professional and forensic duties. We recognize that being both treater and expert for the same person raises important ethical concerns, but we reject notions that professional responsibilities can be divided along any absolute or clean lines. Just as we would not consider forensic evaluations or testimony independent from our clinical training, life experiences, or world-view, we cannot separate the ethics of clinical practice from the additional ethical obligations necessary for forensic practice. Likewise, attempts to exclude personal values that inform family, community, and political life are incongruous to a profession that repeatedly brings its expertise into the public arena. Suggesting it is even possible to ignore core personal or community values truly relegates the expert to the status of automaton or technician.

Consequently the richest model of forensic thinking and report writing brings together the influences acting on examiner, examinee, and community. It recognizes the multiple subjectivities of even the most scientific work. The interwoven personal, social, and institutional commitments of the expert can then be united to offer an ethic of wholeness or intactness, rather than one of splintering or splitting. This brings us to a discussion of professional integrity as a necessary component of report writing.

Ethicists Miller and Brody (1995) provided the model of professional integrity that is most relevant to the complexity of forensic report writing. They recognized the necessity of (1) a set of well-regarded personal principles that remain somewhat stable over time and are coherent, (2) verbal expression of those values and principles, and (3) consistency between what one says and what one does.

This was a model that acknowledged professionals' personal values, the importance of their open declaration, and their manifestation in behavior. It was the expression of values in word and deed that made professional integrity a truly communitarian endeavor (Candilis 2009). Expert and community could now set definitions and expectations, explore their subjectivities, discuss their priorities and values, and arrive together at a robust ethic for professional practice. Added to the concern for the evaluee's culture and narrative, practitioners now had a more complete ethical picture of the forensic encounter. It is in this integrated view that Wynia's "professionalism defined in terms of moral relationships" sees its full meaning. If professionalism is a protective, stabilizing force in society, it must be related in some way to elemental community and personal values. Moreover, if vulnerable values and individuals are to be protected, there must be recognition of the profession's commitment to that ethic.

The importance of protecting vulnerable individuals has gained recent traction in the debate over use of psychiatrists and psychologists in the interrogations of Guantanamo Bay detainees (Lewis 2005; Margulies 2007). Some commentators accepted the role of these mental health professionals outside their usual ethic by positing a kind of splintering of professional duties known as "exceptionalism" (see the discussion in Freedman & Halpern 1998). These professionals could practice outside foundational professional values as long as their role was as clear as reasonably possible, and they were consulting directly to a specific institution (Phillips 2005). Yet this was an exception that ignored the moderating influences of the primary profession, of traditional societal expectations, and historical narratives from the Nazi doctors to the Soviet psychiatrists (Candilis 2009). It was not a role acceptable to an integrated professional ethic that served as a morally protective force. If we allowed a moral exception for this kind of forensic involvement, then all forensic work could be subject to skepticism. The integrity of the profession would be undermined.

As surprising as it may seem, avoiding ethical pitfalls in report writing requires the same habits and practices as avoiding the pitfalls of consulting at Guantanamo Bay. Integrating multiple values and perspectives into a forensic report requires a set of behaviors that operationalizes the moral relationships found in all forensic work. A robust professionalism consequently requires that practitioners familiarize themselves with Griffith's cultural formulation, recognize role conflicts in their interviews, and attend to the vulnerabilities of evaluees. It requires that they be self-reflective and self-aware, noting the personal and contextual influences on their work, and the limits of their expertise. It requires them to explore a case from all perspectives, seeking its strengths and weaknesses so as to present the best report possible. It requires them to practice openness and transparency in their reasoning to expose their thinking and logic as well. These are the tools of robust report writing as they are the tools of a robust professionalism.

4.6 Conclusion

The debate over whether we are primarily physicians in the courtroom (recall Bernard Diamond), or some other breed of professional that incorporates strong duties to society and the court (recall Paul Appelbaum) will continue. However, we argue that all forensic reports must at least reflect the values contained in the AAPL ethical guidelines. Against this backdrop we recognize that a robust professional obligation includes the recognition that none of our work is relevant unless we understand that it arises from human beings engaged in moral relationships. Therefore, we posit the following interpretation of principles for guiding forensic reports:

1. Respect for persons. All evaluees should be regarded in the written report with respect and professional fairness. Even the defendant who has committed horrendous acts warrants a professional demeanor, appropriate confidentiality warnings, and self-reflection that guards against counter-transferential prejudice. It is important that

forensic reports are written in a manner that does not go beyond the data nor claim to settle the legal question (although we recognize that some jurisdictions require such opinions), but rather provides non-inflammatory data that are useful to the court in its social responsibilities.

2. Respect for privacy and confidentiality. While there are limitations to this value in the forensic setting, social responsibility, honesty, and truth do not require unnecessary and gratuitous information that is irrelevant to the legal question. Balance and perspective are critical practices here.

3. Respect for consent processes. This is reflected when information is obtained through proper disclosure and consent procedures. Reports that provide information obtained without proper consent are unethical on their face, independent of any new data discovered or the quality of the narrative.

4. Commitment to honesty and striving for objectivity. Reports must reflect the author's commitment to these principles, often applied in resisting the "hired gun" phenomenon. Point of view and how the report is written can be particularly revealing here. Reports that demonize and oversimplify motive and intention are particularly suspect. Rather, the finding of humanity or compassion in the encounter (Norko 2005) can be useful. Thoroughness, collateral sources, avoiding shortcuts, refusing to distort information or opinions based on the wishes of the retaining party, insisting that all relevant information be provided for assessments and incorporated into the report, avoiding all contingency arrangements, and avoiding simple conflicts between treating and forensic roles are all part of this commitment. In the event that personal values strongly inform one's professional judgments (e.g., in death penalty cases, or in the presence of defense/prosecution biases), they must be handled transparently, not hidden in the narrative.

We believe that forensic report writing, as a major and consistent product of forensic practice, is one of the most important reflections of our professional ethics. Reports should reflect the values intrinsic to forensic practice. In order for these values to guide and shape reports, forensic practitioners must first have a clear understanding of their complex role and its underlying ethical influences.

As a profession, we have duties and obligations that are rooted in the recognition that we are engaged in clear moral relationships. We have obligations to ourselves, the evaluees, the persons to whom we submit our expert assessment, the social forum itself, and to our fellow professionals. When we evaluate, assess, and record our findings, we are ethically bound to balance both duties to the profession and those we serve, while simultaneously upholding aspirations toward high moral standards. We consequently argue for a "robust professionalism" that recognizes our common human commitments, our obligations as physicians, and our unique struggle to understand and integrate the conflicting duties that mark the nature of forensic work and its reports.

References

American Academy of Psychiatry and Law Governing Council (2005) Ethics guidelines for the practice of forensic psychiatry. The American Academy of Psychiatry and the Law. Available from: http://www.aapl.org/ethics. htm. [Accessed September 15, 2009.]

Appelbaum, P. S. (1997) A theory of ethics for forensic psychiatry. *Journal of the American Academy of Psychiatry and the Law* **25**: 233–247.

Beauchamp, T. L. & Childress, J. F. (2001) *Principles of Bioethics*, 5th edn. Oxford, New York: Oxford University Press.

Booth, W. C. (1983) *The Rhetoric of Fiction*, 2nd edn. Chicago: University of Chicago Press.

Candilis, P. J. (2009) The revolution in forensic ethics: narrative, compassion, and robust professionalism. In Ethics in psychiatry: a review. *Psychiatric Clinics of North America*, guest ed. L. W. Roberts and J. G. Hoop. **32**(2): 423–435.

Candilis, P. J., Martinez, R., & Dording, C. (2001) Principles and narrative in forensic psychiatry: toward a robust view of professional role. *Journal of the American Academy of Psychiatry and the Law* **29**: 167–173.

Candilis, P. J., Weinstock, R., & Martinez, R. (2007) *Forensic Ethics and the Expert Witness*. New York: Springer.

Chambers, T. (1999) *The Fiction of Bioethics: Cases as Literary Texts*. New York and London: Routledge.

Diamond, B. L. (1959) The fallacy of the impartial expert. *Archives of Criminal Psychodynamics* **3**: 221–236.

Diamond, B. L. (1992) The forensic psychiatrist: consultant vs. activist in legal doctrine. *Bulletin of the American Academy of Psychiatry and the Law* **20**: 119–132.

Freedman, A. M. & Halpern, A. L. (1998) Forum – psychiatrists and the death penalty: some ethical dilemmas. *Current Opinion in Psychiatry* **11**: 1–15.

Gilligan, C. (1982) *In a Different Voice: Psychological Theory and Women's Development*. Cambridge: Harvard University Press.

Griffith, E. E. H. (1998) Ethics in forensic psychiatry: a response to Stone and Appelbaum. *Journal of the American Academy of Psychiatry and the Law* **26**: 171–184.

Griffith, E. E. H. & Baranoski, M. V. (2007) Commentary: the place of performative writing in forensic psychiatry. *Journal of the American Academy of Psychiatry and the Law* **35**(1): 27–31.

Gutheil, T. G., Bursztajn, H. J., Brodsky, A., et al. (1991) *Decision-making in Psychiatry and the Law*. Baltimore: Williams & Wilkins.

Lewis, N. A. (2005) Interrogators cite doctors' aid at Guantanamo Prison Camp. *The New York Times* June 24, p. A1.

Margulies, J. (2007) *Guantanamo and the Abuse of Presidential Power*. New York: Simon & Schuster.

Martinez, R. (2009) Narrative ethics. In *Psychiatric Ethics*, 4th edn., ed. S. Bloch & S. A. Green. Oxford: Oxford University Press.

Martinez, R. & Candilis, P. J. (2005) Commentary: toward a unified theory of personal and professional ethics. *Journal of the American Academy of Psychiatry and the Law* **33**: 382–385.

Miller, F. G. & Brody, H. (1995) Professional integrity and physician-assisted death. *Hastings Center Report* **25**: 8–17.

Nagel, T. (1986) *The View from Nowhere*. Oxford, New York: Oxford University Press.

Norko, M. A. (2005) Commentary: compassion at the core of forensic ethics. *Journal of the American Academy of Psychiatry and the Law* **33**: 386–389.

Phillips, R. T. M. (2005) Expanding the role of the forensic consultant. *Newsletter of the American Academy of Psychiatry and the Law* **30**(1): 4–5.

Pollack, S. (1974) *Forensic Psychiatry in Criminal Law*. Los Angeles: University of Southern California Press.

Simon, R. I. (2007) Authorship in forensic psychiatry: a perspective. *Journal of the American Academy of Psychiatry and the Law* **35**(1), 18–26.

Stone, A. A. (1980) Presidential address: conceptual ambiguity and morality in modern psychiatry. *American Journal of Psychiatry* **137**: 887–891.

Stone, A. A. (1984) The ethical boundaries of forensic psychiatry: a view from the ivory tower. *Bulletin of the American Academy of Psychiatry and the Law* **12**: 209–219.

Strasburger, L. H., Gutheil, T. G., & Brodsky, A. (1997) On wearing two hats: role conflict in serving as both psychotherapist and expert witness. *American Journal of Psychiatry* **154**: 448–456.

Toulmin, S. (1982) How medicine saved the life of ethics. *Perspectives in Biology and Medicine* **25**: 736–750.

Toulmin, S. & Jonsen, A. (1988) *The Abuse of Casuistry: A History of Moral Reasoning*. Berkeley: University of California Press.

Weinstock, R. (1988) Controversial ethical issues in forensic psychiatry: a survey. *Journal of Forensic Sciences* **33**: 176–186.

Weinstock, R. (1989) Perceptions of ethical problems by forensic psychiatrists. *Bulletin of the American Academy of Psychiatry and the Law* **17**: 189–202.

Weinstock, R. (2001) Commentary: a broadened conception of forensic psychiatric ethics. *Journal of the American Academy of Psychiatry and the Law* **29**: 180–185.

Weinstock, R., Leong, G. B., & Silva, J. A. (1990) The role of traditional medical ethics in forensic psychiatry. In *Ethical Practice in Psychiatry and the Law*, ed. R. Rosner & R. Weinstock. New York: Plenum Press.

Weinstock, R., Leong, G. B., & Silva, J. A. (1991) Opinions by AAPL forensic psychiatrists on controversial ethical guidelines. *Bulletin of the American Academy of Psychiatry and the Law* **19**: 237–248.

Wynia, M. K., Lathan, S. R., Kao, A. C., Berg, J., & Emanuel, L. (1999) Medical professionalism in society. *New England Journal of Medicine* **341**: 1612–1616.

Chapter

5

Writing a narrative

Ezra E. H. Griffith, Aleksandra Stankovic, and
Madelon V. Baranoski

… what everybody wants in life: to control the narrative … the efforts people make to gerry-
mander the story to suit their interests …

Menand (2007, p. 64)

In recent years, the specialized discipline of forensic psychiatry has undergone substantial change. Where once upon a time psychiatrists who practiced in this field were being challenged to articulate what constituted their work, there is no question now that the subspecialty presently has a place as a specialized form of psychiatric practice. Forensic psychiatry specialists at this time are expected to have studied for a year in a didactic fellowship program and to pass a certification examination after having completed the subspecialty training. Furthermore, the plethora of academic journals in the area and the demand for forensic psychiatry expertise from courts, lawyers, ethics committees, prison administrations, and other entities have helped solidify the identity of the forensic subspecialist.

With forensic psychiatry's evolution into a form of specialized practice, two key practice elements have emerged as arenas of activity that demand core competency. One element is the writing of forensic psychiatry reports; the other is the oral presentation of written findings in an adversarial context such as expert testimony. Both forms of presentation demand the ability to present ideas in a forum that anticipates critical analysis, disagreement, and even verbal confrontation or cross-examination. Under such scrutiny, both forms of presentation should be seen therefore as acts of performance, requiring a degree of cogent argumentation and artistry (Griffith & Baranoski 2007).

The mastery of written performance is fundamental to forensic psychiatry for several reasons. The written report is the practice-product of forensic psychiatry. While in other medical specialties the written record often documents the product (the surgery, the treatment, the assessment for treatment), in forensic psychiatry the written record itself is the product. It represents the assessment, formulation, and opinions that the expert was contracted to provide. Therefore, mastery at producing that product is required. In addition, the written document (alone or in combination with testimony) may in some cases have substantial influence on the outcome of the legal conflict (Silva et al. 2003).

The forensic psychiatrist writes for others, for those outside the profession. Legal professionals may not share the education, language, or professional mission of medicine.

The Psychiatric Report, ed. Alec Buchanan and Michael A. Norko. Published by Cambridge University Press. © Cambridge University Press 2011.
This chapter is based on the article written by the same authors: "Conceptualizing the forensic psychiatry report as performative narrative" published in *The Journal of the American Academy of Psychiatry and the Law*, Volume 38, Number 1, 2010.

Therefore, the forensic psychiatrist has the burden of crafting a document that can be under-stood by the culture of the law – and to some extent the public. Forensic psychiatrists must do more than record facts accurately, conduct comprehensive assessments, and apply the science and art of the specialty. They must write to protect against the corruption of transla-tion, unintended bias of language, and unhelpful ambiguity. O'Grady (2004) suggested that the report writer must translate from psychiatry into law such that the court can understand psychiatric findings in its own terms.

Forensic reports are in themselves the product of the expert rather than the record of the psychiatric work; forensic report writers do not simply recount their clinical findings as though they were at the usual medical rounds. In their forensic reports, writers must organize information pulled from clinical examinations, interviews, laboratory tests, and documents and rework it all into a coherent narrative. It is this act of remaking and of trans-formation that Peterson and Langellier (2006) consider performative and describe as "mak-ing a to do" about a story. As a result, the written psychiatric forensic report is a study in narrative complexity for several reasons. First, forensic psychiatrists do not simply recount the objective data of blood pressure readings, the findings elicited on examination of an indi-vidual, or the individual's account of past medical and psychiatric diagnoses and treatment. Forensic psychiatrists gather information from different sources and meld it into a coherent narrative. The second reason for the complexity of the narrative comes both from the nature of psychiatry as a medical specialty and from the role psychiatry plays in the forensic arena – to see beyond the data to infer their meaning. The science and art of psychiatry are to make sense out of senseless behavior and to create a structure within which the data and collateral sources can be included. The third reason for the complex narrative in forensic psychiatry is that the task of writing the report is to persuade the readers of the report that the writer's story is cogently argued, buttressed by data, and objectively presented.

We shall focus in this chapter on narrative in the written forensic psychiatry report, its cen-tral role in the work of forensic psychiatry, and techniques and pitfalls in telling the story for the legal audience. A narrative is necessary to address the complex task of explaining a behav-ior isolated in time, a decline in function, or an unanticipated reaction to an event. Psychiatry has the burden of creating an integrated explanation that cannot be captured through the sum of discrete lists of factors under the usual headings found in clinical records. The additional requirement for analysis and interpretation that includes the person's own view of the past and reason for it demands a different writing form than that which simply describes and justi-fies a diagnosis. The weaving of fact and interpretation into a story is the form that allows the audience to understand the psychiatric formulation. However, the narrative of the forensic psychiatrist does not have the latitude of a fiction where creative invention of detail shapes the story and the author has no responsibility to its characters in the story and the written prod-uct serves to entertain the reader. The narrative in the forensic psychiatric report is held to the ethical standards of truth-telling and respect for person and it has impact on lives and on the profession. Therefore, the construction of the forensic psychiatric narrative requires attention to form and content as well as the risks inherent in telling a truthful story.

5.1 The construction of narrative

Forensic psychiatric reports answer questions posed by the law through the explication of individuals' thinking and their behavior and how individuals came to carry out their actions. In any forensic case, the parties involved compete to have their perspective accepted as the one that determines the outcome. Each involved party creates a narrative that reflects a particular perspective and purpose. The adversarial legal process itself rests on the foundation of competing perspectives and objectives. For example, in the context of a criminal trial, the state has the perspective of the event, an isolated moment in time, and focuses the story on the offense as perpetrated by the defendant. The victim is evidence of the crime and has a narrative about suffering and loss.

When the defense concedes the facts of an act and mounts a psychiatric defense or mitigation, it argues for a different perspective, one that places the moment of the crime into the context of a life, a complicated interplay between a disturbed psyche and a malevolent act. It is the role of the forensic psychiatrist to highlight and give name to that disturbance, explicate its origins, and explain its role in the crime as either substantial or irrelevant. The psychiatric perspective is determined by psychiatric expertise and data, not by the circumscribed role of defense or state or plaintiff. Indeed, the expert psychiatric opinion may end up being discordant with the perspective and purpose of the requesting party. Melton et al. (2007) have succinctly made the distinction between the goals: "above all, clinicians should be effective advocates for their data, whether or not that makes them effective advocates for the party that calls them to court" (p. 578).

Assuming that the sides refrain from manufacturing evidence, no perspective represents more truth than the other; each perspective has its own truth. For the state, the defendant is the crime; for the defense, the defendant is an unfortunate player caught in difficult circumstances; for the forensic psychiatrist, the task is to explain the event within the context of a person's life, using psychiatric, psychological, cultural, and sociological constructs to find meaning. Ultimately that meaning must resonate as "truthful" to all of the players in the legal drama – defense, prosecution, court, jury, professional colleagues, and defendant.

As we continue our focus on the criminal context, we are suggesting that the prosecution and the defense tend to suggest perspectives that are sometimes too simplistic. Borrowing language from Felman and Laub (1992), the forensic psychiatrist must offer "new articulations of perspective" by more richly contextualizing the incident that has placed the defendant in court. This is done by creating multilayered visions of what has led to the incident in question. In this way, there is a yielding of "new avenues of insight" that borrow from a number of different realities: political, historical, biological, biographical, and cultural, among others (Felman & Laub 1992, p. xv).

Once the narrator has set out clearly in the report's Introduction what the purpose of the narrative will be, the sources from which information has been pulled, and the person who has been examined, the narrator then turns to present the data in the second major section of the report. It is in trying to make sense of the information and framing it with an eye on the purpose and objectives of the report that narrators will first confront the concept of voice as articulated and defined by Lawrence-Lightfoot and Davis (1997). If we continue our emphasis on a report that addresses a problem in the criminal context, it is evident that narrators will have to contend with the multiple and varying, even contradicting, narratives of the criminal event put forth by the prosecutor, defense attorney, eye-witnesses to the event, and perhaps even third parties who have an interest in how the criminal case is resolved.

In presenting the data sections of the report, the expert must present these narratives because they provided information that shaped the formulation. We call the myriad voices that contribute the data, which the forensic psychiatrist will use to reach the answer to the legal question, the expository narratives. Including these in the report serves to establish the expert's objectivity in collecting and evaluating all of the relevant data. Expository narratives are, however, more than a record of data points. They represent the perspectives of invested parties who wish their view to be understood and taken seriously. In their accounts they "seize voice," that is, make an effort to have their versions taken seriously. The task for the forensic psychiatrist narrator is to sort through these different perspectives to find cogency and integration that will be represented in the conclusion and formulation of the case. The written report includes an account of that process in order to prepare the reader for the psychiatrist's narrative and opinion.

One challenge for the psychiatrist is how to include the voices of the expository narratives that, more than an objective account of the data, reflect the attitudes and experience of the reporter. For example, a police report describing an arrest and behavior will reflect the officer's understanding of what transpired as well as a record of the physical facts. Consider the report of an arrest of a person who has just beaten his wife, is incoherent, and needs to be restrained by police. An officer sympathetic to what he considers signs of mental illness might describe the attack as "a scene of chaos where Mr. Doe was out of control and clearly disturbed and resisted arrest." Another officer, who views psychiatric disorders as a pretense for avoiding responsibility for bad behavior, may produce a different narrative: "After viciously beating his wife, Mr. Doe turned on this officer." In the written report, the forensic psychiatrist may be tempted to rework (or transform) either police report to include only the factual account of the beating and resisting of arrest. However, an expository narrative requires that the voice of the police be included regardless of whether it supports or contradicts the final conclusion. The presentation of the expository narratives is important for several reasons. First, including the exposition as reported allows the reporter (in this case the police officer) to be heard and documents that the psychiatrist considered that narrative in full. Second, it shows respect for person, acknowledging the opinion as expressed. Finally, it allows the psychiatrist to avoid the accusation of "sanitizing" information to fit the conclusion, an allegation that could, for example, distract the jury from the formulation during cross-examination. Although our recommendation is controversial in the field, we recommend that the expository narratives include as much of the reporter's voice as respectfully possible in order to demonstrate the complexity of the analysis, the diligence of the expert, and richness of the data collected.

The inclusion of the expository narratives regardless of their relevance to the final conclusion is also a factor that distinguishes the ethical expert from the hired gun who formulates the case when first engaged and frames the data simply to support his or her position. To the hired gun, the data voices are distracting annoyances that need to be emphasized or extinguished as the predetermined conclusion demands. For the forensic psychiatrist practicing according to the ethics of the discipline, the final opinion is crafted through systematic attention to each voice and the extent to which each voice represents credible information that is relevant to the final narrative, what we call the formulation narrative, expressed in the psychiatrist's own voice to be presented in the report.

As Lawrence-Lightfoot and Davis (1997) described it, the narrator brings experience and professional training to the work of creating the story and eventually acquires the technique of synthesizing competing voices that will lead to the final narrative. This story will emerge in its full form as the narrative progresses to the Discussion section. Of course, on occasion, the expert may be unable to formulate a narrative because the competing voices are too contradictory or because essential data are missing. For example, consider a criminal case in which the psychiatrist is asked to evaluate the state of mind of the defendant at the time of the offense, but the defendant cannot recall the event or the time surrounding it. Although other information may confirm a past history of psychosis and witnesses may describe deteriorating function in the person in the days leading up to the event, the psychiatrist may justifiably decide not to prepare a report, concluding that the question about state of mind could not be answered without the critical data on what the person was thinking at the time. For a state of mind evaluation, some psychiatric experts consider the person's account of the event as critical to the formulation. Of course psychiatric experts vary in their approach to missing or conflicting data, but the construction of a formulation narrative assumes that the expert has enough information to do so.

The ethics-based imperative of truth-telling fits well with the role of forensic psychiatrist as expert who forms an objective opinion based on an honest and comprehensive review of all available and relevant information. That opinion may at times be deemed unhelpful by those hiring and paying the fee, because the psychiatrist's narrative may do nothing to advance their objective in the legal context.

5.2 Language and narrative

Language and writing style are critical elements in the forensic report. Resnick (2006) has argued that bad grammar and typographical errors diminish the effectiveness of the report. He has also pointed out that employing words such as "suspect," "possibly," and "supposedly" weaken the report. Resnick offers four principles of good writing: clarity, simplicity, brevity, and humanity, expressed through respect for both the subjects of the report and their words and perceptions. The latter principle makes clear that the use of quotations animates the writing, humanizes the subject of the narrative, and facilitates the author's attempt to speak directly to the reader. Collectively, these principles indicate that the writing of a report requires sophisticated judgment and reflection, and the writing process requires formalized consideration of how one uses words in the creation of the report. Consequently, even in setting out the Introduction, the author must be judicious in the selection of vocabulary (See Chapter 6 for further discussion of these ideas.)

Resnick's approach in his lectures is amply supported by the writings of Gerald Lebovits (Lebovits 2008a, 2008b), author of "The Legal Writer," a regular column in the *New York State Bar Association Journal*. (See columns in January, February, March/April, May, September, and October 2008 issues.) Lebovits cautioned that errors in grammar and punctuation weaken the effectiveness and appeal of legal texts. Examples he explicated included use of incorrect idioms such as "abide from a ruling" instead of "abide by a ruling." Although Lebovits writes to the legal community, his suggestions are relevant to forensic psychiatrists who adopt legal jargon in order to communicate more directly with their colleagues in the law. Lebovits also makes a distinction between two forms of writing in a legal case: one that is neutral in the objective memorandum of facts and the other that is persuasive in the legal brief where some facts are emphasized and others deemphasized with the goal of convincing the audience of a particular perspective. Without using narrative terminology, Lebovits presents the task of creating the story and the methodology of performative writing. He also emphasizes that the writing should communicate the client's humanity, a point supported by Resnick (2006). Lebovits (2008a) recommended that attorneys humanize their clients in legal writing. As a telling example, he reminded us of how the parties were presented in the case of Paula Jones against Bill Clinton. Ms. Jones's attorneys presented her as a lowly paid government employee, while Clinton's lawyers made clear that he was the President of the United States. In applying these principles to the task of forensic report writing, the forensic psychiatrist is being urged to think of ways to make his subjects appear as functional human beings.

However, the forensic psychiatrist's narrative is different from that of the attorney who humanizes or dehumanizes the client to persuade the audience to accept a simplified account of complex circumstances. Within the adversarial context of American justice, the humanization of the client (whether perpetrator, victim, plaintiff, or defendant) serves the legal purpose of winning the dispute. In contrast, the psychiatrist's narrative humanizes the examinee without regard for which side of the legal case requested the examination; the psychiatrist writes to explain a complex life. Consequently, in a drug case, the psychiatrist does not choose to describe his subject as a victim of drug addiction or one who engages in the purposeful abuse of substances based on the legal side that hired him, but rather on the circumstances that account for the person's use of drugs, the extent of the addiction, and other psychiatric and psychological factors.

Lebovits emphasized that the best way to be persuasive was to engage in storytelling, which clearly indicated his recognition that narrative was an important reference point for him as he conceptualized how to present legal writing persuasively. He also noted that "all legally significant facts, even those unfavorable to the client, must be stated in the brief" (Lebovits 2008a, p. 66). Scheub (1977), addressing the task in oral performance, identified several points useful to the conceptualization of performative writing. First, Scheub noted that language is a creative medium like paint is to art and sounds are to music. He further described language as culturally nuanced as color and musical notes and rhythms. Consequently, written narrative is comparable to other aesthetic forms of making stories. Second, in telling a story, the narrator is engaged in using words to arrange images and patterns that are understood by the reader, because they represent meaning embodied in the culture of narrator and reader. These images, if presented aesthetically enough by the writer, can have an impact that is seen, heard, and even felt. Scheub's ideas make sense when seen in the light of Blanchard's contributions (Blanchard 1991). The latter pointed out that in the construction of narrative, we use language as a system of verbal signs, while at the same time relying on their metaphorical coherence. That is, the language of the written report imparts information through the words, but also creates a connection between the writer and reader and reader and subject that can convey attitude and evoke, for example, empathy or abhorrence, acceptance or alienation.

Of course, it is a serious error for forensic psychiatrists to believe that they alone are engaged in this narrative process, bent on persuading the audience that one explanation is superior to the others. Forensic psychiatrists are regularly engaged in an adversarial legal process, and others are, therefore, in the marketplace attempting to sell their own narratives, their own versions of what has occurred in the criminal, civil, or administrative context. As a result, others are also looking to construct their stories with an eye to persuading the audience.

Hudgins (1996) articulated one of the most intriguing warnings about the traps that await us as we utilize language in the construction of a narrative; that is, the inadvertent "lying" that occurs as the product of artistic expression. In reflecting on his views, we think it useful to reemphasize the conceptualization of a forensic report as the construction of a work of art, as the act of writing the report requires the translating of actual events onto the page. And while it is possible to characterize this art form as a kind of visual art, let us for the moment think of it as a literary activity. This facilitates our understanding of what Hudgins had to say. In performing the act of writing the forensic report, the forensic

Box 5.1 Common contextual lies in narratives

Lie of cogency

Leaving out details
  To simplify the story
  To avoid confusion by contradictory facts
  To protect the dignity of the client
  To honor requests of others (family, lawyer)

Lie of texture

Embellishment and emphasis
  To fill in gaps of missing data
  To enhance coherence
  To humanize the subject
Biased tone of report to favor one side
  To persuade according to the legal side
  To meet attorney demands

Lie of emotional evasion

Omission of underlying theme
  To avoid controversial area (such as race, religion, sexual orientation)
  To protect the dignity of the subject
  To control the attention of the audience

---

specialist transcribes actuality onto the page, even as he is urged, or tempted if you prefer, to recreate the actuality selectively and imaginatively. Hudgins hints at what the forensic report writer confronts: the act of transcribing the actuality of a human life and explaining a human act can never be accomplished without imagination. Indeed, in a criminal case, the forensic psychiatrist is forced to imagine what might have happened in the past and then convince others that that reconstruction is the one most likely to have occurred. The psychiatrist is armed with the science, practice, and art of a medical specialty, and then must make the language and the words work to convey that expertise. It is in the process of converting psychiatric expertise into a comprehensible and persuasive explanation of a complex act within a complex life that the inadvertent "lies" occur. Hudgins argues that transcription and imagination "enjoy their uneasy congress only by lying to each other" (Hudgins 1996, p. 542), and these lies take several forms that are relevant to the forensic report (Box 5.1).

The *lie of narrative cogency* was defined by Hudgins as "clearing out the narrative underbrush, so the story ... can be more easily seen and appreciated" (Hudgins 1996, p. 542). In forensic psychiatry reports, this type of "lie" can occur under several circumstances. The first is when collateral data are dismissed as irrelevant because they do not fit into a coherent narrative that leads naturally and easily to the conclusion. Often the information may not even be collected in the evaluation. For example, instead of asking the person to clarify exact names and locations of the ten elementary schools he attended during his formative years, it is easier to condense the schools into one or two and have the story proceed. Whether this omission creates a substantive lie depends on the circumstances. If the subject went on to achieve an advanced degree at an Ivy League college and the early education contributed nothing of relevance to the event of interest that occurred when the man was 50 years of age, then the omission may have little consequence to the psychiatric report and be of little interest to the opposing side. However, taking short cuts on details related to the dynamics of the event in question can result in a biased narrative that, although more neatly packaged in prose, will fall short of accurate reporting. Consider, for example, a subject who attended ten different public and parochial elementary schools as a consequence of misbehavior and who later is arrested for arson of a church. The early school experience in this case may indeed not be clutter, but the first seeds of the evolving life.

Sometimes the forensic psychiatrist chooses to clear out the underbrush for the ethics imperative of respecting the person, a second circumstance that calls for ignoring information in the write-up. Including in the report pejorative or embarrassing information that is irrelevant to the legal issue might demonstrate a completeness of interview, but it does so at the cost of the client's dignity. For example, consider a woman in her fifties who is charged with embezzlement of funds to pay off gambling debts incurred by her ailing husband. The psychiatrist would need to weigh very carefully whether the benefit of including in the report her having had an abortion at the age of 19 when she first entered college, a deed that she has never divulged to her strict Catholic family, outweighs the impact that information will have on her, her family, and her trust in psychiatry. The cost-benefit analysis will necessarily be different for a woman with the same history who has been arrested for killing her newborn.

Another circumstance of the cogency lie occurs when a psychiatrist is asked to omit information. When an attorney asks to have information omitted, the psychiatrist must critically analyze the basis of the request. We believe that the most ethical and productive framework for deciding is the extent to which the data in question are essential to the formulation. Essential in this case means that the data either support the formulation or contradict it, since both types of data must be considered by the psychiatrist in order to formulate an opinion; exclusion would weaken the credibility of the report and raise questions about the ethics of the psychiatrist.

There are no easy solutions, and experts will have different recommendations. What is clear is that the inclusion or exclusion of data in the forensic report is neither a facile decision nor one without significant consequences. What we recommend without hesitation is critical consideration, consultation with colleagues, and repeated conferences with the attorney.

Hudgins identifies another category of "lie" relevant to the writing of forensic reports – the *lie of texture*. He noted that "the accumulation of precise and telling details is what makes the story, scene, image, line vivid in the reader's imagination" (Hudgins 1996, p. 544). In forensic reports, the lie of texture is one of embellishment. Of course we do not include here the unethical act of making up material; the lie of texture is a subtler filling of gaps and tying of loose ends to enhance understanding and interest. Although such enhancement may make the narrative more convincing, it creates an artificial coherence that may obfuscate the depth of chaos or complexity. Indeed, cases become forensic in the psychiatric sense when there is confusion of perspectives; such confusion cannot be remedied by completing the story with plausible but created detail. The embellishment also leaves the psychiatrist open to questions about credibility and ethics.

Consider an example of a forensic pre-sentence report describing a woman who lost her husband after a protracted illness but continued illegally to collect his pension. The psychiatrist builds the narrative on the woman's dependence and depression after her husband's death, embellishing the woman's mental anguish around his deteriorating health that prevented her from focusing on any other part of her life. The woman provided scant detail about her thinking or emotions no matter how the psychiatrist probed, but the evidence of her depression was clear to the psychiatrist who corroborated the woman's loss of weight, absence from social events, and avoidance of family. To communicate the depth of her depression for the legal audience, the psychiatrist embellished details of mental anguish. It made a better story than the void of emotion that arose from her depression. The prosecuting attorney, however, used interviews with work associates who described the defendant's behaviors as not that different from usual. The psychiatrist had also interviewed the associates but had never resolved the conflict between his richly textured account of her mental suffering and the associates' perspective that little had changed. The psychiatrist's report was discredited because his embellished account had created such a strong contrast to what appeared to the fact finders to be the more objective account of others.

Sometimes, the lie of texture is one of emphasis. Because collateral information is rarely uniformly useful and consistent, highlighting data supportive to the formulation leads the audience to the psychiatrist's conclusion. Although the idea of selective emphasis may seem similar to the lie of narrative cogency described before, it differs because of the intent of the psychiatrist. In the lie of texture, the psychiatrist emphasizes some details over others to control the attention of the audience and set the foundation for the ultimate formulation. In the lie of narrative cogency, the psychiatrist attempts to remove distractors from the story or to exclude data that have no relevance to the formulation. Competing narratives by the opposing side will likely emphasize a different set of facts. To the extent that the psychiatrist has not acknowledged the contradictory information and explained why it does not negate the formulation, the report can be discredited as biased and incomplete. For example, in a criminal case of a young mother who killed her 10-year-old son, her elementary school history and collateral information from her educated parents supported the psychiatrist's narrative of a woman with a long history of low intelligence and limited coping skills who was overwhelmed by the demands of parenting a child with learning and emotional difficulties, especially after being deserted by her husband. The report barely acknowledged that she had attended a community college, traveled abroad on her own, and had researched and purchased the drugs that she used to overdose her son. The majority of the data did support the psychiatrist's assessment, but by emphasizing one side of the data and not discussing the other information as unexpected and outlying – thereby attesting to her complex state of mind and disorder – the doctor produced a narrative that could not accommodate the facts.

The *lie of emotional evasion* is worth mention, as we know this appears in forensic reports quite regularly. It is what Hudgins called the "sin of omission" (Hudgins 1996, p. 545). Subjects will engage in this maneuver as they talk about their lives and try to sidestep areas that cause them emotional difficulty. But we recognize these omissions in, for example, the report of a forensic specialist writing about a custody fight between a black husband and a white wife over their child with no mention of the implications of race in the marital struggle. Any reader must ask how such an omission could occur. The reasons for this type of omission vary. The psychiatrist might wish to avoid a controversial subject that he or she believes has little to do with the case. For example, in the case just described, the psychiatrist may find that race was not the relevant issue, but the societal view of race as a problem requires that the psychiatrist address the matter. In other cases, the psychiatrist may be avoiding the obvious in deference to the subject's dignity or safety. Consider, for example, the case of a man arrested in an assault of a prison guard that occurred during an episode of mania in the course of bipolar disorder. The psychiatrist rendered his opinion that the assault occurred as the result of a psychosis, a symptom common during this man's manic episodes, but left out of the report that the man was in prison convicted for a sex offense. In other cases, the psychiatrist may try to divert the attention in the case away from a theme evoked by interesting current social factors. For example, a psychiatrist avoided all mention of a woman's Muslim religion in a report that addressed her mental state when she participated in a bank robbery. Although the goal in each of these cases was to divert attention from what the psychiatrist considers to be irrelevant, avoiding the content often leads to an attack on the psychiatrist's credentials, opinion, and ethics.

These common traps, or in Hudgins' terms lies, are a product of a critical element of forensic report writing – that it is done for an audience. Indeed, performative writing requires regard for the audience. A key aspect of all performance is the interaction between the narrator and the reader. The written forensic report is produced with the goal of engaging the audience in the story and convincing them of its merits. It seems unlikely to us that anyone would want to pay an expert for producing a report that on its face is not expected to persuade the reader.

From the moment that forensic psychiatrists begin in writing to tell the stories of people they have recently examined, they have decided to become engaged with the enterprise of employing language in the service of narrative. That engagement, however, must be predicated on the goal of telling the truth. Creating a persuasive story does not imply a departure from truth-telling; rather, persuasion involves the active use of language to tell the truth in a way that increases comprehension and a buy-in to the conclusions. That is, language is used to persuade one that the truth is, in this case, knowable and captured in the conclusions and formulation. By analogy the psychiatrist has the same task as the expert scientist who has to explain to a public television audience the phenomena of the expanding universe and black holes. Without jargon and with humanized accounts of the discoveries undergirding modern physics, he persuades his audience that the topic is important, knowable, and relevant. He tells a story about astronomy that does not depart from the truth but is comprehensible to his audience. On the other hand, the ethical psychiatrist should not be in the position of the scientist who distorts facts to serve the political agenda for or against global warming. The difference is found in the purpose of the story – to elucidate the psychiatric truth rather than manipulate it for another agenda.

5.3 Safeguards in constructing narrative

The challenges in creating persuasive, truthful narratives can be met through the combination of psychiatric diligence and expertise and literary techniques that facilitate the audience's comprehension of the psychiatrist's formulation and conclusion. This combination produces safeguards against inadvertent distortions of the truth and the discrediting of the psychiatric expertise.

The first safeguard is fundamental to psychiatric assessments – a comprehensive evaluation (Box 5.2). Embedded in a complete evaluation is a second safeguard: diligent attention to collateral sources. How much collateral to include is a prickly issue with no exact answer. The correct amount lies somewhere between "all that is needed" and "all that is available," a wide continuum. When psychiatrists are confident of their formulations, they may find additional collateral information confusing and obfuscating to the story. However, what is enough in a clinical assessment, where diagnosis and treatment are the purpose, may not be adequate in a forensic case, where the aim is convincing others that the psychiatric perspective is valid despite evidence to the contrary.

Box 5.2 Safeguards to truthful narratives

Comprehensive evaluation

  Attention to collateral sources
  Inclusion of expository narratives

Formulation narrative

  Transparency in reasoning from data
  Reasons for rejecting alternative explanations
  Acceptance of limits of the narrative
    Lack of certainty regarding past events
    Tolerance of contradictions, gaps, confusion

Another safeguard is the inclusion of the expository narratives, in which the voices of the various reporters are captured fully in tone and attitude. By including these, the psychiatrist displays the data openly without the distortion that comes through restatement.

The formulation narrative is the final safeguard to the contextual risks in writing a persuasive narrative. It is in the formulation narrative that the psychiatrist seizes voice and presents the expert perspective. Because all of the data are already presented and other voices have been recognized, the formulation narrative can emphasize detail to make a convincing, coherent, and psychiatrically based narrative. The psychiatrist essentially argues: I have laid out all the data, all the collateral information, all the viewpoints, now let me show you how it all fits together into a meaningful story of this person's life that led to these circumstances.

One technique in the formulation narrative that increases persuasion while decreasing the impression of bias is to list the reasons for rejecting an alternative explanation. An extension of the narrative, such an explanation not only leads the audience along the logical path to the conclusion, but displays the psychiatrist's attention to opposing data and the consideration of its merits.

One last protection against creating the Hudgins-type lies in the forensic narrative is the acceptance of the limitations of the story, the subject, the witnesses, and the data. In all evaluations that have the purpose of explaining a past event, the recreation of the circumstances in a written report will have limitations. No one knows for certain all that went into the past events – not even the actors. Being open about the limitations of what is known and what can be inferred highlights the desire to be truthful. It requires the psychiatrist to be tolerant of the contradiction, gaps, and confusion common in crises and real life and to resist creating coherence and clarity where it does not exist.

5.4 Conclusion

We have taken the position in this chapter that written reports in forensic psychiatry are the product of the work of the forensic expert. The most effective means of persuading the audience in a legal matter is through a thoughtful narrative that creates an integrated account of the myriad facts and a comprehensible formulation. The forensic narrator must create a product that meets the ethical requirements of truth-telling and respect for person.

The narrative form is an effective and persuasive tool for psychiatrists. It allows complex ideas to be presented in common terms with real examples from the examinee's life. It leads the audience to understand what led up to a particular point in time and to experience the unfolding of events. Along with the persuasive power it provides to the psychiatrist's report come the risks inherent in the narrative process. Collectively these risks, described as "lies" by Hudgins, serve to improve the narrative at the price of bias or the appearance of such. Distortions that simplify the story, increase the impact, fill in the gaps, and remove the ambiguity may create a readable and convincing report but raise the risk of being viewed as not credible, or even worse, as a hired gun.

The protections against such distortions begin with psychiatric expertise that demands attention to detail and collateral information. But the nature of forensic work demands that the psychiatrist appreciate the audience and the adversarial process and construct a narrative that is psychiatrically sound, truthful and respectful, and thoughtful enough of alternative explanations that it can withstand a rigorous cross-examination.

References

Blanchard, M. (1991) The open grid: focalizing narrative studies. *Modern Philology* **89**: 76–90.

Felman, S. & Laub, D. (1992) *Testimony: Crises of Witnessing in Literature, Psychoanalysis, and History*. New York: Routledge.

Griffith, E. E. H. & Baranoski, M. V. (2007) Commentary: the place of performative writing in forensic psychiatry. *Journal of the American Academy of Psychiatry and the Law* **35**: 27–31.

Hudgins, A. (1996) An autobiographer's lies. *American Scholar* **65**: 541–553.

Lawrence-Lightfoot, S. & Davis, J. H. (1997) *The Art and Science of Portraiture*. San Francisco: Jossey-Bass, Inc.

Lebovits, G. (2008a) Fact vs. fiction: writing the facts – part I. *New York State Bar Journal* September, pp. 58–59, 64.

Lebovits, G. (2008b) Fact vs. fiction: writing the facts – part II. *New York State Bar Journal* October, pp. 57–60.

Melton, G. B., Petrila, J., Poythress, N. G., & Slobogin, C. (2007) *Psychological Evaluations for the Courts. A Handbook for Mental Health Professionals and Lawyers*, 3rd edn. New York: Guilford Press.

Menand, L. (2007) Lives of others: the biography business. *The New Yorker* August **6**, pp. 64–66.

O'Grady, J. C. (2004) Report writing for the criminal court. *Psychiatry* **3**: 34–36.

Peterson, E. E. & Langellier, K. M. (2006) The performance turn in narrative studies. *Narrative Inquiry* **16**: 173–180.

Resnick, P. J. (2006) Principles of psychiatric – legal report writing. In the Course Syllabus

of the Forensic Psychiatry Review Course, American Academy of Psychiatry and the Law.

Scheub, H. (1977) Body and image in oral narrative performance. *New Literary History* **8**: 345–367.

Silva, J. A., Weinstock, R., & Leong, G. B. (2003) Forensic psychiatric report writing. In *Principles and Practice of Forensic Psychiatry*, 2nd edn., ed. R. Rosner. London: Arnold, pp. 31–36.

Suggested reading

Borum, R. & Grisso, T. (1996) Establishing standards for criminal forensic reports: an empirical analysis. *Bulletin of the American Academy of Psychiatry and the Law* **24**: 297–317.

Butts, H. (2002) The black mask of humanity: racial/ethnic discrimination and post-traumatic stress disorder. *Journal of the American Academy of Psychiatry and the Law* **30**: 336–339.

Candilis, P. J. (2007) The place of narrative in the courtroom. Available at http://litsite.alaska. edu/uaa/healing/candilis.html [Accessed January 20, 2007].

Candilis, P. J., Weinstock, R., & Martinez, R. (2007) *Forensic Ethics and the Expert Witness*. New York: Springer Science.

Carter, R. T. (2007) Racism and psychological and emotional injury: recognizing and assessing race-based traumatic stress. *Counseling Psychologist* **35**: 13–105.

Cavallo, S. (2000–2001) Witness: the real, the unspeakable, and the construction of narrative. *Journal of the Midwest*

Modern Language Association **33**: 1–3, Autumn–Winter.

Conroy, M. A. (2006) Report writing and testimony. *Applied Psychology in Criminal Justice* suppl: 237–260.

Giorgi-Guarnieri, D., Janofsky, J., Keram, E., et al. (2002) AAPL practice guideline for forensic psychiatric evaluation of defendants raising the insanity defense. *Journal of the American Academy of Psychiatry and the Law* **30**(2): S1–S40, Supplement.

Gold, L. H., Anfang, S. A., Drukteinis, A. M., et al. (2008) AAPL practice guideline for the forensic evaluation of psychiatric disability. *Journal of the American Academy of Psychiatry and the Law* **36**(Suppl): S1–S50.

Grunebaum-Ralph, H. (2001) Re-placing pasts, forgetting presents: narrative, place, and memory in the time of the Truth and Reconciliation Commission. *Research in African Literatures* **32**: 198–212.

Hoffman, B. F. (1986) How to write a psychiatric report for litigation following a personal injury. *American Journal of Psychiatry* **143**: 164–169.

Hollander, J. (1996) Legal rhetoric. In *Law's Stories: Narrative and Rhetoric in the Law*, ed. P. Brooks & P. Gewirtz. New Haven, CT: Yale University Press, pp. 176–186.

Morse, S. J. (2008) The ethics of forensic practice: reclaiming the wasteland. *Journal of the American Academy of Psychiatry and the Law* **36**: 206–217.

Mossman, D., Noffsinger, S. G., Ash, P., et al. AAPL practice guideline for the forensic psychiatric evaluation of competence to stand trial. *Journal of the American Academy of Psychiatry and the Law* **35**(suppl): S1–S72.

Noffsinger, S. G. & Resnick, P. J. (1999) Insanity defense evaluations. *Directions in Psychiatry* **19**: 325–338.

Pollack, S. (1974) *Forensic Psychiatry in Criminal Law*. Los Angeles: University of Southern California Press.

Wettstein, R. M. (2005) Quality and quality improvement in forensic mental health evaluations. *Journal of the American Academy of Psychiatry and the Law* **33**: 158–175.

Chapter

Draftsmanship

6

Phillip J. Resnick and Sherif Soliman

6.1 Introduction

A survey of industrial accident commissioners in California showed that compared with reports by other physicians, psychiatrists' reports were seen as weaker, less understandable, more subjective, more complicated, and more unscientific (Pollack 1969). It is essential for forensic psychiatrists to express ideas clearly and succinctly in written reports. This is challenging because psychiatrists, who are trained to think, speak, and write in medical terms, are here writing for a legal audience. Forensic psychiatrists are similar to foreign ambassadors bridging medical and legal worlds. You bring medical expertise to bear on a legal issue in order to assist the trier of fact. In order to be helpful to a legal audience, this information must be communicated free of jargon.

The key to writing an effective report is to focus from the beginning on the legal question. Merely adding a psycho-legal opinion at the end of a clinical report is not adequate. In order to accomplish this task, you must organize each report around the legal question. Rather than applying a single structure to all reports, you should individualize each report to suit its particular purpose. You must fully understand the legal question and legal standard before drafting your report. Of course, you must also be certain that the retaining party wants a written report.

The stages of report writing are planning, writing, and editing. This chapter will discuss each of these stages.

6.2 Planning

As with any endeavor, effective planning is critical to success. Although errors in grammar or typing can be easily corrected during the editing phase, errors in organization or addressing the wrong legal question are more likely to seriously undermine your report's effectiveness. The planning stage can be subdivided into gathering data, considering the audience, organizing, and outlining.

6.2.1 Data gathering

All of the necessary information should be collected before writing the report. This includes notes from interviews, referral letters, medical records, depositions, police reports, and relevant literature. If you are sent a summary of progress notes by a past therapist, you should seek the therapist's complete notes.

The Psychiatric Report, ed. Alec Buchanan and Michael A. Norko. Published by Cambridge University Press. © Cambridge University Press 2011.

You should keep a list of all sources of information. This list will eventually be integrated into the written report. In the meantime, it keeps track of information and helps you to determine whether additional documents should be requested. The list should be numbered (Guthiel 2009). It can be organized chronologically or by the types of information. For example, all medical records or all depositions can be grouped together.

Each listed item should be described in sufficient detail. For example, a clinical interview should include the date of the interview, the place, and the duration. In describing medical records, the dates, author and/or institution should be identified. Instead of listing, "Mr. Smith's past medical records," specify, "Mr. Smith's medical records from Smallville General Hospital from January 2, 2009 until January 8, 2009."

When listing sources of information, avoid using vague terms to describe sources such as "various medical records." Such language makes you appear careless and will make it difficult for you to testify about what you reviewed without referring to the original records. A complete list of sources of information makes the expert appear precise and facilitates testimony months or sometimes even years after your report has been prepared.

Any professional literature cited in your report should be listed as a source of information. When citing articles, be sure you are familiar with the latest literature in the area. Your entire report can be undermined if the literature cited is obsolete or has been contradicted by subsequent authority. When referring to textbooks, be sure to cite the most recent edition. Even if the authority is cited to support information that has not changed, the use of an older edition can make you appear out of touch with new developments in the field (Babitsky & Mangraviti 2002).

6.2.2 Consider the audience for your report

Even the most carefully prepared report is useless if it does not effectively convey information to the target audience. Thinking carefully about how best to communicate to the recipient of your report early in the planning stage will make your report more effective. Reports prepared for different readers may require different structures and content. For example, a report to an employer addressing fitness to return to work should not contain personal information that is not relevant to the question of whether the employee is able to do the job. While providing some background information helps provide context, excessive details that are not relevant to the legal question should not be included.

Forensic psychiatric trainees are taught to define medical terms and describe the purpose of all medications mentioned. This is good practice in writing for a legal audience. However, we have sometimes encountered reports prepared by forensic psychiatrists consulting to treating physicians that described the purpose of prescribed medications. For example, "You are currently treating Mr. Smith with the antipsychotic medication olanzapine." This language is superfluous at best and may even be viewed as condescending. Even a generally sound practice can lead to a flawed report when the audience is not considered.

6.2.3 Organizing the report

In *The Elements of Style*, Strunk and White (2000) advise authors to "choose a suitable design and hold on to it" (p. 15). The design, the basic skeleton of your report, is dictated by the purpose of the report. In selecting a design, you should decide which data are important and how to convey that information in a clear manner. A report prepared to address a defendant's sanity at the time of the act should include a description of the alleged offense and the symptoms the defendant was experiencing at the time of the offense. These data will inform the psychiatrist's opinion regarding the sanity issue. In contrast, the core of a report addressing competence to stand trial is the defendant's current mental state and their ability to understand the proceedings and work effectively with an attorney.

6.2.4 Outlining

Outlines are particularly useful when dictating reports because they impose an organization upon the writer. The outline may be detailed. It may contain each heading in the report and the data to be discussed in each section. For example, an outline of the section addressing Educational History could include points about behavioral problems, special education, highest level of education attained, and academic performance.

The use of headings to break up the body of the report into smaller sections allows the reader to easily find information within your report. Attorneys strongly favor the use of headings. For example, instead of a single large section labeled "Personal History," it is more reader friendly to subdivide the history into sections such as "Educational History," "Relationship History," "Employment History," and "Legal History." The choice of headings should be tailored to address the particular legal issue. For example, appropriate headings in a sanity report might include the defendant's relationship to the victim, events preceding the crime, the defendant's account of the offense, and the defendant's mental state at the time of the offense. Having a heading labeled "Defendant's Account of the Crime" also reduces the need to continually begin sentences with "The defendant stated …"

The outline is an appropriate place to organize your opinions and reasoning. Each opinion should be listed along with subpoints of supporting evidence. A carefully prepared outline will help you state your opinions and reasoning in a clear, crisp manner.

6.3 Writing the report

If you have spent adequate time and thought in planning the report, the writing stage should go smoothly. The four principles of good writing are clarity, simplicity, brevity, and humanity. We will offer specific suggestions to apply these principles to forensic psychiatric report writing.

6.3.1 Clarity

Achieving clarity begins with good formatting. Babitsky and Mangraviti (2002) recommend using a 12-point font and one and a half-line spacing to make the report easy to read. They also suggest numbering the pages to indicate the total number of pages in your report; for example, "Page 8 of 10." In a complex report, consider adding a table of contents. You should use clear attribution throughout your report so the reader can determine where each piece of information came from.

Reports should be self-sufficient. Consequently, you should consider summarizing any records in the body of your report that you rely upon in forming your opinion. Without referring to other documents, the reader should be able to understand how your opinion was reached from the data in the report.

Avoid ambiguity in word choice and sentence construction. For example, "The plaintiff has discussed your proposal to fill the drainage ditch with his partners." Contranyms should be avoided. Contranyms are words that have two opposite meanings. For example, sanction may mean both to "give permission" or to "disapprove."

Use the correct verb tense. In the report of your interview put things in the past tense. For example, "Mr. Jones described his father as passive and weak." Your mental status observations should also be in the past tense. For example, "Mr. Jones was neatly dressed and cooperative." Your opinion section should be in the present tense. For example, "It is my opinion with reasonable medical certainty that Mr. Jones is competent to stand trial." Your review of medical records is also usually best put in the present tense because they were just read. For example, "The doctor's progress note on January 4 states …"

Make correct word choices. For example, "feel" is often incorrectly used, such as in, "The defendant felt he was unjustly arrested." Feel refers to visceral descriptions. So it is proper to say that the defendant felt dizzy and nauseated. "Think," "believe," and "state" refer to intellectual statements. Thus, the above statement should say, "The defendant believed that he was unjustly arrested." "Guilty" carries a stronger connotation of blameworthiness than "liable." One is guilty of a crime but liable for a civil wrong (Lebovits 2005).

Serial commas refer to the commas that separate a series of three or more words or phrases. The last comma in the series – the serial comma – is optional. Serial commas reflect a natural pause in spoken English and promote clarity. Example: "Yesterday the police arrested five criminals, two robbers, and three burglars." The serial comma makes it clear that the police arrested ten criminals (Lebovits 2008c).

It is useful to clarify inconsistent data in your report. For example, "Although Mr. Jones stated that he was diagnosed with PTSD while in Elsewhere Hospital in 2009, the discharge summary from Elsewhere Hospital dated June 13, 2009 reported only a diagnosis of malingering. When Mr. Jones was confronted with this inconsistency, he said he must have been mistaken in his recollection."

6.3.2 Simplicity

Simplicity is conveyed in the voice and language of the report. Always use the active voice because using the passive voice makes your report harder to read. For example, instead of saying "the psychiatrist was repeatedly interrupted by the evaluee," say "the evaluee repeatedly interrupted me." Refer to yourself in the first person. Some psychiatrists refer to themselves in the third person. This is awkward and, as Babitsky and Mangraviti (2002) point out, the cross-examiner can use this language to make the expert look silly or pompous. Plain language should be used in your report. Do not use archaic language such as "aforementioned." Instead of "enclosed *herewith* please find …," say "I enclose …" Avoid formalisms such as "the instant case" (Lebovits 2008e, p. 60). The use of overly formal language both confounds the meaning of your report and communicates a lack of confidence.

Multi-syllable words reduce readability, tax the reader, and decrease comprehension. Sentences of 20 to 25 words have the greatest readability. Use common words. Rather than writing "remuneration," use "salary" instead. Instead of saying, "subsequent to," say "after." Many jurors are confused by the phrase "subsequent to." In constructing sentences, eliminate meaningless introductions. Do not write, "It is possible that …" or "There are …" For example, do not write, "There are two basic rules that psychiatrists should follow in preparing reports." Instead write, "Psychiatrists should follow two basic rules in preparing reports."

Simplicity means forgetting the jargon that you spent eight years learning in your medical training. While medical terminology facilitates communication among medical professionals, it obfuscates communication with the non-medical reader. Instead of stating, "Mr. Smith's mood was euthymic with a full affect. His thought process was linear," write, "Mr. Smith's mood was neither depressed nor elevated and he displayed an appropriate range of emotional expression. He responded relevantly to my questions and his thoughts were logical and easy to follow." When medical terms cannot be avoided, they should be clearly defined. Even terms that seem basic to you can be misleading to attorneys. For example, schizophrenia is commonly misunderstood by the public to mean having multiple personalities.

The lay reader is not likely to be familiar with prescribed medications. Therefore, the first time a medication is mentioned, you should describe its use and route of administration (if not oral), and you may characterize the dose being given as low, average, or high. For example, instead of stating, "sertraline 150 mg qd," write "sertraline 150 milligrams daily (antidepressant, average dose)."

Avoid acronyms unless they are widely known. Although acronyms may appear to shorten your report, they force the reader to retrace their steps to find definitions (Lebovits 2008e). Don't use periods for acronyms. Acronyms take the first letter from a series of words to form a pronounceable word that stands for something. For example, "AIDS" stands for acquired immune deficiency syndrome. Periods may be used for abbreviations. In abbreviations, you pronounce each individual letter; for example, F.B.I. (Lebovits 2008a). (However, in other countries such as the UK, periods are not usually included in abbreviations.)

Avoid embellishments like *italics*, <u>underlining</u>, or **bold font**. These techniques suggest that you want to emphasize a fact but you don't know how to do so. They also shout at the reader. It is better to express your thoughts through content, not style (Lebovits 2008d).

6.3.3 Brevity

Reports should be long enough to address the legal issue and no longer. Although lengthy reports are sometimes necessary in complex cases, you can usually be brief. The two primary strategies to achieve brevity are eliminating unnecessary words and eliminating unnecessary information.

Strunk and White (2000) admonish writers to "omit needless words." They state, "A sentence should contain no unnecessary words, a paragraph no unnecessary sentences, for the same reason that a drawing should have no unnecessary lines and a machine no unnecessary parts" (p. 23). Avoid unnecessary words and redundancy. Here is an example: "The lack of confidentiality of this interview was explained to the defendant by the undersigned as well as the fact that a report of my findings would be prepared and submitted to the court." This could be stated briefly as follows: "I explained to the defendant that this interview was not confidential, and that I would submit my findings to the court."

The data contained in your report should be relevant to the legal issue being addressed. Information that does not relate to the referral issue should be kept to a minimum. For example, a detailed review of the evaluee's relationships and sexual practices in a competency to stand trial report is often useless. On the other hand, such information may be highly relevant in a sanity report about a sex crime. Including unnecessary information makes the report unwieldy and even worse, sometimes results in unnecessary disclosure of unfavorable information about the evaluee.

The decision to include or omit a piece of information is sometimes fraught with legal and ethical pitfalls. Both the language chosen and the data presented may indicate overt or subtle bias. Some decisions about omitting data are relatively straightforward. The fact that a 40-year-old police officer used marijuana on one occasion at the age of 16 is not likely to be relevant to his current fitness for duty. Such information may prove embarrassing to the officer without contributing to the formulation of your opinion. However, some decisions are more complicated. For example, in a sanity report about a mother who killed her two children due to a delusional belief that she was saving them from damnation, would it be appropriate to mention that she had an abortion 4 years earlier? In deciding whether to include information that is damaging or embarrassing, carefully weigh the probative value of the information against its prejudicial effect.

6.3.4 Humanity

While we strive to be objective and dispassionate, we must not lose sight of the fact that we are writing not about concepts or objects but about human beings. As Griffith and Baranoski (2000) observed, "Forensic reports must contend with several human voices seeking to be heard." The humanity of those voices can be conveyed without using dramatic language. There is no need to say, "At the time of the tragic events of the August 1, 2007 …". Using quotations of the evaluee's language animates writing. They allow the person quoted to speak directly to the reader. Using quotations is particularly important in conveying the defendant's account of the crime.

In a quotation that contains a factual, spelling, or usage error, use "[sic]," meaning "thus," after the error. However, if the context makes it clear that the mistake was in the original don't add "[sic]." Overusing "[sic]" suggests that you are embarrassing the original quotation's author (Lebovits 2008a). Use three-dot ellipses ("…"), all separated by spaces, to show omissions of punctuation or a word or more in the middle of your sentence. Use four-dot ellipses ("….") to show omissions at the end of a sentence if the end of the quotation is omitted (Lebovits 2008b).

One of the easiest ways to maintain humanity is to avoid dehumanizing language. For example, instead of continually referring to the individual being evaluated as "the evaluee," "the defendant," or the "plaintiff," refer to the person by name. Use the person's surname preceded by the appropriate title such as Mr., Ms., or Dr. This approach sends two messages. First, it says that you respect the person being evaluated enough to refer to the evaluee by name. Second, it indicates that your report is individualized rather than a generic report.

Avoid using pejorative language towards the evaluee. Rather than saying, "Mr. Smith is a liar as evidenced by the fact that he told the police he did not rob the store but admitted it an hour later," write, "The fact that Mr. Smith told the police he robbed the store an hour after denying it suggests that he was consciously misrepresenting his role in the offense during his first interview with officers."

6.3.5 Opinion section

The Opinion section will be the most carefully read part of your report and, in some cases the only section read. Thus, it may require 50% of your writing effort and time even if it makes up only 20% of your total report. It is best to label the Opinion section of your report simply "Opinion." Designations such as discussion or formulation sound more like speculation than professional opinions. State each opinion with reasonable medical certainty. After each opinion, our preference is to specify the information supporting it in a numbered list. For example, "It is my opinion with reasonable medical certainty that Mr. Smith has the capacity to consult with his attorney with a reasonable degree of rational understanding. The following evidence supports this opinion."

Each of your supporting points should be based upon solid factual information. Your opinion should be stated in the exact language of the legal standard for that particular jurisdiction. Consider including the data that militates against your opinion and explaining why the weight of the evidence nonetheless supports your opinion.

In organizing the evidence for your opinion, begin with your strongest points. You are likely to testify based on your report. The jury is more likely to remember your first piece of evidence than they are your seventh and eighth. Weak points should be omitted because a cross-examiner can use them to make the entire opinion appear incorrect. For example, if a list of fifteen supporting points contains twelve solid points and three weak points, a cross-examiner can create the impression that your opinion is faulty by focusing on only the three weak points while ignoring the stronger evidence.

It is preferable to start each section of your opinion with a statement and then support it with reasons. Don't begin a sentence with the evidence and conclude with your opinion. For example, rather than saying, "In view of a, b, c, my opinion is x," it is better to say, "My opinion is x. The following evidence supports my opinion: a, b, c."

In planning your Opinion section, you might jot down all your thoughts and then decide how to organize them. This is called mapping your opinion. The following list shows that the defendant knew the wrongfulness of his act in an insanity case. Here are the psychiatrist's initial thoughts in random order:

Hid his gun
Wiped away fingerprints
Apologized to the victim
Waited until dark
Said "sorry" to witness
Cleaned up blood
Wore gloves
Expressed remorse to police
Wore a ski mask

Organizing your reasons will make them more convincing and make them easier for the jury to recall. Upon reflection, these points could be arranged into the following three clusters:

Avoided detection	Removed evidence	Expressed remorse
Gloves	Fingerprints	To police
Ski mask	Cleaned blood	To witness
Darkness	Hid gun	To victim

The reasons supporting your opinions should be fully stated. The reader should not have to use inferences to understand your point. For example, in support of the opinion that a defendant knew the wrongfulness of breaking into the house, you might write, "He wore a ski mask." However, it would be better to say, "The fact that the defendant wore a ski mask before breaking into the house strongly suggests that he did not want to be recognized because he knew that he was going to engage in illegal behavior."

If there are two versions of the facts in a case, you should consider giving alternative opinions. For example, if you are evaluating a malpractice case due to an inpatient suicide, the account of the decedent's wife and the treating psychiatrist may be different as in the following example:

> The decedent's wife stated in her deposition that on the evening that her husband hanged himself, she had told his treating psychiatrist at 4:30 p.m. that her husband was very depressed and talking about suicide. She added that the psychiatrist told her that the staff would keep a very close eye on him. However, the treating psychiatrist in his deposition stated that the decedent's wife never spoke to him on that day. He related that if she had told him that information, he would have placed the decedent on suicide precautions.

In such a case, you may state that if the treating psychiatrist's account is taken at face value, you would have one opinion. However, if the decedent's wife's account is taken at face value, you might offer an opposite opinion about whether the treating psychiatrist fell below the standard of care. Your reasoning for each opinion should be explained in detail. This approach keeps you from usurping the role of the jury in deciding which facts are true.

6.3.6 Practical suggestions

1. Try to dictate or type your report the same day of your evaluation while the material is still fresh in your mind. If the evaluation is done in multiple visits, it is still useful to convert your handwritten notes for each visit into a typed format.
2. When working in the US, use only diagnoses listed in the latest Diagnostic and Statistical Manual of the American Psychiatric Association. Follow each diagnosis with a brief paragraph showing how the symptoms meet the DSM criteria.
3. In the diagnostic section of your forensic report you should never write "rule out." "Ruling out" a diagnosis is appropriate to write upon admission to a hospital. However, the legal reader of your report is not going to rule out any diagnosis. If you have a tentative diagnosis but are not sufficiently confident to state it, you can precede it with the word "probable."
4. In your diagnostic formulation, consider adding a section to show that you considered the possibility of malingering and the reasons you concluded it was or was not present.
5. Put the most important information first. State the general before the specific. Introduce things before you discuss them. Introduce people before you write about them (Lebovits 2008e).
6. Throughout your report there should be a clear separation of factual data from your professional opinions or conclusions. The latter belong only in your Opinion section.
7. To make your report more persuasive, begin sentences with negative clauses and conclude with a positive statement. For example, "Although no appellate cases in this jurisdiction are available, the majority of state supreme courts that have addressed the issue have concluded that there is a duty to protect identifiable victims from foreseeable patient violence."
8. Avoid pregnant negatives. Pregnant negatives are statements of what symptoms are not present rather than statements of which symptoms are present. For example, if you say the evaluee was "not frankly delusional," the reader does not know whether the evaluee had ideas of reference, paranoid personality traits, or some evidence of delusions which did not meet a particular threshold.

9. Avoid hedging statements which weaken writing. For example, avoid saying, "It appears that …" or "In a sense …"

10. Instead of repeatedly saying in your report "the plaintiff said," consider alternatives such as "he added," "he told me," "he described," "he volunteered," or "he related." However, you should avoid using words suggesting bias in the body of your report, such as "he admitted," "he claimed," or "he alleged."

11. Avoid using preambles which weaken writing. For example, in a child custody report, don't say, "I believe that I am being fair to all parties."

12. After your signature block you may add two or three credentials. The signature block should not be an ego trip. In our view, a better approach is to routinely include a copy of your curriculum vitae with your report.

6.3.7 Ten pitfalls

1. *Raising the bar unnecessarily.* The language you use to describe your evaluation can create an unattainably high standard. For example, "In my three hour examination, I obtained a complete and thorough history and have a full understanding of Mr. Smith's mental state." Labeling the evaluation "complete and thorough" makes it easy for a cross-examiner to attack your report by pointing out arcane areas that you did not explore even if they are irrelevant to the referral issue. In addition, the use of the words "full understanding" sets a standard that is impossible to meet. It would be better to simply state, "I interviewed Mr. Smith for three hours."

2. *Using language that appears haughty or pompous.* Never inflate your resumé and avoid describing yourself in haughty terms such as "I am a world renowned expert in schizophrenia, a noted researcher, and a widely published author in the field." If you have a website, be sure it is free of such language also. It is better to objectively spell out your qualifications and let the judge or jury decide how accomplished you are. A better way to state your qualifications is: "I have treated patients with schizophrenia for the past twenty years, authored ten articles on schizophrenia, and have been awarded three research grants to study the genetic origin of schizophrenia." Referring to yourself in the third person or using the "royal we" can make you appear arrogant. A skillful cross-examiner can use such language to distance you from the jury.

3. *Using absolute language.* Using words such as "always" and "never" means that even a shred of contradictory data in the universe of information can be used to impeach your opinion (Babitsky & Mangraviti 2002). For example, "No reasonable psychiatrist would ever prescribe a first generation antipsychotic to a patient with tardive dyskinesia." A more defensible statement would be: "Psychiatrists should carefully consider switching to an atypical antipsychotic medication if a patient has tardive dyskinesia." Attorneys recognize that absolute language is great fodder for cross-examination and it makes the expert appear to be an advocate for the retaining party.

4. *Using hedge words* (Babitsky & Mangraviti 2002). Hedge words or phrases such as "apparently," "possibly," "supposedly," "reportedly," and "I think," imply uncertainty. When used to refer to facts, they indicate that you are guessing about the facts or are imprecise in citing a source of information. There is no justification for using the word "reportedly." Instead, indicate whether the source of information is the evaluee, a collateral interview, or a specific record. Instead of stating, "Mr. Smith was reportedly

admitted to Smallville General Hospital on June 9, 2002," write, "The June 9, 2002 Admission Note by Dr. Jones indicates that Mr. Smith was admitted on June 9, 2002."

When hedge words are used to state an opinion, they imply a lack of confidence in your opinion. Opinions must be stated with reasonable medical certainty (more likely than not in most jurisdictions). Opinions that are not held with at least a reasonable degree of medical certainty are usually legally insufficient. Keeping this standard in mind should eliminate your temptation to precede an opinion with a hedge word or phrase.

5. *Appearing to advocate for the retaining party*. Do not use language in your cover letter that is friendly towards the retaining attorney or imply that you are trying to satisfy the needs of the retaining attorney (Babitsky & Mangraviti 2002). For example, "Dear Bill, I hope this report is useful. XYZ, Inc's conduct was repugnant. They really need to pay for Jerry's injury. P.S., I hope to see you and Joan this Saturday at the country club." The use of such language in your report or a cover letter suggests that you are biased. Even seemingly innocent language such as addressing the retaining attorney by a first name can imply bias. We prefer not to list discussions with retaining counsel as sources or information and you should never imply that your opinion is based on discussions with the retaining attorney.

6. *Labeling the report a "draft," a "work product," or "confidential."* Labeling your report a "draft" alerts the cross-examiner to the fact that there are or were other versions of your report. The opposing attorney may demand to review all previous versions and inquire about the reasons for any changes in your report. If changes have been made at the request of the retaining party, you may be made to appear biased or dishonest. Labeling your report a "work product" or "confidential" can also be made to look like you are trying to hide it from the opposing party or the court (Babitsky & Mangraviti 2002).

7. *Making snide comments about the parties or opposing experts*. Making such comments diminishes your credibility as an expert witness. For example, "Dr. Jones ignored established principles of risk assessment when he gave the opinion that the discharge of an obviously suicidal patient was not below the standard of care. It was egregiously below the standard of care." If the jury credits such a report at all, they will likely consider it a partisan argument rather than unbiased expert opinion. Instead, simply state your opinion with reasonable medical certainty and the reasons supporting it. If you discuss your disagreements with other experts, refrain from any personal attacks or condescending language. Instead, specify the areas of disagreement and list the evidence supporting your opinion.

8. *Using legal terms or using the words "legally" or "legal"* (Babitsky & Mangraviti 2002). The cross-examining attorney is at a disadvantage when discussing psychiatry. However, the tables are turned when discussing the law. Although forensic psychiatrists have knowledge of circumscribed areas of the law, that knowledge pales in comparison with a competent attorney. You should avoid using legal technical terms such as "proximate cause," or "gross negligence." A cross-examiner is likely to ask you the precise legal definition of such terms if you use them. You should also avoid reciting case law or other detailed legal knowledge. It shifts the focus away from the psychiatric issues you are qualified to address.

9. *Using emphasis when expressing your opinion* (Babitsky & Mangraviti 2002). Some examples are using the words "clearly," and "obviously." Using emphasis does not

make an unsupported opinion more persuasive and can make you appear inflexible or arrogant.

10. *Using language that makes your report appear to be the product of a "mill."* Using the phrase "dictated but not read" suggests that the report is one of many produced by experts who are too busy to take the time to edit their own work. In addition, the use of boilerplate language makes a report appear generic. When such language is necessary, individualize it to the extent possible. One example of boilerplate language is the non-confidentiality notice at the beginning of each evaluation. It can be personalized by referring to the evaluee by name rather than as "the subject" and by noting the evaluee's response to the notice. For example, "When I advised Mr. Smith of the non-confidential nature of the evaluation, he laughed and said, 'So I'd better watch what I say, huh, doc?'"

6.4 Editing

The editing phase can be challenging because it requires you to take a critical look at your own work. Sometimes you need to delete or reword sections that you have spent hours writing. As with the planning stage, the editing stage begins by reflecting on whether the report has actually accomplished its purpose. Be certain that the report adequately addresses the referral question and does not go beyond that issue. Rereading your draft report will give you an opportunity to clarify ambiguous sentences. Next, review the organization of the report to be sure that it follows a logical progression and has clear headings. For example, a competence to stand trial report should contain a separate section addressing the defendant's understanding of the basic elements of competence rather than integrating this information into your mental status examination.

Your Opinion section should be reviewed for clarity and logic. Each opinion should be stated clearly and we prefer to have it followed by a list of the supporting information. Carefully review each piece of evidence to be sure there is a factual basis for it and that it actually supports the specific opinion.

Finally, review your report for grammatical and typographical errors. It is sometimes helpful to have a colleague read over the report to be certain that all typographical and grammatical errors have been corrected. Proofreading a report out loud or backwards allows some overlooked errors to be discovered. Reading a report with spelling, grammar, and punctuation errors causes people to assume that a writer who doesn't care about these types of errors will make other mistakes about the facts (Lebovits 2008d). If you have not carefully proofread your report, a cross-examiner might inquire whether you were as careful in reaching your conclusions as you were in the preparation of your report.

6.5 Conclusion

William Zinsser (1988) observed that, "Clear writing is the logical arrangement of thought." No less can be expected in a forensic report. Drafting a forensic psychiatric report consists of planning, writing, and editing. The critical task of planning the report is designing a format that best addresses the specific legal question. Strive to achieve clarity, simplicity, brevity, and humanity in your writing. Be alert to common pitfalls of report writing. Finally, edit the report carefully to be sure it adequately addresses the legal question, is clear and concise, and is free of grammatical and typographical errors.

References

Babitsky, S. & Mangraviti, J. J. (2002) *Writing and Defending Your Expert Report: The Step by Step Guide With Models*. Falmouth, MA: Seak, Inc.

Griffith, E. & Baranoski, M. (2007) Commentary: the place of performative writing in forensic psychiatry. *Journal of the American Academy of Psychiatry and the Law* 35(1): 28.

Guthiel, T. (2009) *The Psychiatrist as Expert Witness*, 2nd edn. Washington, DC: American Psychiatric Publishing, Inc., pp. 95–102.

Lebovits, G. (2005) Problem words and pairs in legal writing – Part III. *New York State Bar Association Journal* May, p. 59.

Lebovits, G. (2008a) Do's, don'ts, and maybes: legal writing punctuation – Part I. *New York State Bar Association Journal* 80(2): 55, 57.

Lebovits, G. (2008b) Do's, don'ts, and maybes: legal writing punctuation – Part III. *New York State Bar Association Journal* 80(4): 54.

Lebovits, G. (2008c) "Do's, don'ts, and maybes": Usage controversies – Part I. *New York State Bar Association Journal* 80(5): 60.

Lebovits, G. (2008d) "Do's, don'ts, and maybes": Usage controversies – Part II. *New York State Bar Association Journal* August, p. 58.

Lebovits, G. (2008e) Plain English: eschew legalese. *New York State Bar Association Journal* November/December: 59, 60.

Pollack, S. (1969) The psychiatrist as expert witness: Cross examination of the psychiatrist. Presented to First Annual Practicing Law institute, Criminal Advocacy Institute, "Are Your Techniques Obsolete?" January 25, 1969.

Strunk, W. & White, E. B. (2000) *The Elements of Style*, 4th edn. London: Longman.

Zinsser, W. (1988) *Writing to Learn*. New York: Harper & Row, Publishers, p. viii.

Report structure

Chapter

7

Alec Buchanan and Michael A. Norko

7.1 The design of this section of the book

Each chapter in Section 2 describes the content of a type of psychiatric report. To do this, all of the chapters use a single report structure. This is shown in Table 7.1.

Obviously, many different structures are capable of contributing to a good report. That contained in Table 7.1 is presented partly to avoid repetition: while the content of a report differs according to the setting and the question being answered, many of the elements, such as the provision of background information and a description of the mental state findings, are nearly always present. Working from a single structure also serves to highlight the differences between reports written for different purposes and between the styles of different authors.

Each chapter in Section 2 also addresses aspects of preparing a report that are essential to or inseparable from the writing. These include the conduct of the psychiatric evaluation, the antecedents and outcomes of writing, and the questions frequently asked of report writers in cross-examination. The written report is not a static document confined to a preset inquiry; it is the product of forethought, planning, and execution of a range of relevant details pertinent to a unique set of circumstances, and it anticipates questions relevant to legitimate inquiry in the adversarial process in order to meet adequately the demands of the legal system.

The elements of Table 7.1 are the results of choices made by the editors: models of reports offered for use by social workers and psychologists can look very different (see Perry 1979; Enfield 1987). The content of Table 7.1 is not arbitrary, however. Certain themes have been evident in the evolution of the psychiatric report since East (1927) listed his five headings 80 years ago. These themes are reflected in Table 7.1 and described in the next section of this chapter. Finally, following any outline will not always be feasible. Many US states require reports for use in civil commitment proceedings to follow a prescribed structure, and some states provide guidelines for other reports also (see Conroy 2006).

7.2 The structure of a psychiatric report

Reviews of style and content in psychiatric writing take a range of positions on basic questions such as whether a report should be couched in the first person and the value, or otherwise, of stating a diagnosis (see Scott 1954; Group for the Advancement of Psychiatry 1991; Rix 1999). By contrast, the report structure has been relatively stable, and recent suggestions resemble those of East (see Wettstein 2004). Reviews of report writing note the value of

Table 7.1 Structure of the psychiatric report

1. **Preliminary and identifying information**
2. **Introduction**

   Why the report is being written, the circumstances of the request and the questions that are being addressed

   Dates and duration of interviews with the subject

   Sources of information used in the report

   Information given to the subject at time of interview, including information regarding confidentiality

   List of appended material

3. **Body of report**

   Background information

   Current events (the crime in a sentencing report; the events leading to the claim in a civil action), the circumstances surrounding those events, and relevant sequelae

   Findings on examination

   Psychological and other test results

4. **Opinion**
5. **Concluding material**

   Signature of author

   Name, qualifications, and current post

   Date of signing

structure to both reader and author. Structure helps an author to ensure that all relevant areas are covered and can provide a familiar, and therefore more easily used, framework on which to base a report's conclusions.

Structure can also help the author achieve balance. Decisions as to what to include and how to present information are central to the way a report is understood. As such, those decisions are potential sources of unwanted bias. Structuring the report is one way of seeking to minimize bias and ensure, for instance, that information suggesting a different conclusion is not improperly excluded. To protect such intangible qualities Lord Woolf (1996) suggested the author testify to a report's being "complete" and "accurate." In criminal cases, Scott (1954, p. 91) recommended the author ask, "Could I substantiate all the facts mentioned if I were to be cross-examined upon them, and is the whole report strictly fair to the offender?"

7.2.1 Preliminary and identifying information

Most reports will start with the name and date of birth of the person being evaluated. Depending on the nature of the case, some authorities recommend providing additional information at the outset. One review, noting that the legal position is unclear, suggests that heading the report "Private and Confidential" may limit the reporter's liability following improper disclosure (see Bowden 1990). Where the report concerns ensuing psychological harm, Hoffman (1986) includes the date of the accident. Some reports for criminal proceedings list the charges (Bluglass 1979). Pollack (1974) includes the court number; Trick and Tennant (1981), the author's credentials.

7.2.2 Introductory material

A number of reviews note that the safest approach to describing why the report has been written is to quote from a written request or court order. If this is impractical, or for other reasons the legal instructions are to be summarized, it will sometimes be helpful to confirm with the person commissioning the report that the summary is accurate.

Examples of material typically included under Sources of Information include police reports, statements made by the evaluee, and interviews with informants. The number and length of any interviews will usually be described (Group for the Advancement of Psychiatry 1991); some reporters include the dates (Conroy 2006). Civil litigation reports sometimes include in the Introduction a description of the incident on which the claim is based (see Hoffman 1986).

The report will usually describe the explanation that the reporter provided to the client. This explanation will usually have included: (1) the purpose of the evaluation and the expert's role, (2) the option not to participate, (3) the limits to confidentiality, and (4) an assessment of whether the client understood each of these (Bluglass 1995; Wettstein 2004; American Acadamy of Psychiatry and the Law 2005; Royal College of Psychiatrists 2008). The way in which the information is presented should take into account the capacities of the client.

Finally, the introductory material should list any materials that are appended, such as the author's curriculum vitae, if this has been requested and has not already been supplied, and reports of psychological testing.

7.2.3 Body of the report

Many authors provide subheadings under "Background" (see Table 7.1) for areas such as family history, personal history, past medical history, and psychiatric history. Whether or not this is done, the aim will be to create a coherent narrative preparatory to answering the legal question. If that question relates to criminal sentencing and the defendant has a history of mental illness, for instance, the report will usually emphasize the temporal relationship between symptoms and the behavior of concern. Depending on the case, the sequence of subheadings may change.

Some authors make it easier for the reader to distinguish the sources used by including information from each collateral in a separate section, often towards the end of a report (see Hoffman 1986). This has the additional advantage of preserving the internal coherence of each account. One disadvantage of such an approach, particularly when there are numerous collateral sources, is that it can leave unclear what the author of the report thinks happened. An alternative is to incorporate all relevant information into a single narrative, making clear the areas of agreement and disagreement. Whichever approach is adopted, by the end of the report it should be clear to which version, or versions, of the facts the Opinion refers.

The usual position regarding the inclusion of psychological and other test results was stated by the Group for the Advancement of Psychiatry (1991, p. 97): "A summary of any test results should be reported in terms that are clear to the lay audience. The complete test report should be appended to the report." Jargon should be avoided (see Gibbens 1974). Other approaches to the inclusion of test results are discussed in Chapter 15.

7.2.4 Opinion

Some authors insert a summary of the Opinion at the start of the report, often immediately preceding the Background section. Most Opinions will briefly summarize the background before addressing the questions listed in the introductory material. Reviews are unanimous that no new material should be introduced at this stage. Facts used to support the Opinion should already have appeared in the Background. The author's reasoning should be easy to follow. There seems no single best way to present the arguments. Gutheil (2009) distinguishes "conclusion-first" from "conclusion-last" approaches, noting that neither has been shown to be superior. Pollack (1974) recommends stating an opinion, then providing the reasoning.

7.2.5 Concluding material

The Group for the Advancement of Psychiatry (1991) suggests a report should end with the expert's "current position, title and professional credentials" and most reviews see this as an acceptable minimum. Some authors place the date of signing below their signature; others place it at the start of the report. Mendelson (1999) notes that signatures should only include membership of colleges, institutes, or academies where these memberships are officially recognized or where they amount to a medical qualification.

7.3 Length

Reviewers differ greatly in their recommendations regarding length. The length of the report will vary with the question, the circumstances, and the writer. Three points seem important. First, the report should provide sufficient data to support the Opinion. Second, the purpose of the report is to present that Opinion. Transparency is now a virtue, although this was not always the case (see, "Never give your reasons. Your decisions will probably be right. Your reasons will probably be wrong"; Mullins 1944, p. 180). But because not everything is relevant, simply adding more information will usually not help. Third, the information contained in a report can have consequences for the client or others that the author does not intend. When the information is superfluous, those consequences are harder to justify.

References

American Academy of Psychiatry and the Law (2005) *Ethics Guidelines for the Practice of Forensic Psychiatry*. American Academy of Psychiatry and The Law: Bloomfield, CT.

Bluglass, R. (1979) The psychiatric court report. *Medicine, Science and the Law* **19**: 121–129.

Bluglass, R. (1995) Preparing a medico-legal report. *Advances in Psychiatric Treatment* **1**: 131–137.

Bowden, P. (1990) The written report and sentences. In *Principles and Practice of Forensic Psychiatry*, ed. R. Bluglass & P. Bowden. Edinburgh: Churchill Livingstone, pp. 183–197.

Conroy, M. (2006) Report writing and testimony. *Applied Psychology in Criminal Justice* **2**: 237–260.

East, N. (1927) *An Introduction to Forensic Psychiatry in Criminal Courts*. New York: William Wood.

Enfield, R. (1987) A model for developing the written forensic report. In *Innovations in Clinical Practice: A Source Book*, vol. 6, ed. P. Keller & S. Heyman, Sarasota, FL: Professional Resource Exchange, pp. 379–394.

Gibbens, T. (1974) Preparing psychiatric court reports. *British Journal of Hospital Medicine* 278–284.

Group for the Advancement of Psychiatry (1991) *The Mental Health Professional and the Legal System*. New York: Brunner Mazel.

Gutheil, T. (2009) *The Psychiatrist as Expert Witness*, 2nd edn. Washington, DC: American Psychiatric Publishing.

Hoffman, B. (1986) How to write a psychiatric report for litigation following a personal injury. *American Journal of Psychiatry* **143**: 164–169.

Mendelson, G. (1999) Writing a psychiatric medico-legal report. *Australasian Forensic Psychiatry Bulletin* **16**: 5–18.

Mullins, C. (1944) *Crime and Psychology.* London: Methuen.

Perry, F. (1979) *Reports for Criminal Courts.* Ilkley, UK: Owen Wells.

Pollack, S. (1974) *Forensic Psychiatry in Criminal Law.* University of Southern California: Los Angeles, CA.

Rix, K. (1999) Expert evidence and the courts 2. Proposals for reform, expert witness bodies and "the model report". *Advances in Psychiatric Treatment* **5**: 154–160.

Royal College of Psychiatrists (2008) *Court Work. College Report CR147.* London: Royal College of Psychiatrists.

Scott, P. (1954) Psychiatric reports for magistrates' courts. *British Journal of Delinquency* **4**: 82–98.

Trick, K. & Tennant, T. (1981) *Forensic Psychiatry: An Introductory Text.* Pitman: London.

Wettstein, E. (2004) The forensic examination and report. In *Textbook of Forensic Psychiatry,* ed. R. Simon and L. Gold. Washington, DC: American Psychiatric Publishing, pp. 139–164.

Woolf, H. (1996) Access to Justice: Final Report to the Lord Chancellor on the Civil Justice System in England and Wales. London: HMSO.

Criminal litigation

J. Richard Ciccone and Joshua Jones

8.1 Introduction

8.1.1 General

"The psychiatric report for legal purposes is the closest professional link between the two disciplines of psychiatry and law," wrote Seymour Pollack in 1968. Despite this, few empirical studies have looked at the format or process of preparing the report.

In the criminal domain, the studies that have been done have demonstrated significant inadequacies. Hess and Thomas (1963) reviewed the records of 77 patients with court-ordered commitments to a state hospital. They found that the standards for competence to stand trial and criminal responsibility were often confused with each other. They also found that only rarely were the grounds for the psychiatrist's opinion presented in the report, thus putting the court in the position of accepting or rejecting the report on an arbitrary basis. Geller and Lister (1978) found that psychiatric reports written for the purpose of giving opinions on both competence to stand trial and criminal responsibility frequently did not address one or the other of the ultimate issues. Sixty-five percent of the reports did not address the issue of competence to stand trial and 93% of the reports did not address the issue of criminal responsibility. On the other hand, 55% of the reports offered a prediction of dangerousness even though the court did not request an opinion on that issue.

Writing a forensic psychiatric report begins with understanding that the referral source is asking a question. This may not be clear from written communication and a direct request for clarification is often necessary. Psychiatrists with consultation-liaison experience will find this dynamic familiar, as clarifying the referring physician's question is part and parcel of hospital consultation. While the forensic psychiatric report occurs within a different system, the principles applicable to the consultation of the psychiatrists elsewhere in the hospital are applicable to the work of the forensic psychiatrist. Of special note is that the work of the forensic psychiatrist requires knowledge of the needs, procedures, and language of the legal system.

8.1.2 Writing for the audience

The audience of the criminal forensic psychiatric report may be a judge, probation department, prosecuting or defense attorney, or jury. The audience, and the purpose for which the audience will use the report, will help dictate the nature and length of report.

The Psychiatric Report, ed. Alec Buchanan and Michael A. Norko. Published by Cambridge University Press. © Cambridge University Press 2011.

From a questionnaire survey at a conference of California judges, an attempt was made to systematically study the deficiencies of psychiatric forensic reports from the standpoint of the judiciary. The judges were critical of the length and wordiness of reports and of those reports that repeated information otherwise available to them. They also looked askance at psychodynamic terminology, technical psychiatric terms, and psychoanalytic jargon (Pollack 1974). The overly lengthy report – although interesting to the author – may burden the reader and impair the capacity to clearly transmit the relevant information. This difficulty can be addressed using the structure of the report if the conclusions are clearly labeled and other sections of the report which the reader may choose to skip or peruse are clearly labeled also.

The most important function of the forensic psychiatric report is to communicate clearly. All is lost if thoughtful reasoning and conclusion are buried under poor writing. Forensic psychiatrists who do not have a substantial command of written English should obtain a consultation regarding the language, grammar, and phrasing of the report. Psychiatrists fluent in written English may also benefit from such input, as years of writing in medical shorthand can influence the ability to communicate clearly with non-physicians.

8.1.3 Distribution

The forensic psychiatrist will want to understand who will have access to the report. In certain circumstances the report will be available to the judge and attorneys on both sides, whereas in other jurisdictions just the judge may have access. Informing the examinee of who will have access to the report is part of the consent to examination that the forensic psychiatrist is obliged to obtain before conducting the evaluation. This should be reviewed with the subject at that time of the initial evaluation, and the consent to examination is generally documented in the forensic report.

When a psychiatrist is examining for the prosecution in a criminal matter there is obviously no confidentiality in terms of the defense attorney's knowledge of the examination. When examining for the defense, it may well be possible for the existence and content of the forensic examination to remain confidential unless the defense attorney requests a written report. The defense attorney may only want a verbal conference after the evaluation instead of a written report that could become a subject of discovery.

As a general principle, a written report in legal matters should be assumed to be or to be liable to become available to all relevant parties. Gratuitous information or inflammatory characterizations included in the report that are not vital to the opinion and reasoning may be embarrassing or hurtful to the subject or others. Tact and diplomacy in writing the report will serve to avoid alienating any potential readers unnecessarily.

8.1.4 Length

In forensic reports, including criminal reports, the length should match the function of the report. One size does not fit all, and the reports may range from one to over one hundred pages.

It is perfectly reasonable to have a brief, even one-page report that adequately summarizes the nature of the examination and conclusions. Brief reports may not even have section headings, but may be composed of several paragraphs as the style of the writer or purpose of the report dictates. These are frequently used in competency to stand trial examinations. Reports to town and city courts may also fall into this category. An abundance of raw data is not the goal of these reports, as they may be widely disseminated in city or town courts. The focus is on the conclusions and recommendations. Another example of a brief report is the one-page summary report that leaves out potentially incriminating details provided to the prosecution in US Department of Defense Sanity Board evaluations.

Most typically, reports will be in the range of six to eight pages. This format generally allows for a reasonable inclusion of the relevant data. We suggest that to have a report over eight pages requires a well-thought-out rationale.

At times the forensic question will be so complex and the data will be so massive as to require a very long report that can range from 50 to 100 or more pages. If deciding to write an extensive report, the forensic psychiatrist should consider the scope of the questions being asked, the necessity of including such a volume of information in the report, and the gravity of the potential consequences of the outcome of the proceedings for the subject. These reports can be especially difficult for the reader to comprehend and it is helpful for all reports of this size to include a table of contents.

Construct extensive reports cautiously. One hazard with extensive reports is that the intended audience – usually attorneys and judges – are accustomed to identifying the opinion of a report up front, and focusing on the conclusions. It may improve the impact of such reports to introduce the opinion at the front of the report and clearly identify it in the table of contents. Other hazards with extensive reports include the sheer volume of data that may distract from the primary focus of the report and may provide much more potential material on which to be cross-examined.

8.1.5 Style and content

The report is essential communication that shares the forensic examiner's conclusions and reasoning with the criminal justice system. The nature of the question being answered and the circumstances that spawn the question play a role in dictating the specific length, style, organization, and content of the report. Since the report may be read by a number of people including the defendant it behoves the report writer to use not only clear but also tempered language. No matter the length of the report, it should contain the referral question, the nature of the examination, and the conclusions and reasoning of the examiner.

As with all written communication the author must keep in mind the purpose and intended audience of the work. Some psychiatrists assume that their reports for legal purposes should follow the same format as reports for medical purposes. The format of the medical report is dictated by the empirical approach to medical practice and therapeutic goals of the report. The forensic psychiatric report on the other hand provides data and conclusions that are to be used by the legal system to decide a course of action. Of special importance is the explanation of the reasoning that underlies the conclusions of the forensic psychiatrist. The organization of the forensic psychiatric report should be determined by the legal system's style of logical reasoning rather than by the empirical approach used in medicine (Pollack 1968).

Legal decisions are characterized by a statement of the issue, the finding, the underlying fact pattern, and the reasoning behind the finding. The format of the forensic psychiatric report therefore is structured to meet the legal system's logical style. The inclusion of certain information may not be relevant to the task at hand. For instance, the description of psychopathology and elaboration of psychodynamics have little to no role in the forensic psychiatric report unless they can be logically related to the legal issue. The psychiatrist's reasoning and clarity with which that reasoning incorporates the data significantly adds to the credibility of the report. Ultimately it is the psychiatric reasoning that will influence the weight that the fact finder will give the psychiatric opinions.

The report format should reinforce and not detract from the purpose of the report: providing the reader with the nature of the examination, the findings, the expert's opinions, and the reasoning used to arrive at the opinions. Personal style should not be overlooked in organizing a report, and many forensic psychiatrists believe their own personal modification of the standard report format makes their reports more powerful. Also do not neglect that a personal report style may change over time as the needs of the referral source change, continuing professional education informs on alternative styles, and the professional experience of the psychiatrist accumulates.

8.2 Special considerations for criminal reports

8.2.1 Conduct of the evaluation

Clarifying the consultation question is a vital component of effective forensic psychiatric report writing. Attorneys' questions as asked may be well crafted and focused, or can confuse the psychiatric issue at hand, or can be unanswerable by a forensic psychiatrist. Clarifying the questions to be answered and at times helping to restructure the question into a more appropriate or readily answerable question is the first step to undertaking the forensic psychiatric evaluation. The agreement on the goals of the evaluation may help to avoid the bewilderment and disappointment that attorneys or courts may experience after receiving a report that does not answer the question they thought they were asking.

Part of the agreement with the attorney is how soon a report is expected after the examination is performed. This can range from immediately afterwards to months hence. The attorney may ask for findings to be discussed before the attorney makes a decision about whether or not to seek a written report. The writing of the report will depend on an individual's particular style, whether it be handwritten, dictated, or directly typed into the computer. The report may go through several drafts. Many recommend that drafts, as a general rule, be destroyed and that only the final product is kept.

There is some controversy over whether the referring attorney should have the opportunity to review a draft of your report. This practice can give the attorney an opportunity to correct factual errors, provide additional information received after the examination, and point out problems with terms or phrases that may be unexplained psychiatric jargon. This practice contrasts with the recommendation that the discussion with the attorney precede the draft of the report to avoid undue influence in crafting the psychiatric opinion.

In the legal system, the forensic report exploits the exception to the hearsay rule and permits the introduction of expert opinions in written form that can then be expanded upon during testimony.

8.2.2 Content of the report

Criminal competencies

Purpose of criminal competency reports

The evaluation of a specific criminal competency follows the same general paradigm as evaluation for any capacity determination. That is, the examiner must understand the specific abilities required by the reigning jurisdiction to perform a specific function within the criminal justice system. The psychiatric evaluation is conducted to determine whether or not the defendant has a mental disorder and if, as a result of that disorder, there is significant impairment of one or several of the abilities required to meet the applicable standard of competence. The issue of competence can be raised at virtually any point in the criminal process, from arrest to ultimate sentencing (Mossman et al. 2007).

Competence to give a confession

The particular area of interest in this specific evaluation is the person's mental condition at the time of the interrogation. Police reports and witness statements are valuable sources of information regarding the person's mental condition shortly before and during the time that they were taken into custody and questioned. Understanding and detailing the nature of the interrogation is important to understanding the context of the confession. Information describing the length and circumstances of the interrogation will inform the necessary review of recordings and any written documents.

The defendant may have been provided Miranda rights in a way that they could not understand. Obviously, any existing language barrier (including complete unfamiliarity with a language, partial fluency, and sign language needs) is one concern. Beyond language comprehension is the ability to factually and rationally understand individual rights. Many psychiatric disorders can – but do not necessarily – impact understanding. Subjects should be evaluated for evidence of a delirium or dementia and whatever cause may be underlying those conditions. The individual may have had psychotic symptoms that either prevented them from having a rational understanding that they were, in fact, confessing or they may have been delusionally compelled to confess.

Usually the issue of competence to give a confession would be raised by the defense. The usual report structure should be modified to include sections that focused on the specific task of confessing, and may include descriptions of the interrogation and the circumstances of the custody. Special attention should be paid to the mental status examination at the time of the confession and impairments should be identified that may or may not affect the defendant's competence. In pre-trial competence evaluations of any nature, the data supporting the reasoned conclusions should stay limited to that which is relevant to the question at hand as jurisdictions vary as to how the data from competence evaluations may be used at any subsequent trial.

Competence to stand trial

Unlike competence to give a confession, competence to stand trial is a dynamic state that may change over time. The examination may be asked for before, during or after a trial, or at sentencing, by the defense, prosecution, or *sua sponte* (a judge's order made without a request by any party to the case). While the standards for competence to stand trial remain the same no matter how the issue is raised, in each of these circumstances there are particular challenges.

Most commonly, a competence to stand trial evaluation is requested prior to the trial. Some examiners use rating scales to guide the evaluation and if a rating scale is used it may be useful to append it to the report. In some jurisdictions, the report is in a standardized format that provides for limited information that is specific to the task at hand and carefully avoids providing additional information for the court, especially if the defendant proceeds to stand trial. If the person is not competent to stand trial, the report may be more extensive. It may include relevant history, mental status examination, and diagnosis as well as a discussion of how the defendant's mental disorder specifically impairs their competence to stand trial.

The request for an evaluation in the midst of a trial may put pressure on the examiner to conduct the examination and provide a report quickly. The requirements of the examination and the report are no less demanding than a pre-trial competency evaluation. The examiner should avoid being pressured into producing a report that contains a premature conclusion. In choosing between opining "competent or "not competent," do not fear opining, "Further observation and evaluation is required" if the available data do not support a definitive conclusion. If more time or data are necessary to form an opinion about competence, the psychiatrist may opine in the report that the defendant may need to be sent to a forensic facility.

An evaluation of the defendant's competence to stand trial that is requested after the trial is completed challenges the examiner with a retrospective evaluation rather than a contemporaneous one. Focus should be on the mental status of the defendant during the trial, and not on his or her presentation at the time of the examination. The report may include a section on the defendant's conduct during the trial, both in the courtroom and while in custody. A subsection of "Sources of information" highlighting collateral interviews of people who observed the defendant in the courtroom and while in custody may be appropriate.

The Supreme Court found in *Godinez* v. *Moran* (1993) that accepting a guilty plea required no greater competency than standing trial. As such, the evaluation for competence to stand trial includes an evaluation of the defendant's capacity to enter a plea. However, at times, the psychiatrist may wish to highlight this capacity with an extended discussion, e.g., when the request for a competence to stand trial evaluation is prompted by a plea bargain offer. At these times, the report should specifically emphasize the defendant's understanding of the rights being waived, the defenses available, and the consequences of the guilty plea. It may be especially important to highlight portions of the mental status examination that concern paranoia, delusions, and insight. If a person with serious mental illness lacks insight into having that illness, they may be unable to rationally appreciate the option of taking a not guilty by reason of insanity (NGRI) plea in those jurisdictions in which this is available.

Competence to go *pro se*

A criminal defendant competent to proceed to trial with an attorney may not be competent to proceed without one. Evaluating a defendant for competence to go *pro se* requires that the examiner understand the legal standard for going *pro se* in the applicable jurisdiction. The US Supreme Court in *Edwards* v. *Indiana* (2008) ruled that the standard for being competent to go *pro se* can be different from the standard to be competent to stand trial. These evaluations can present a significant challenge to the examiner. For instance, the delusional and paranoid defendant who wants to go *pro se* may sound coherent and rational at first blush. Or, a defendant who has hypomania that leads to an assuredness and certainty of purpose may appear to the court simply self-confident, but the "self-confidence" may be the result of significant affective illness. The report must clearly present the examiner's findings that may seem to fly in the face of common sense. Particular attention should be made in the report to mental status examination findings that may be subtle but eminently illustrative in demonstrating impaired thinking underlying the defendant's wish to go *pro se*. These reports may be helped by subheading each part of the mental status examination to highlight the specific impairment.

Competence to be executed

The forensic psychiatrist may be asked to provide an opinion and report on whether an inmate with a capital sentence is competent to be executed. Deciding whether to provide an opinion in these cases, as in any forensic case, is an individual choice the forensic psychiatrist must make, adhering to the professional ethics of the medical profession and psychiatric specialty (American Medical Association Council 2008–2009). In *Ford* v. *Wainwright* (1986) the Supreme Court found that the Eighth Amendment prohibits the execution of an "insane" person, but did not provide a definition of competency to be executed. Justice Powell wrote that a person who was "unaware of the punishment they are about to suffer and why they are to suffer it" would not be competent. In *Panetti* v. *Quarterman* (2007), the Supreme Court found that "[a] prisoner's awareness of the State's rationale for an execution is not the same as a rational understanding of it." The authors suggest that reports on competence to be executed should focus on the inmate's current mental status, specifically his factual and rational understanding of the reasons for the punishment and the means and result of execution.

Criminal responsibility

Criminal responsibility: general

Reports on criminal responsibility take the same general form as other criminal forensic reports. One major difference shared by all criminal responsibility reports is that a section detailing the evaluation subject's detailed recount of the events is included, most reasonably prior to the mental status exam (Giorgi-Guanieri et al. 2002).

Not guilty by reason of insanity

The not guilty by reason of insanity defense is rarely put forth, rarely reaches trial (60% are reached via plea agreement), and even more rarely successful (less than 1% of felony prosecutions) (Milton et al. 2007). The challenge for the examiner is to construct a report that clearly conveys the psychiatrist's opinion whether there is a mental illness, and if so, when it began and what role it played in the alleged crime.

The beginning point of providing an opinion on whether a person is not guilty by reason of insanity is having an understanding of the legal definition of NGRI in the relevant jurisdiction. It can be helpful to include that definition in the report, identifying the law in the Introduction to the report and referring to the law as written in the Conclusion or Opinion section.

While we have mentioned the importance of record review earlier, the retrospective nature of NGRI examinations cannot be stressed enough. The report will necessarily stress record review and collateral interviews.

Assessment of malingering is important in all forensic evaluations. It is of heightened importance in a report regarding criminal responsibility due to the great stakes usually involved in these cases. The prosecution is most likely to question whether a defendant is malingering, and indeed the prosecution has a responsibility to the public to ensure criminals do not escape punishment by malingering mental illness and wrongfully asserting lack of criminal responsibility. One strategy for the report is to put an opinion on the presence or absence of malingering in the Conclusion section, along with reasoning supporting the stance.

Extreme emotional disturbance/diminished capacity

The extreme emotional disturbance (EED) defense and, in those jurisdictions that recognize the concept, the diminished capacity defense, are complex tests that consider the defendant's subjective mental state and an outsider's (in most cases, a juror's) objective view of the defendant's behavior. The report addresses not just the defendant's mental state at the time of the crime but also provides, as clearly as possible, a description of the circumstances and events leading up to the alleged crime. The Opinion section of the report requires a discussion of whether or not the defendant meets the legal standard for EED or diminished capacity.

Mens rea

In states that do not have an NGRI defense, the defendant can still claim that they lacked the requisite *mens rea* to commit the alleged crime. Similarly to NGRI reports, the *mens rea* report focuses on the retrospective review of records and collateral interviews, although if a relatively static condition is suspected to have prevented the defendant from forming *mens rea*, the current mental status examination may be useful to highlight as well. *Mens rea* reports should also have a discussion of how the mental illness precluded formation of intent in the Conclusion or Opinion section.

Dangerousness evaluation report after not guilty by reason of insanity verdict

In most jurisdictions, after an individual is found NGRI statutes provide for a forensic evaluation to determine the individual's dangerousness. This evaluation is usually done in a psychiatric hospital, but may be done on an outpatient basis as determined by the court. "Dangerousness" in this context is defined by statute or case law and reference to the standard being applied is advisable in these reports. Of particular importance in most of these assessments is a comparison of the evaluee's current recount of the offense compared and contrasted against the (presumably accurate) documents that detail the offense, such as police reports, witness statements, etc. Risk assessments, often using standardized checklists or actuarial instruments, are frequently used in these reports. Detailed history sections and recent mental status examination can be highlighted, and if the referral source or governmental organization requires, checklists or other forms that are used should be attached. It is not simply enough to attach these forms. Any instrument used should be discussed in the body of the report and results incorporated into the Conclusion or Opinion section.

Sentencing

When preparing a pre-sentence investigation report where the crime is a misdemeanor, the probation department may seek a forensic psychiatric evaluation. The court is generally interested in whether or not the misdemeanant has a mental disorder and would benefit from psychiatric treatment while serving his sentence or as a condition of probation. These reports are frequently one to two pages. Diagnosis and a discussion of the nature of the treatment that the person requires or would benefit from is important.

These reports may be brief like misdemeanor reports, or longer depending on the nature of the crime and the circumstances of the evaluation. Felons receive a sentence of a year or more in prison and may receive treatment there. On arriving at the prison facility, medical personnel screen the felon and the forensic psychiatric report conducted as part of the pre-sentence investigation can be forwarded to the prison medical department for review. Early identification of psychiatric illness and the need for treatment by the forensic psychiatrist can help flag these felons and alert prison mental health personnel. This is a further example of keeping the potential audience in mind when preparing the report.

Providing additional material

Some cases will call for psychological and neuropsychological testing. Unless the psychiatrist is specifically trained in the administration and interpretation of these tests, the authors recommend asking a psychologist or neuropsychologist to perform those vital functions. The psychologist will often provide an independent report that may be referenced by the psychiatrist in the forensic report, and summarized in this section. The raw testing data provided by the psychologist should not, except in highly unusual circumstances, be part of the psychiatrist's report.

Appendices in forensic reports are other existing reports that have been referenced or summarized in the main report or specific rating scales or actuarial instruments that may be included at the end of a report. Some referral sources may require these rating scales or instruments; at other times, the psychiatrist may include them at their discretion. References are tricky. We have seen reports that have included references to journal articles or book chapters. These references can appear authoritative. They can also be used to cross-examine the psychiatrist, however, and can be seen as diluting the value, knowledge, and experience of the expert witness. We do not recommend them.

8.3 The report

The elements of the psychiatric report that were described in Chapter 7 and that warrant distinctive treatment in reports on criminal litigation are shown in Box 8.1.

Box 8.1 Topics warranting distinctive treatment in criminal litigation reports

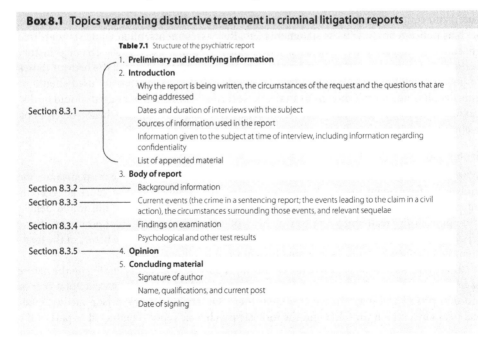

Table 7.1 Structure of the psychiatric report

1. **Preliminary and identifying information**
2. **Introduction**

Section 8.3.1
- Why the report is being written, the circumstances of the request and the questions that are being addressed
- Dates and duration of interviews with the subject
- Sources of information used in the report
- Information given to the subject at time of interview, including information regarding confidentiality
- List of appended material

3. **Body of report**

Section 8.3.2 — Background information

Section 8.3.3 — Current events (the crime in a sentencing report; the events leading to the claim in a civil action), the circumstances surrounding those events, and relevant sequelae

Section 8.3.4 — Findings on examination
- Psychological and other test results

Section 8.3.5 — 4. **Opinion**

5. **Concluding material**
- Signature of author
- Name, qualifications, and current post
- Date of signing

8.3.1 Introduction to report

In this section the examinee is identified and the legal data that form the forensic psychiatric question are explained. The writer next outlines the steps taken to obtain informed consent to examine the defendant. Our preference is to describe this in a separate section, titled "Consent to Examination". If the subject chose not to participate in an interview, that fact can be stated at this point. Forensic reports are still often prepared even if the individual did not choose to participate; non-participation may or may not mean that the findings of the forensic psychiatrist may be limited.

It is our practice also to include within the Introduction a separate section titled "Sources of Information." Here the site and duration of the examination is stated; for example, "I interviewed Mr.X on July 7, 1999 for 4.5 hours at the Local Medical Center." The section also includes a list of all persons interviewed or consulted, materials reviewed, and materials that were requested but not made available. Finally, we include here any collateral interviews or consultations. Collateral interviews may be of family members, witnesses or treating clinicians. Consultations may include other experts, including psychologists to interpret any relevant psychological testing.

Relevant lists of records in a criminal case frequently include the indictment, police reports, witness statements, ambulance or first-responder reports, and emergency department and hospital records. The subject may have relevant jail records and jail medical records. Records of the individual's educational history, medical history, psychiatric history, work history, legal history, pharmacy history, and military history may all be relevant. While the examining psychiatrist should request these, invariably some will not be available. Requesting, in writing, all relevant documents in general – and specific documents that the psychiatrist wants given the particulars of the case – can mitigate difficult cross-examination should the case go to trial. The phrase, "Please send all the relevant records relating to the case, including but not limited to …" is one the authors use frequently. The records requested but not received may be included as a separate section to indicate the thoroughness of the psychiatrist's search for relevant data.

8.3.2 Background

In some reports, a single section briefly describing the subject's personal history may suffice. In others, a more comprehensive and well-delineated breakdown of the personal history into separate sections will provide clarity and detail necessary to support more complex conclusions. Here, the psychiatrist will recognize many components of a clinical psychiatric evaluation. Some common subheadings include:

- Early developmental history: relevant information about early life experiences should be included here. Collateral interviews with family members are often helpful.
- School or education history: the subject's highest level of academic achievement, any special educational needs, and any repeated grades are important to include here. Particular attention should be paid to disciplinary history and behavior concerns in school. School records, although sometimes difficult to obtain, can be troves of information establishing early patterns of behavior.
- Social history: number, type, length, and dynamics of relationships with significant others and children may be documented here. Discrepancies or agreements between

social history given by the examinee and collateral sources may be important to highlight.

- Family history: as would be the case for a clinical assessment, detailing the personal histories of members of the family of origin can be important in the forensic context. Familial patterns may inform an understanding of the examinee's behavior.
- Sexual history: this section may not be included unless relevant. Clearly for a sexually-based crime, sexual history is important. Earliest sexual experience, a history of sexual abuse, prior arrests for sexual behavior, and any treatment for sexual disorders or paraphilias are vital to include. If a sexual history is relevant to the evaluation, record review and collateral interviews are necessary as self-report of sexual behaviors is often unreliable in the criminal context.
- Military history: the examinee's account of his military service can be given here. Military records should be requested even if a person has spent little time in the service. Asking about and looking for evidence of disciplinary actions can give a good indication of how a military career progressed. Of course, if the subject was discharged for medical or psychiatric reasons, or under any conditions other than "Honorable," these records are vital as well.
- Legal history: the examinee's arrest and conviction record, involvement in litigation, time incarcerated, and current probation or parole status are items that may included in the section.
- Medical history: various medical conditions can be included here, and if complicated these conditions can be described, avoiding medical jargon, for the non-medical audience of the report.
- Psychiatric history: the need for this section is obvious. One problem arises when the examinee has numerous hospitalizations, rehabilitations, or outpatient treatment courses, and organization and distillation of the large volume of data becomes paramount. A chronological numbered or bulleted list of each treatment course and a brief summary including outcome of each can be helpful for the author and reader.

Again, personal styles will differ in the organization, titles, and content of these sections. Allow flexibility in formatting of these sections to meet the specific needs of the individual case.

8.3.3 Description of alleged offense

The description of the alleged or adjudicated offense is usually undertaken in two parts. The first section may provide the description of events as obtained from a review of relevant records, including police reports, witness statements and interview of defendant (perhaps on video or audio recording). This description can be followed by the defendant's account as told at time of the psychiatric evaluation.

8.3.4 Findings on examination

The mental status examination should be painstakingly tailored to the purpose of the report. The depth of this section may range from a brief description of the appearance and behavior of the subject to an itemized, detailed, formal psychiatric mental status examination. It may be helpful to include moment-by-moment descriptions of behaviors or speech that the psychiatrist finds especially illustrative of the exam. Even when describing the mental status examination in detail, it is important to avoid jargon. Do not assume that even the most sophisticated non-medical reader is versed in psychiatric vocabulary.

8.3.5 Conclusions and recommendations

The conclusion section is the psychiatrist's opinions in written form. One format for this section is to state the diagnostic impression as the first of a number of opinions. Listing opinions and their supporting reasoning, instead of using paragraph format, highlights each opinion and may make it easier for the reader to follow the most important part of the report. Subsequent opinions may address the basis for the diagnostic impression, provide responses to the legal referral questions, and delineate the reasoning underlying the forensic responses to the legal issues.

Diagnostic impression

The DSM-IV-TR or the most current DSM is the standard diagnostic system used in the United States and Canada and we recommend using this system in forensic reports. If the psychiatrist uses another diagnostic schema other than those within the DSM framework, we view it as the obligation of the forensic psychiatrist to clearly explain why they choose not to use the format and definitions of the DSM. Unless legally required, requested by the referral source, or dictated by the complexity of the case, including Axes III, IV, and V of the DSM multi-axial diagnosis may not be necessary.

Responses to legal questions and reasoning behind responses

The remaining conclusions are the responses to the legal questions that initiated the report in the first place. These responses, and especially the reasoning supporting those responses, are perhaps the most crucial parts of the forensic report. Stating a response to a legal question is more straightforward than providing strong reasoning. In responding to the legal questions, be clear and unequivocal when the data and reasoning can support the opinion; e.g., "In my opinion, within a reasonable degree of medical certainty, the defendant is not competent to stand trial."

The reasoning behind the opinion needs to be clear and supported with data. Data-driven, logical reasoning will add greater credibility to the psychiatrist's report. Whether those data will be repeated in other parts of the report will depend on the type and length of the report. Brief reports may only introduce the supporting data in the reasoning section or paragraph.

Malingering

Defendants have an obvious interest in malingering in a criminal setting. As described in DSM-IV-TR, "Malingering is the intentional production of false or grossly exaggerated physical or psychological symptoms, motivated by external incentives such as … evading criminal prosecution …" In criminal forensic report writing, it is often helpful to discuss the presence or absence of malingering in the Conclusion or Opinion section. Consistency among the sources of information, clinical examination, and psychological test results supports the finding that the defendant is not malingering. If malingering is suspected the author of the report may wish to deal with the credibility of the defendant by discussing inconsistencies between the record review, psychological test results, and the clinical examination.

8.4 Conclusion

No chapter or book can anticipate every possibility in writing a forensic psychiatric report in a criminal context. The unusual circumstance may well arise. We recommend using this chapter as a starting point for the writing of the criminal forensic report, but acknowledge the need for flexibility and encourage the forensic psychiatrist to adapt their report to the specific context of the referral, evaluation, jurisdiction, and personnel involved in each case. When the forensic psychiatrist is considering using an unusual format for constructing a report, we encourage consultation with a trusted colleague.

The forensic psychiatric report allows the expert witness to perform a teaching function using their psychiatric education, training, and experience to put psychiatric information and conclusions in a legal context. In forensic report writing in a criminal context – like psychiatric consultation in medical settings – making a diagnosis is not enough. The forensic psychiatrist uses the report to explain to the legal system how the specific manifestations of the mental illness affect or affected the subject's thinking, judgment, and behavior.

References

American Medical Association Council on Ethical and Judicial Affairs (2008) *Code of Medical Ethics: Current Opinions and Annotations, 2008–2009*. Chicago, IL: American Medical Association Press, pp. 20–25.

Edwards v. Indiana 554 US 208 (2008).

Ford v. Wainwright 477 US 399 (1986).

Geller, J. L. & Lister, E. D. (1978) The process of criminal commitment for pretrial psychiatric examination: an evaluation. *American Journal of Psychiatry* **135**: 53–60.

Giorgi-Guanieri, D., Janofsky, J., Keram, E., et al. (2002) AAPL Practice guidelines for forensic psychiatric evaluation of defendants raising the insanity defense. *Journal of the American Academy of Psychiatry and the Law* 30: 53.

Godinez v. Moran 509 US 389 (1993).

Hess, J. & Thomas, H. E. (1963) Incompetency to stand trial: procedures, results, and problems. *American Journal of Psychiatry* **119**: 713–720.

Melton, J. B., Petrilla, J., Poythress, N. G., & Slobogin, C. (2007) *Psychological Evaluations for the Courts: A Handbook for Mental Health Professionals and Lawyers*, 3rd edn. New York: Guilford Press, pp. 202–203.

Mossman, D., Noffsinger, S., Ash, P., et al. (2007) AAPL Practice Guideline for the Forensic Evaluation of Forensic Evaluation

of Competence to Stand Trial. *Journal of the American Academy of Psychiatry and the Law* **35**: 53.

Panetti v. Quarterman 551 US 930 (2007).

Pollack, S. (1968) Consultation with the Courts. In *The Psychiatric Consultation*, ed. M. Mendel & P. Solomon. New York: Grune & Stratton, p. 149.

Pollack, S. (1974) *Forensic Psychiatry in Criminal Law*. Los Angeles, CA: University of Southern California, p. 120.

Materials of interest

Ackerman, M. J. (2006) Forensic report writing. *Journal of Clinical Psychology* **62**: 59–72.

Allnutt, S. H. & Chaplow, D. (2000) General principles of forensic report writing. *Australian and New Zealand Journal of Psychiatry* **34**: 980–987.

Babitsky, S. & Mangraviti J. J., Jr. (2002) *Writing and Defending Your Expert Report*. Falmouth, MA: SEAK, Inc.

Damer, T. E. (2005) *Attacking Faulty Reasoning*, 5th edn. Belmont, CA: Thomson Wadsworth.

Garrick, T. R. & Stotland, N. L. (1982) How to write a psychiatric consultation. *American Journal of Psychiatry* **139**: 849–855.

Griffith, E. E. H. & Baranoski, M. V. (2007) Commentary: the place of performative writing in forensic psychiatry. *Journal of the American Academy of Psychiatry and the Law* **35**: 27–31.

Hoffman, B. F. (1986) How to write a psychiatric report for litigation following a personal injury. *American Journal of Psychiatry* **143**: 164–169.

Melton, G. B., Petrila J., Polythress, N. G., & Slobogin, C. (2007) *Psychological Evaluations for the Courts*, 3rd edn. New York: Guilford Press.

Rosner, R. (2003) *Principles and Practice of Forensic Psychiatry*, 2nd edn. London: Arnold.

Simon, R. I. (2007) Authorship in forensic psychiatry: a perspective. *Journal of the American Academy of Psychiatry and the Law* **35**: 18–26.

Civil litigation

Patricia Ryan Recupero and Marilyn Price

9.1 Introduction

Psychiatric reports may be useful in numerous types of civil litigation. Several of the more common types of cases include civil commitment proceedings (see Chapter 10), professional competency and fitness for duty (see Chapter 11), evaluations for child custody disputes (see Chapter 12), and employment litigation, such as sexual harassment or disability evaluations (see Chapter 13). This chapter introduces the general principles of forensic report writing for psychiatrists involved in civil cases as well as particular considerations for several specific types of evaluations in civil litigation, including medical malpractice, personal injury (psychic harm), and civil competencies such as testamentary capacity. Because there are so many contexts in which a forensic report might be required, there is no overall general rule for what the report must address for civil litigation per se. As always, it is important to identify with the referring source the precise questions to be answered and the relevant legal standards to be applied.

In medical malpractice proceedings, a psychiatrist may be asked to review the medical records of an individual who committed suicide to assess whether or not a treatment provider was negligent in the care of the decedent. An individual injured by the negligent driving of a psychiatric outpatient might file suit alleging failure to warn of the dangers of operating a motor vehicle while taking antidepressants or other psychotropic medications (Hollister 1992), and a psychiatric report may help inform the court as to the standards for informed consent and clinical outpatient treatment. In addition to focusing on liability and the duty of care, assessments in many civil cases require evaluation of current disability, prognosis, and expected costs of medical treatment. Psychiatrists may also be asked to assess a number of different civil competencies including whether an individual requires a guardian of the person or a guardian of the estate. During a will contest, a psychiatrist may evaluate medical records and interview collateral sources to determine whether or not the testator possessed testamentary capacity or was subject to undue influence at the time the will was created. The principles of professional forensic psychiatric report writing apply equally to all of these types of cases.

9.2 Special considerations for civil litigation reports

9.2.1 Conduct of the evaluation

Before agreeing to complete a report for civil litigation, the forensic psychiatrist must consider the ethical aspects of participation in the legal proceedings. Forensic experts should not

The Psychiatric Report, ed. Alec Buchanan and Michael A. Norko. Published by Cambridge University Press. © Cambridge University Press 2011.

agree to perform an evaluation and write a report outside their area of expertise (Weinstock & Gold 2004). It is also important not to proceed with an evaluation and report when the psychiatrist's objectivity may be impaired by, for example, a prior relationship that existed with the evaluee (Wettstein 2004).

The forensic psychiatrist must pay attention to the potential of bias when conducting an evaluation. Weinstock and Gold (2004, p. 99) warn forensic psychiatrists about the risk of advocacy bias, defined as "the pressure to conform opinions to assist the retaining attorney." Other dangers include retrospective bias in medical malpractice (the tendency to oversimplify "a complicated clinical situation, especially the uncertainties surrounding clinical judgment at the time of the alleged negligence"[Simon 2005, p. 11]) and hindsight bias in retrospective assessments for personal injury (the tendency to overestimate foreseeability and causation) (Knoll & Gerbasi 2006; LeBourgeois et al. 2007). In reports for testamentary capacity and guardianship, bias may arise from overidentifying with the evaluee or another party whose interests are at stake or by substituting one's own personal beliefs for the evaluee's intent or best interests.

An evaluation may entail conducting a psychiatric examination of a living person (e.g., assessing competency for a guardianship proceeding) or possibly only completing a retrospective review of medical records and other documents (as in some cases of alleged malpractice or will contests). In a face-to-face psychiatric examination, the evaluee should be advised of the purpose of the examination and the limits of confidentiality. Collateral sources of information, such as interviews and documents, are helpful in prospective analyses and crucial in retrospective assessments.

The evaluator may also conduct interviews with persons having knowledge of the evaluee, such as family members, friends, medical care providers, business associates, and others (Shulman et al. 2005; Melton et al. 2007). It is especially critical for the examiner to request all of the depositions, answers to interrogatories, and other relevant documents in the case. Oftentimes, attorneys may not be aware that the information contained in depositions may have relevance to the psychiatrist's understanding of the case.

Differences in laws among various jurisdictions will affect the conduct and goals of the forensic evaluation. The report and evaluation must be structured to address jurisdiction-specific inquiries. The examining psychiatrist should clarify the exact circumstances that led to the request for the evaluation, and the report should be sensitive to the legal context of the psychiatrist's involvement in the case. For example, several states have adopted ante-mortem probate statutes which allow wills to be probated prior to the death of the testator (Shuman 2004). In states lacking these statutes, a prudent attorney may recommend an evaluation of testamentary capacity at the time of execution of the will, particularly when there is evidence of mild to moderate dementia or other factors that may increase the likelihood of a legal dispute, such as when the testator plans an unusual distribution of assets (Champine 2006; Melton et al. 2007).

9.2.2 Content of the report
Medical malpractice

The report's content will vary depending upon the type of litigation and the type of information being sought by the retaining party. A common error in the composition of forensic reports for civil litigation is a failure to fully address the questions asked by the referral source. It is also important to avoid including content which does not address the relevant questions and which may detract from the authority and relevance of the report. Written reports should avoid explicit speculation about ultimate questions that the court may need to answer, such as whether the defendant's conduct was the proximate cause of the plaintiff's injury, or whether the plaintiff's claim of harm is legitimate. Unlike reports created for medical malpractice related to a wrongful death, reports addressing psychic harm typically require discussion of what treatment is needed, the associated costs, and the prognosis.

At later stages, such as during or after the drafting of the report, retaining attorneys may request revisions to the report in order to more strongly support the retaining party's objective. As numerous experts have explained, making substantive changes (i.e., beyond minor typographical or factual errors) to a report at the request of the retaining attorney is usually to be avoided (Sadoff 2004; Wettstein 2004). Such changes may be unethical and make the report and the expert's opinion especially vulnerable to impeachment.

In a forensic psychiatric evaluation for medical malpractice, the psychiatrist should record in the report the relevant standard of care and whether the defendant physician or entity (such as a hospital) conformed to that standard. Clinical practice guidelines (CPGs), academic literature on evidence-based medicine, up-to-date textbooks, training or policy manuals, and similar resources for professional clinicians often contain suggestions and risk management advice relevant to the standard of care. The psychiatrist may find it useful to refer to the exact language in such documents in order to give the forensic report more precision. However, CPGs and related resources do not set the standard of care. As Simon (2005, p. 8) notes, they "set forth practice parameters that may or may not apply to a fact-specific case in litigation." Meyer and Simon (2004) identify the following considerations in formulating the standard of care: (1) the physician's level of expertise; (2) different schools of thought regarding treatment; (3) scientific advances, including recent discoveries relevant to the standard of care; and (4) the existence and availability of CPGs. Additional factors to consider are the standards and policies at the facility in which the patient received treatment, the role of other medical or mental health care providers (such as Primary Care Providers and therapists), the patient's legal status (involuntary versus voluntary), the provider's ethical obligations, and the duration of treatment.

In a review of medical records for civil litigation, but particularly in cases of alleged malpractice, the psychiatrist should examine the medical record carefully for evidence of the quality and nature of care provided. For an inpatient stay, accreditation standards and guidelines produced by regulatory bodies (such as the Joint Commission) and other certifying authorities may provide a guide to the standard of care (Recupero 2008). The CMS State Operations Manual includes a set of Interpretive Guidelines and Survey Procedures for Psychiatric Hospitals that can be especially helpful in structuring the inquiry when using medical records, particularly in inpatient treatment (US Dept. HHS/CMS 2009) (see Table 9.1).

Other issues to be noted in a record review include risk assessments, both for self-harm and harm to others, inconsistencies in reports, and lapses in communication.

Psychic harm

Psychic harm may arise in a variety of civil cases, and the forensic psychiatrist may be asked to evaluate the claimant's level of disability or impairment (Gold et al. 2008). Typical cases of psychic harm claim ongoing disability resulting from inappropriate sexual relations with a treatment provider, discrimination or harassment in employment, or life-threatening traumatic events, such as a posttraumatic stress disorder (PTSD) that emerges after an

Table 9.1 Suggested areas of inquiry for the evaluation of medical records

Documentation of the patient's psychiatric history and the course of the illness

Substance abuse history

Medical history including allergies and comorbid medical conditions

Results of any physical examinations

Results of the mental status examination

Results of any laboratory tests or other testing requested

Documented risk assessments for changing observation levels, granting a pass, and discharge planning

The treatment plan, including short-term and long-term goals of treatment; the specific treatment modalities to be applied; and the roles and expectations of the patient, treatment providers, family members, and others

Changes in treatment, observation status, or medication, including the rationale for such changes

Evidence of the patient's informed consent (if appropriate), including whether the patient was admitted on a voluntary or involuntary basis for an inpatient stay

Diagnoses at admission (provisional) and discharge

A comprehensive, individualized treatment plan designed to address the patient's particular needs, strengths, and disabilities

Progress notes and psychotherapy notes

The medication administration record

Discharge summary including discharge diagnosis and recommendations, the degree to which treatment goals have been met, changes in functioning from admission to time of discharge, and the post-discharge plan for follow-up

automobile accident. In these cases it is usually possible for the forensic psychiatrist to examine the claimant directly. A court-ordered examination may be needed if the psychiatrist is not retained by the evaluee's counsel. The psychiatrist should document a comprehensive evaluation, with particular sensitivity to issues of somatization, pre-existing conditions, personality disorders, and malingering, as appropriate (Gerbasi 2004). In conjunction with the psychiatric examination, the psychiatrist may also find that a criminal background check is helpful.

Civil competencies

Competency or legal capacity is a legal status referring to the quality or condition of being legally qualified to perform an act and/or make decisions. "Capacity is difficult to define globally and therefore is generally defined in law in reference to a specific task (e.g., capacity to execute a will)" (ABA & APA 2009, p. 149). There has been a trend for probate courts to consider capacity as being task specific rather than global (Moye et al. 2007a; Naik et al. 2008; ABA & APA 2009). As a result, in guardianship proceedings there can be recognition of impairment in one area of decision-making with retention of capacity in another. Examples of civil competencies that have been recognized are given in Table 9.2. The report should clearly identify the capacity being addressed.

Table 9.2 Civil competencies

Competency
Competence to make treatment decisions
Competence to live independently
Competence to consent to research
Competence to consent to a sexual relationship
Competence to vote
Competence to drive
Testimonial competence
Competence to handle financial affairs
Competence to make a will (testamentary capacity)
Competence to execute a durable power of attorney or health care advance directive
Competence to convey real property
Competence to enter into a contract
Competence to make a gift (donative competency)
Professional competency

There are various terms used by states to describe guardianship of person and guardianship of property, such as conservatorship for guardianship of property (Marson 2001). In the past 20 years there has been a shift to a limited guardianship model that preserved autonomy in areas of decision-making that are intact (ABA & APA 2009) and consideration of the least restrictive alternative. There is great diversity in the statutes governing guardianship. Many states have developed templates that offer guidance in completing the assessment consistent with the relevant standard (Moye et al. 2007a; Naik et al. 2008; ABA & APA 2009) with the goal of encouraging more limited orders by courts based upon a functional assessment across a range of capacities (Moye et al. 2007b).

It is the role of the psychiatric evaluator to identify impairment related to a psychiatric disorder and describe how that impairment impacts the specific competency-related function (Slovenko 2004). There has been a recommendation that competence assessments follow a nine-part framework (ABA & APA 2009): (1) be familiar with the applicable legal standard; (2) examine the specific functional elements associated with meeting the standard; (3) offer a medical diagnosis that can explain the functional impairments; (4) evaluate cognitive functioning; (5) consider psychiatric/emotional factors; (6) appreciate the individual's values; (7) identify risks related to the individual and situation; (8) consider means to enhance the individual's capacity; and (9) make a clinical judgment of capacity. The forensic report should address the relevant issues associated with each element.

A testamentary capacity evaluation can be requested at the time of the execution of the will to provide some assurance against challenges after death or as a retrospective assessment. The report should address the testator's capacity at the time of the execution of the will. In prospective civil competency evaluations, the evaluee's capacity to consent to the evaluation as well as their consent should be documented in the report. The report of a prospective evaluation for testamentary capacity should include the testator's descriptions of the purpose of the will, what is meant by making a will, and why the testator is considering making a new will at that time (Marson 2004). The retrospective assessment of testamentary capacity seeks to answer similar questions, relying primarily upon collateral sources of information to conduct the evaluation. In a retrospective assessment there are times when examination of the will versus the testator's known assets can indicate deficits in cognitive functioning. For example, the testator may leave an office building to a daughter yet may not have owned the property for 20 years (Melton et al. 2007). States vary in the specific legal criteria used for establishing testamentary capacity and undue influence. Thus psychiatric evaluators should have a clear understanding of the relevant standards of the jurisdiction and list them in the report.

9.3 The report

The elements of the psychiatric report that were described in Chapter 7 and that warrant distinctive treatment in reports on civil litigation are shown in Box 9.1.

9.3.1 Introduction to the report

Psychiatric reports in civil litigation serve different purposes depending upon the type of case in question. In medical malpractice, the report typically seeks to define the relevant standard of care and to support the expert's opinion regarding whether the appropriate standard of care was upheld or breached. In cases alleging psychic harm, such as in personal injury litigation, the report typically serves to document and explain the existence of any psychiatric impairment in the claimant and its relationship (if any) to

---

Box 9.1 Topics warranting distinctive treatment in civil litigation reports

Table 7.1 Structure of the psychiatric report

	1. **Preliminary and identifying information**
Section 9.3.1 ———	2. **Introduction**
	Why the report is being written, the circumstances of the request and the questions that are being addressed
	Dates and duration of interviews with the subject
Section 9.3.3 ———	Sources of information used in the report
Section 9.3.2 ———	Information given to the subject at time of interview, including information regarding confidentiality
	List of appended material
	3. **Body of report**
Section 9.3.4 ———	Background information
Section 9.3.5 ———	Current events (the crime in a sentencing report; the events leading to the claim in a civil action), the circumstances surrounding those events, and relevant sequelae
Section 9.3.6 ———	Findings on examination
	Psychological and other test results
Section 9.3.7 ———	4. **Opinion**
	5. **Concluding material**
	Signature of author
	Name, qualifications, and current post
	Date of signing

the incident alleged to have caused the injury. In cases requiring evaluation of civil competency, such as proceedings regarding testamentary capacity or guardianship, the purpose of the psychiatric report is to explain the results of the psychiatric evaluation and any findings regarding the evaluee's task-specific capacities and disabilities. The examining psychiatrist should clarify the exact purpose of the evaluation and the report in the introduction.

9.3.2 Description of warning regarding confidentiality

When the evaluation requires a psychiatric examination of a living person, the evaluee should be clearly informed of (and should understand): (1) the reason for the evaluation; (2) the fact that a report will be produced following the evaluation; (3) that the psychiatrist is not providing treatment in the evaluation and that the evaluee is not the psychiatrist's patient; (4) that there is no doctor–patient relationship in place between the evaluee and the physician doing the assessment; (5) that the psychiatrist may have a legal obligation to report real or suspected abuse and to intervene in the event that the evaluee discloses suicidal ideation or violent intentions; (6) that the results of the examination will be shared in a written report with the requesting party; and (7) that anything said might be disclosed in a deposition or at court or under other appropriate circumstances. An agreement form can help to document that the evaluee has been adequately informed of the purpose and circumstances of the evaluation and that the evaluee understands and agrees to the terms of the evaluation. The forensic report should document that the evaluee received, understood, and agreed to these warnings.

9.3.3 Sources of information

A good report includes an inventory of each item reviewed during the course of the preparation of the expert's opinion. Each source of data upon which the expert has relied should be specifically recorded somewhere in the report. The report should itemize all documents reviewed and note any additional materials that were unavailable but might have been informative. Some forensic psychiatrists fully summarize all documents reviewed, but a complete summary is not usually necessary.

If an evaluee has been examined, it is prudent to document the length of the interview(s), the location in which the interview was conducted, who initiated the evaluation, who transported the evaluee, and whether any other persons were in the room during the interview. For retrospective evaluations, the forensic psychiatrist will need to carefully document that there was no personal interview with the evaluee. Some experts recommend recording the evaluation for reference when the forensic psychiatrist composes the report and for documentation of the interview should questions later arise. The report should note all sources of information the psychiatrist consulted in preparation, including any recorded evaluations.

Psychiatrists should attempt to review relevant medical or psychiatric records including office notes, consultations, neuropsychological testing, hospital records, and visiting nurses' assessments (Shulman et al. 2005; Melton et al. 2007). In evaluations for civil competencies, legal documents should be examined, including previous wills and powers of attorney as well as financial records. Personal records, such as correspondence, diaries, and family films, can be especially useful sources of information in the evaluation. The retainer agreement with the referral source can be drafted to include a provision that all relevant records be made available to the evaluating psychiatrist (Gutheil & Simon 2002).

Table 9.3 Potential sources of information in malpractice litigation

Administrative records of observation maintained by a hospital (separate from an individual patient's clinical records) in order to comply with requirements for accreditation by the Joint Commission or the Centers for Medicare & Medicaid Services (CMS)

Records maintained by state departments of health and medical boards

The National Practitioner Data Bank

Records for Medicare debarment

Employment or school records

Police reports

Ambulance records

Pharmacy records

Attendance records from the evaluee's employer or school

Any relevant court documents, including responses to interrogatories, depositions, relevant materials produced for inspection, and statements of witnesses or other third parties having knowledge of the circumstances

The forensic expert should request and review all pertinent medical records, including psychiatric treatment records as well as general medical charts. Current medical and mental health records are especially important to examine if the claimant is currently in treatment. Obtaining extensive and complete medical records may be a challenge, but conducting a thorough review of these records is often crucial. The scope of the investigation of collateral materials will vary depending upon the circumstances of the alleged wrong. Additional documentation may be found outside of the individual patient's medical record, and these documents may be especially useful sources of information in the report. For reports in malpractice litigation, several additional sources of information may be considered (Table 9.3).

9.3.4 Background

The report should describe the course of events leading up to the claim. Information about the evaluee's background, including developmental, family, social, and occupational history, as well as psychiatric and general medical history, can be critical to situating the events within the appropriate context. Any pre-existing problems should be identified in the report. Such problems may help to clarify questions of causation and damages, or they may illustrate an evaluee's vulnerability to harm, such as exploitation through boundary violations in the context of malpractice litigation (Binder & McNiel 2007) or undue influence in the execution of a will or other legal documents.

It is important for the psychiatrist to consider aspects of the evaluee's functioning prior to the incident in question. For example, litigants with head injury often exaggerate their pre-injury intellectual functioning (Greiffenstein et al. 2002). Because the forensic psychiatrist typically does not have any acquaintance with the person prior to the events that prompted the legal dispute, it can be very difficult to compare the evaluee's past psychological functioning to current levels of functioning. The report should describe how the psychiatrist assessed prior functioning and detail other relevant factors in the evaluee's background.

The psychiatric expert should address the passage of time from the event in question (e.g., incident of alleged malpractice or injury, or execution of a will) to the subsequent evaluation. It is often useful to present the sources of information in chronological order in the report. A timeline can help to document the course of events and changes throughout the relevant time period in a case. In reports for determinations of civil competency, for example, documenting information received from collateral sources in such a timeline can illustrate the speed of the deterioration of cognitive functioning or may demonstrate indices of undue influence preceding the execution of a will.

In addition to background information about the evaluee who is the subject of the evaluation, the report may also provide important background information about other individuals or entities that are involved in the litigation, such as family members of a person being evaluated for civil competencies in guardianship proceedings. The report should present only such background information as is directly relevant to the legal proceedings and the purpose of the psychiatrist's report.

9.3.5 Current events and circumstances

In malpractice litigation, it is important for the report to clarify the basis of the claim against the provider. Just as a report for criminal prosecution must address the crime described in a sentencing report, a report for medical malpractice litigation must address the nature of the physician's alleged negligence, which may involve errors of fact or errors of judgment. The distinction between these two types of errors is relevant to the report's discussion of the events and circumstances of the case:

> Courts look much more harshly on errors of fact than on errors of judgment. Psychiatric errors of fact usually arise from a failure to gather relevant data about a patient; examples include not inquiring about suicidal thoughts or not obtaining medical records from a previous hospitalization. (Tsao & Layde 2007, p. 310)

A complaint of psychic harm generally argues that the negligent event has resulted in impaired functioning. In reports for personal injury litigation, the discussion of current events and circumstances should describe the evaluee's day-to-day functioning as well as his or her current treatment. Hoffman recommends describing the event of alleged negligence in the evaluee's own words, verbatim, to help courts understand the evaluee's subjective point of view regarding the incident, including realistic as well as distorted perceptions of the danger (Hoffman 1986).

The forensic report should address the possibility of other issues or events that could be contributing to an evaluee's disability, such as divorce or the death of a parent. The discussion of the circumstances in the case should address whether or not symptoms of a psychiatric disorder predated the event in question. Traumatic events have different impacts upon different victims. Someone with a history of childhood sexual abuse by a family member may be especially vulnerable to the psychic harm inflicted when a therapist crosses professional boundaries and becomes sexually involved with the client. In the report, the psychiatrist should clarify why and how the incident in question relates to the litigant's current disability.

Since in most will contests the testator is deceased, the evaluator should attempt to describe in detail the circumstances that led to the litigation. Information obtained from both sides of the dispute should be noted. Information from parties who are not beneficiaries of the will may be particularly helpful. Shulman and colleagues (2007, p. 723) identified several situations which raise suspicion about the validity of the will including "a radical change from previous consistently expressed wishes; evidence of a mental or neurological disorder that may affect cognition, judgment, impulsivity or reality testing; a dependent situation whereby the testator is vulnerable to undue influence, or the testator makes multiple changes in the will as a means of controlling individuals who are perceived as necessary for the testator's support or independence." These types of circumstances should be discussed in reports regarding testamentary capacity.

9.3.6 Examination findings

In reports for civil litigation, the nature and extent of the "examination" will vary depending upon the circumstances of each particular case. The report should describe the outcomes of any testing conducted during the examination, including the mental status examination, any laboratory testing completed or ordered by the examining psychiatrist, and the findings from any neuropsychiatric testing, which may help to confirm the psychiatrist's diagnostic formulation and explain any deficits noted during the interview (Marson 2001; Roked & Patel 2008). In examinations for civil competencies, deficits in semantic memory, verbal abstraction, comprehension abilities, and language skills may be relevant (ABA & APA 2009). The report's examination findings should also document any symptoms of mood disorder, psychotic symptoms such as delusions, and personality traits or disorders which may be relevant to the psychiatrist's professional opinion.

Just as the report must describe findings of any physical or cognitive examination, the "examination findings" should also discuss the results of the document review as well as information collected from other collateral sources, such as interviews with third parties. The relevant findings vary depending upon the type of civil litigation in question. In medical malpractice, the comprehensive forensic report will evaluate the medical record, commenting at least on any elements that are found to be inadequate, explaining the deficiencies and why they are significant. The "findings" should comment on all relevant components of the record, detailing the presence, absence, and quality of care the patient received. When a psychiatric diagnosis is requested or relevant to the report, the examination findings should include a detailed diagnostic formulation, following "[the current] DSM ... multiaxial format" (Firestone 2004, p. 275). The report should identify relevant relationships between Axis I or Axis II psychiatric diagnoses and Axis III medical conditions and Axis IV psychosocial functioning. The psychiatrist should explain the reason for assigning a particular Global Assessment of Functioning (GAF) score in Axis V. Litigation can be very stressful for both plaintiffs and defendants, so the report should identify any litigation-related exacerbations of psychiatric symptoms (Gerbasi 2004).

Hoffman (1986, pp. 168–169) suggests the following options for explaining the examination findings in personal injury cases:

> (1) There has been no change in the patient's behavior or emotions following the accident ...
> (2) The patient's posttraumatic behavior and emotions are a reasonable psychological response to real physical trauma and pain ... (3) The symptoms following an accident are related to difficulties coping with developmental tasks ... (4) The posttraumatic course is an accentuation of normal premorbid personality traits ... (5) The posttraumatic course is an accentuation of pathological premorbid personality patterns ... (6) The accident has precipitated the emergence of a full-blown psychiatric disorder independent of premorbid health ... (7) The posttraumatic course was influenced by the development of an unrelated independent syndrome or illness.

In addition to documenting the usual elements of a forensic evaluation including a detailed mental status exam, a testamentary capacity report should have a section documenting a task-specific competency examination which corresponds to the relevant legal standards. Despite some variability in state statutes, the following factors tend to be accepted in most jurisdictions (Shulman et al. 2007), and the report findings should comment on testators' knowledge (1) that they are making a will; (2) of the nature and extent of their property; (3) of the natural objects of their bounty; and (4) of the general dispositive scheme.

Wills can be challenged on the basis that due to mental illness or a neurological condition the testator had impairments in understanding the above elements or had an insane delusion. Persons with a major mental illness characterized by delusion may nonetheless retain testamentary capacity. To invalidate a will, the delusion must specifically and materially compromise testamentary capacity, as for example when the testator falsely believes that his daughter has been poisoning him and therefore should not be a beneficiary. The report should discuss any delusions in the context of the specific state standard of testamentary capacity. Wills can also be challenged by claims that the testator lacked capacity and/or was subject to undue influence (Scalise 2008). For a challenge based on undue influence to succeed, courts have generally required that the following elements be present (Frolik 2001):

1. confidential relationship between testator and influencer
2. relationship was used to change the estate's distribution
3. change in estate plan was unconscionable or did not reflect the testator's true intentions
4. testator was susceptible to undue influence.

While many elements of undue influence can be established through fact witness testimony, the psychiatric evaluator may be asked to provide an expert opinion concerning whether the testator was susceptible to being influenced because of a mental or physical condition.

9.3.7 Conclusions and recommendations

The expert's conclusions and recommendations form a critical part of the report for civil litigation. The conclusions should reflect back upon the report's purpose as originally described in the introduction. Specific recommendations should address the particular questions the psychiatrist was requested to answer in the report. The types of conclusions and recommendations in the report vary depending on the questions to be answered.

To succeed in a medical malpractice claim, the plaintiff must show "by a preponderance of the evidence (more likely than not)" (Meyer & Simon 2004, p. 186) that each of four elements of malpractice has been met. The forensic psychiatrist is often called upon to assist the court in determining whether the requisite conditions have been met. The four major elements are: (1) the existence of a duty of care toward the claimant, (2) the breach of that duty of care, (3) proximately resulting in (4) harm to the claimant. Each jurisdiction may have different standards of liability and definitions of the physician's duty of care. Therefore, the report should reflect an understanding of the standard of care appropriate in the jurisdiction and the facts that support the report's conclusions.

A good forensic report does not merely state that the doctor conformed to a reasonably prudent standard of care. The report must review each alleged breach of duty and explain why each action did or did not adhere to the relevant standard of care; each alleged deviation must be addressed separately. Furthermore, the forensic professional should remain cognizant of proximate cause concerns. For example, failing to obtain a patient's past medical record from a previous hospitalization may constitute a deviation from the standard of care, but the failure to request that record might not be the proximate cause of the plaintiff's injury

(Knoll & Gerbasi 2006). The report may also address the degree to which the physician met, exceeded, or deviated from the standard of care. Gross negligence may be required in some cases (*Naidu v. Laird*, 1988).

One error to avoid, particularly in conducting retrospective assessments of care, is to establish a duty of perfect care and then find that the duty was breached. The law does not require perfect care but rather adherence to a reasonably prudent standard of care. Another problem to avoid involves applying one's own personal ideas regarding the appropriate standard of care ("It's what I do, therefore it must be okay"); this error implies that the evaluating psychiatrist establishes the standard of the reasonably prudent physician based not on a professional standard but on idiosyncratic principles. Knoll and Gerbasi (2006) discuss problems in the forensic evaluation of psychiatric malpractice, paying particular attention to the risk of applying the inappropriate standard of care in case analysis. The conclusions and recommendations in a forensic psychiatric report for negligence proceedings should evidence a careful review of the appropriate standard of care in the case.

In personal injury and related cases, the claimant's expected future impairment or functioning should be considered. If additional treatment is necessary in order to effect a meaningful change in the evaluee's symptoms or level of disability, this need should be clear in the psychiatric report's conclusions and recommendations. Occasionally, the consulting psychiatrist may not have enough information about the claimant to give a final conclusion about the claimant's condition and expected prognosis. In such cases, the conclusion and recommendations may include a recommendation for ongoing re-evaluation, including the possibility of further psychological or neuropsychological testing, monitoring, or further personal interviews.

In evaluations of civil competencies the expert should focus on describing the task-related capacities and the areas of retained capacity and relate the deficits to the underlying condition. In a prospective evaluation of testamentary capacity, the psychiatric evaluator's opinion is based on the testator's level of functioning at the time of the execution of the will. Shulman et al. (2005, p. 66) noted, "As part of a retrospective assessment, the psychiatrist or expert should be able to interpret for the Courts relevant intellectual and cognitive functions in terms of their relationship to the legal criteria for testamentary capacity." A diagnosis of a neurological or psychiatric condition will help to explain the deficits revealed during the mental status, neuropsychological testing, and the specific testamentary capacity measures. In retrospective assessments, collateral information can be used to describe the level of impairment at the time of the execution of the will. This would include evidence of cognitive impairment as well as the presence of an insane delusion. For situations in which there are allegations of undue influence the conclusion should review the factors that would render the testator more vulnerable to undue influence such as cognitive impairment, mood disorder, psychotic symptoms, or personality style/traits/disorder as well as evidence regarding the presence of situational indices of undue influence.

9.4 Frequently asked questions in cross-examination

Although this textbook focuses on written *reports* rather than expert witness testimony, many aspects of the report may be vulnerable to a *Daubert* challenge or interrogation during cross-examination if there is a trial. The expert who composed the report may be called upon to defend the report and the opinions and arguments it contains. Claims in psychiatric reports should not be speculative but should be supported by scientific evidence: "[E]xpert opinions … should be formed with the expectation of meeting the standards and potential challenges expressed by US Supreme Court decisions in *Daubert … Joiner …* and *Kumho Tire*" (Meyer & Simon 2004, pp. 191–192). These cases have been discussed extensively elsewhere in the legal and forensic psychiatry literature (see, e.g., Gutheil & Bursztajn 2003; Note 2003), and a full explanation of their importance to the psychiatric report is beyond the scope of this chapter. Fortunately, as Meyer and Simon (2004, p. 192) note, "The diagnostic classification system of [the DSM-IV-TR], many of the psychological tests used in forensic psychiatry, and many therapeutic interventions in psychiatry meet specific criteria noted in *Daubert*. They can be cited as sources of information in expert reports and testimony to assist the expert in meeting court admissibility criteria."

Cross-examination, like forensic reports, will vary depending upon the type of case in civil litigation. In medical malpractice proceedings, attorneys for either side of the case may challenge the expert witness's knowledge regarding the standard of care. Unfortunately, as Simon (2005, p. 9) notes, "[t]here is no stock answer to the question: what is the standard of care? The courts apply reasonable standards to fact-specific cases." Typical questions during cross-examination might include, for example, "Doctor, would you please explain to the court how you know what the relevant standard of care is?" In order to strengthen a report, the expert may quote the exact language of the statutory law or case law that defines the standard of care for that jurisdiction (Meyer & Simon 2004, p. 188). The evaluator should consider whether the opinion can be supported by references to peer-reviewed scientific publications.

Forensic experts may differ on the citation of literature in a report. One good solution to this conundrum is to keep careful records of the literature upon which the expert relied and to maintain a file of the literature for later reference should it become necessary to testify in deposition or in court. At such occasions an update of the research is appropriate, but one should always keep in mind that it is the literature and standard of care at the time of the event that should form the basis of the opinion. The decision not to reference published literature in the report avoids the issue of those sources being deemed authoritative by virtue of their citation. Cited sources may be used in cross-examination to narrow the basis for the expert's opinion and then to discredit the expert through another witness or in argument. All reports should be replete with support directly from the medical record, legal record, relevant collateral sources, and the examination of the claimant (when applicable). These references may be included in the report for convenience should testimony be required. Moreover, citation to the specific data strengthens the report.

Particular caution is warranted regarding the citation of (and reliance upon) clinical practice guidelines in the context of malpractice proceedings. However, attorneys for either side in a malpractice case may introduce CPGs into the court record as evidence through the learned treatise exception (Recupero 2008), so the report should provide background information about the available CPGs that apply in the plaintiff's case. As noted previously in this chapter, CPGs do not set the standard of care; the report should therefore clarify that CPGs and similar professional clinical resources can provide detail about different schools of thought and the ethical responsibilities of the treatment provider but cannot alone define the relevant standard of care.

Observations and opinions expressed in a report can form the basis for cross-examination. The psychiatrist's report is particularly vulnerable to cross-examination if differential diagnoses were not addressed or explained in the report. If the evaluee's symptoms are associated with other diagnostic findings, the psychiatrist should explain which other diagnoses were considered and why they were rejected. One common problem in reports for capacity evaluations is the failure to document task-specific capacity. Another is to equate diagnosis with loss of functional capacity, especially in patients suffering with dementia (Marson et al. 2004). The report should acknowledge the limitations of the assessment but at the same time provide a strong foundation for the opinion. The evaluator should determine whether they have been able to correct for bias.

In reports based on retrospective evaluations, one can expect challenges to opinions bearing on the lack of direct contact with the evaluee. Simon (2004) has developed a checklist that can be used both for the preparation of the report and for later deposition or testimony in retrospective evaluations. He recommends that the report contain sufficient information to support any retrospective diagnosis. In reports regarding testamentary capacity, the examiner should be clear about the legal standard and should demonstrate understanding of the concepts of duress, coercion, and undue influence in the jurisdiction. The psychiatric expert should be able to relate cognitive and volitional impairments to the legal standard. When appropriate, a distinction between intentional and volitional behavior and between persuasion and coercion should be noted. Since the evaluation is being performed to document capacity at the time of the execution of the will, questions may arise if family members who may benefit from the new provisions of the will are present.

9.5 Conclusion

In writing reports for civil litigation, the forensic psychiatrist must tailor each report in order to address the specific question being asked. A report for alleged negligence in treatment would appear quite different from a report for testamentary capacity or guardianship. The forensic evaluator must be clear at the outset what specific question(s) the report is expected to answer as well as which jurisdiction is concerned and what governing law applies to the particular case. Experts should also remain cognizant of the ethical and professional limitations of their skills. For further guidance on questions of style, ethics, and professionalism in the production of psychiatric reports, the reader is referred to Section 1 of this volume.

References

American Bar Association and American Psychological Association (2009) *Assessment of Older Adults with Diminished Capacity: A Handbook for Psychologists.* ABA/APA Assessment of Capacity in Older Adults Project Working Group. Accessed September 27, 2009. http://www.apa.org/pi/aging/capacity_psychologist_handbook.pdf.

Binder, R. L. & McNiel, D. E. (2007) "He said – she said": the role of the forensic evaluator in determining credibility of plaintiffs who allege sexual exploitation and boundary violations. *Journal of the American Academy of Psychiatry and the Law* **35**: 211–218.

Champine, P. (2006) Expertise and instinct in the assessment of testamentary capacity. *Villanova Law Review* **51**: 25–85.

Firestone, M. (2004) Personal injury and the legal process. In *Textbook of Forensic Psychiatry*, ed. R. I. Simon & L. H. Gold. Washington, DC: American Psychiatric Publishing, Inc., pp. 263–285.

Frolik, L. A. (2001) The strange interplay of testamentary capacity and the doctrine of undue influence. Are we protecting older testators or overriding individual preferences? *International Journal of Law and Psychiatry* **24**: 253–266.

Gerbasi, J. B. (2004) Forensic assessment in personal injury litigation. In *Textbook of Forensic Psychiatry*, ed. R. I. Simon & L. H. Gold. Washington, DC: American Psychiatric Publishing, Inc., pp. 231–261.

Gold, L. H., Anfang, S. A., Drukteinis, A. M., et al. (2008) AAPL practice guideline for the forensic evaluation of psychiatric disability. *Journal of the American Academy of Psychiatry and the Law* **36**(Suppl.): S3–S50.

Greiffenstein, M. F., Baker, W. J. & Johnson-Greene, D. (2002) Actual versus self-reported scholastic achievements of litigating postconcussion and severe closed head injury claimants. *Psychological Assessment* **14**: 202–208.

Gutheil, T. G. & Bursztajn, H. (2003) Avoiding ipse dixit mislabeling: post-Daubert approaches to expert clinical opinions. *Journal of the American Academy of Psychiatry and the Law* **31**: 205–210.

Gutheil, T. G. & Simon, R. I. (2002) *Mastering Forensic Psychiatric Practice*. Washington, DC: American Psychiatric Publishing, Inc.

Hoffman, B. F. (1986) How to write a psychiatric report for litigation following a personal injury. *American Journal of Psychiatry* **143**: 164–169.

Hollister, L. E. (1992) Automobile driving by psychiatric patients (letter). *American Journal of Psychiatry* **149**: 274.

Knoll, J. & Gerbasi, J. (2006) Psychiatric malpractice case analysis: striving for objectivity. *Journal of the American Academy of Psychiatry and the Law* **34**: 215–223.

LeBourgeois III, H. W., Pinals, D. A., Williams, V., & Appelbaum, P. S. (2007) Hindsight bias among psychiatrists. *Journal of the American Academy of Psychiatry and the Law* **35**: 67–73.

Marson, D. C. (2001) Loss of competency in Alzheimer's disease: conceptual and psychometric approaches. *International Journal of Law and Psychiatry* **24**: 267–283.

Marson, D. C., Huthwaite, J. S., & Hebert, K. (2004) Testamentary capacity and undue influence in the elderly: a jurisprudent therapy perspective. *Law and Psychology Review* **28**: 71–94.

Melton, G. B., Petrila, J., Poythress, N. G., & Slobogin, C. (2007) *Psychological Evaluations for the Courts: a Handbook for Mental Health Professionals and Lawyers*, 3rd edn. New York: Guilford Press.

Meyer, D. J. & Simon, R. I. (2004) Psychiatric malpractice and the standard of care. In *Textbook of Forensic Psychiatry*, ed. R. I. Simon

& L. H. Gold. Washington, DC: American Psychiatric Publishing, Inc., pp. 185–203.

Moye, J., Butz S. W., Marson D., et al. (2007a) A conceptual model and assessment template for capacity evaluation in adult guardianship. *The Gerontologist* **47**: 591–599.

Moye J., Wood S., Edelstein B., et al. (2007b) Clinical evidence in guardianship of older adults is inadequate: findings from a tri-state study. *The Gerontologist* **47**: 604–612.

Naidu v. *Laird*, No. 77, 1987; 539 A.2d 1064 (Del. 1988).

Naik, A. D, Teal, C. R., Pavlik, V. N., Dyer, C. B., & McCullough, L. B. (2008) Conceptual challenges and practical approaches to screening capacity for self-care and protection in vulnerable older adults. *Journal of the American Geriatrics Association* **56**: S266–S270.

Note (2003) Reliable evaluation of expert testimony. *Harvard Law Review* **116**: 2142–2163.

Recupero, P. R. (2008) Clinical practice guidelines as learned treatises: understanding their use as evidence in the courtroom. *Journal of the American Academy of Psychiatry and the Law* **36**: 290–301.

Roked, F. & Patel, A. (2008) Which aspects of cognitive function are best associated with testamentary capacity in patients with Alzheimer's disease? *International Journal of Geriatric Psychiatry* **23**: 552–553.

Sadoff, R. L. (2004) Working with attorneys. In *Textbook of Forensic Psychiatry*, ed. R. I. Simon & L. H. Gold. Washington, DC: American Psychiatric Publishing, Inc., pp. 165–182.

Scalise, R. J. (2008) Undue influence and the law of will: a comparative analysis. *Duke Journal of Comparative and International Law* **19**: 41–107.

Shulman, K. I., Cohen, C. A., & Hull, I. (2005) Psychiatric issues in retrospective challenges of testamentary capacity. *International Journal of Geriatric Psychiatry* **20**: 63–69.

Shulman, K. I., Cohen, C. A., Kirsh, F. C., Hull, I. M., & Champine, P. R. (2007) Assessment of testamentary capacity and vulnerability to undue influence. *American Journal of Psychiatry* **164**: 722–727.

Shuman, D. W. (2004) Retrospective assessment of mental states and the law. In *Retrospective Assessment of Mental States in Litigation*, ed. R. I. Simon & D. W. Shuman. Washington, DC: American Psychiatric Publishing, Inc., pp. 21–46.

Simon, R. I. (2004) Retrospective assessment of mental states in criminal and civil litigation: A clinical review. *In Retrospective Assessment of Mental States in Litigation*, ed. R. I. Simon & D. W. Shuman. Washington, DC: American Psychiatric Publishing, Inc., pp. 1–20.

Simon, R. I. (2005) Standard-of-care testimony: best practices or reasonable care? *Journal of the American Academy of Psychiatry and the Law* **33**: 8–11.

Slovenko, R. (2004) Civil competency. *Textbook of Forensic Psychiatry*, ed. R. I. Simon & L. H. Gold. Washington, DC: American Psychiatric Publishing, Inc., pp. 205–261.

Tsao, C. I. & Layde, J. B. (2007) A basic review of psychiatric medical malpractice law in the United States. *Comprehensive Psychiatry* **48**: 309–312.

United States Department of Health and Human Services, Centers for Medicare & Medicaid Services (2009) *State Operations Manual*, Rev. 1, 05–21–04, Publication #100–07. Appendix AA: Psychiatric Hospitals: Interpretive Guidelines and Survey Procedures. Baltimore, MD: Centers for Medicare & Medicaid Services, 2009. Accessed March 17, 2009 from http://www.cms.hhs.gov/CFCsAndCoPs/downloads/som107ap_aa_psyc_hospitals.pdf.

Weinstock, R. & Gold, L. H. (2004) Ethics in forensic psychiatry. In *Textbook of Forensic Psychiatry*, ed. R. I. Simon & L. H. Gold. Washington, DC: American Psychiatric Publishing, Inc., pp. 91–115.

Wettstein, R. M. (2004) The forensic examination and report. In *Textbook of Forensic Psychiatry*, ed. R. I. Simon & L. H. Gold. Washington, DC: American Psychiatric Publishing, Inc., pp. 139–164.

Chapter

10

Civil and sex-offender commitment

Debra A. Pinals, Graham D. Glancy, and
Li-Wen Grace Lee

10.1 Introduction

This chapter addresses forensic reports related to two forms of commitment: civil commitment to psychiatric hospitals based on mental illness and civil commitment to a variety of facilities for a person who, after serving a sentence for a criminal sexual offense, is found to be a risk to society as a result of some form of "mental abnormality" (the latter such persons are labeled differently across jurisdictions with terms such as sexual predator or sexually dangerous person).

Societies have over the years dealt with individuals with mental illness by banishing them, keeping them at home, often in deplorable conditions, or by sending them to jails and prisons (Deutsch 1945). The mid-eighteenth century saw a wave of reform regarding the care of the "insane," which included the establishment of long-term and acute hospitals. Over time, legal cases shifted the standards for involuntary hospitalization and shaped the commitment process. The key issues and rulings are summarized in Table 10.1. They have been reviewed by Stone (1984) and Appelbaum (1994).

Sex-offender commitment laws were present in over half of US states in the 1960s but pessimism over the prospects for rehabilitation led to most being repealed in the 1980s. Similar legislation reemerged in the 1990s with the passing of a Washington statute that defines a "sexually violent predator" as an individual who has been convicted or charged with a sexually violent offense and who has a mental abnormality "which makes the person likely to engage in predatory acts of sexual violence if not confined in a secure facility." These individuals may be committed for an indeterminate period, until deemed safe (Washington Code 71.09.010). In *Specht* v. *Patterson* (1967) the US Supreme Court applied most criminal procedural safeguards to sexual offender commitment hearing including: full judicial hearing, assistance of counsel, the right to confront and cross-examine witnesses, and the right to present evidence. Sex-offender commitment laws and related statutes have evolved in large part as a result of case law. The key cases are summarized in Table 10.2.

10.2 Special considerations in commitment reports
10.2.1 Conduct of the evaluation
Civil commitment

The ethical guidelines of the American Academy of Psychiatry and the Law (2005) identify civil commitment proceedings as an exception to the rule that psychiatrists should not offer expert testimony concerning their own patients (see Strasburger et al. 1997). Treating

The Psychiatric Report, ed. Alec Buchanan and Michael A. Norko. Published by Cambridge University Press. © Cambridge University Press 2011.

Table 10.1 Summary of the evolution of landmark cases relevant to civil commitment for persons with mental illness

Case	Issue	Ruling
Lake v. *Cameron* (1966)	Appropriate setting for care	Least restrictive alternative
Lessard v. *Schmidt* (1972)	Legal protections in civil commitment proceedings	Due process safeguards similar to criminal proceedings, including proof beyond a reasonable doubt
O'Connor v. *Donaldson* (1975)	Criteria for ongoing commitment	Non-dangerous patients able to survive in the community may not be involuntarily committed
Addington v. *Texas* (1979)	Standard of proof in civil commitment	"Clear and convincing" adequate; beyond a reasonable doubt not required
Foucha v. *Louisiana* (1992)	Criteria for ongoing commitment of insanity acquittees	Clear and convincing evidence of mental illness and dangerousness both required

Table 10.2 Summary of the evolution of landmark cases related to the civil commitment of sex offenders

Case	Issue	Ruling
Specht v. *Patterson* (1967)	Indefinite detention in absence of hearing	Most criminal procedural safeguards necessary
Allen v. *Illinois* (1986)	Whether proceedings are civil or criminal in nature	Proceedings are civil: goal is to provide treatment to address dangerousness due to mental disorder
In re Young & Cunningham (1993)	Civil versus criminal nature of statute. Determination of dangerousness	Civil nature affirmed. Exerts allowed to testify on prediction of dangerousness beyond recent acts, and least restrictive alternatives must be considered
Kansas v. *Hendricks* (1997)	Commitment challenged on *ex post facto* and double jeopardy grounds	Statute reaffirmed as civil in nature, and civil commitment can be used to segregate those who are dangerous to the public and unable to control themselves
Kansas v. *Crane* (2002)	Necessity of lack-of-control determination	Must have proof of serious difficulty in controlling behavior, but absolute lack of control not required

psychiatrists often testify in these proceedings. When an independent evaluator undertakes a case, it should be made clear to the patient for whom the evaluator is working.

Though a routine part of psychiatric inpatient care, commitment proceedings have a tremendous impact on the lives of those affected. There are no instruments to assess whether someone meets commitment criteria. Clinicians must consider risk of harm in a variety of domains. Assessment of suicide and violence risk is critical and methods to do so have been delineated elsewhere (American Psychiatric Association 2003; Pinals et al. 2009). Scales such as a scale of suicide intent (Beck et al. 1979), the HCR-20 (Webster et al. 1997; Douglas et al. 2001), and the Classification of Violence Risk (COVR) (Monahan et al. 2005) may be useful adjuncts to the clinical evaluation of risk in particular cases. Their use in evaluations for sex-offender commitment is discussed below.

Sex-offender evaluations

Many states in the United States require pre-referral assessments to inform prosecutors whether there is a reasonable prospect of a commitment application succeeding. These assessments are often performed by correctional or state employees. In the second stage of the process, pre-commitment assessments, both the state and the respondent may retain their own experts. The experts should be clear on the issue of who the retaining party is and how the information will be used.

A clinical interview should be performed whenever possible (Zonana 2000; Boer 2006). If the assessor is denied access to the person being assessed, efforts at gaining access should be clearly documented. Any denial of access to the client should be explicitly stated in the conclusions as a cautionary caveat and possible limitation.

A review of the limits of confidentiality is critical. Given the high stakes and potential for the broader use of the information obtained in these assessments, other aspects of the evaluation should be reviewed also with the respondents. It is imperative that the interviewer is clear in identifying the agency requesting the assessment and the intended nature and purpose of the assessment. It should also be made clear whether or not a report will be prepared, the form of this report (verbal or written), and to whom the report is being submitted. If the assessment is for legal purposes as opposed to clinical or treatment purposes, this should be stated. It is also important that the respondent understand what will happen to the report, if any, and this may include a warning that there could be cross-examination and that the press may be present.

Corroborating data should be considered essential in the assessment of sexual preda-tors. In collecting these data, the evaluator should be mindful of the issues related to mental abnormality and sexual offending. Specific family issues and dynamics may be helpful in understanding the person and would, therefore, be paramount in a treatment plan. Police synopses of the offenses, court transcripts, victim statements, and evidence and probation and parole reports are also helpful. Records of treatment, counseling, or other contacts with mental health agencies can also reveal valuable information.

Considering the magnitude of the issue under question when assessing sexual predators, testing should be as comprehensive as possible. General as well as specific testing related to sexual preferences and attitudes are important. Most psychometric testing, though not all, requires a licensed clinical psychologist. Some of the more general tests such as a Minnesota Multiphasic Personality Inventory-2 (MMPI-2) and Millon Clinical Multiaxial Inventory-III (MCMI-III) can be most helpful in determining the personality profile of the offender and are helpful also in assessing validity and credibility. In addition, a neuropsychological screen can assist in identifying neuropsychological contributors. Langevin and Watson (1996) and Zonana (1999) outline the most relevant tests related to these assessments.

Sexual preference testing is a specialized field that should only be attempted with the requis-ite experience and qualifications. Three forms of such testing should be considered. Penile tumescence testing (PTT or phallometry) is the single best indicator of a paraphilia (Langevin

& Watson 1996). It involves the measurement of penile volume or circumference when the individual is exposed to a variety of standardized stimuli. It is primarily a clinical technique and caution should be exercised when using this test in the legal context (Zonana 1999).

In Canada PTT is routinely used in clinical and psycho-legal assessments of sexual offenders referred to forensic services. In other jurisdictions, it is more often used as part of a comprehensive treatment approach (Scott 1994). The test can be valuable in confronting "non-admitters." Some courts have ruled it inadmissible for the purpose of placing a person (e.g., an incest offender) in a group who would likely commit a sexual offense (Glancy & Bradford 2007; Federoff et al. 2009). PTT should therefore only be considered as one part of a comprehensive assessment. It should be performed by a recognized laboratory, using standardized test materials, in an appropriate setting, whilst ensuring a procedure respecting the dignity of the client. Results should be scrutinized for faking, taking into account the client's mental state, his age and any physical illnesses such as diabetes or prescribed medicine that may affect the results of testing.

Visual reaction time testing (VRT; Abel et al. 1998; Abel & Wiegel 2009) has some advantages over phallometry. It can be administered in an hour with a laptop computer and does not require naked stimulus material. High figures for sensitivity and specificity have been reported (Johnson & Listiak 1999; Letourneau 2002) but concern remains over the level of independent replication and whether it has reached the accepted standard for admissibility in court (Krueger et al. 1998; Abel & Wiegel 2009). Polygraphy (or the lie detector) is another test that has been used during the assessment and treatment of sex offenders. This, again, has not usually been held to be admissible in court but can be used as an adjunctive test in some circumstances (Zonana 1999).

Sex-offender evaluations for commitment under sexual predator laws also require an estimation of risk. Table 10.3 describes the process of risk assessment in these cases. The assessment must be thorough and completed by someone with relevant expertise. The outcome of the assessment has profound implications for individual liberty and community safety and the results of these assessments are vigorously argued in the courts. In recent years, considerable attention has focused on the development of actuarial and "structured professional judgment" measures to predict risk of future danger in general (see above relevant to dangerousness among persons with mental illness) and sex offending risk in particular. Table 10.4 summarizes several tests that are used along with comments on some of their strengths and weaknesses.

Some studies have suggested that actuarial tools may be more accurate than clinical judgment alone (Grove & Meehl 1996) and some experts suggest that actuarial tests should be used alone without the confusion of clinical judgment (Quinsey et al. 1998b). Others have suggested that the assertion that actuarial tests should be used in the absence of a clinical interview is unsupported by data (Zonana 2000; Boer 2006).

10.2.2 Content of the report

Civil commitment

Civil commitment proceedings often take place without a formal written report. An affidavit or a brief petition to the court requesting a hearing serves as the written data that set the stage. Depending on the state, petitions require a summary of the symptoms and how they link to the commitment criteria.

After the petition is received, testimony of the witness is the primary basis upon which the court relies to render a decision regarding commitment. In some jurisdictions, report

Table 10.3 Aspects of assessment for sexual predators (modified from Glancy & Regehr 2004)

Clinical interview

Limits of confidentiality

Historical factors

Dynamic factors

Corroborating data

Family

Legal data

Previous treatment records

Testing

Psychometric

MMPI/MCMI

Neuropsychological

Tests for malingering

Biomedical

Neuroimaging

Endocrine

Sexual preference

Penile plethysmography

Visual reaction time

Polygraphy

Attitude and history

Clarke Sexual History (SHQ-R) (Langevin & Paitic 2005)

Abel & Becker Cognition (Abel et al. 1984)

Attitudes Towards Women Scale (Check 1988)

Burt Rape Myth Scale (Burt 1980)

Michigan Alcoholism Screening Test (Selzer 1971)

Substance Abuse Subtle Screening Inventory-III (Miller & Lazowski 1999)

Drug Abuse Screening Test (Skinner 1982)

Predictive tests*

RRASOR

Static 99/Static 2002

SONAR

MnSOST

SVR-20

Risk Matrix 2000/Sexual

PCL-R

SORAG/VRAG

* Described further in Table 10.4.

Table 10.4 Summary of actuarial prediction tests for sex offenders (modified from Glancy & Regehr 2004)

Actuarial prediction test	Strengths	Limitations
Violence Risk Assessment Guide/Sex Offender Risk Assessment Guide (VRAG/ SORAG; Quinsey et al. 1998a) VRAG – 12 items plus the Psychopathy Checklist-Revised (PCL-R; Hare 1991) SORAG – 13 items plus the PCL-R	Moderate ability to predict violence Good for mentally disordered offenders	Requires training for PCL-R Includes any form of minor violence Standardized on small number of high-risk offenders No dynamic factors
Minnesota Sex Offender Screening Tool (Revised) (MnSOST(R); Epperson et al. 1998) 16 items	Some dynamic factors Easy to score	Validation sample too small
Rapid Risk Assessment for Sexual Offender Recidivism (RRASOR; Hanson 1997) 4 items	Easy to score Moderate ability to predict sexual violence Well validated	Simplistic No dynamic factors
Static-99 (Hanson & Thornton 2000) 10 items Static 2002 (Hanson & Thornton 2003) 14 items	Easy to score Moderate ability to predict sexual violence Static-99 is well validated Static 2002 designed to improve on weakness of Static-99 New validation studies are promising relevant to Static 2002, though recidivism predictive accuracy may differ across populations	No dynamic factors
Sex Offender Needs Assessment Rating (SONAR; Hanson & Harris 1998) 9 items	Considers dynamic factors May predict short-term and long-term risk of sexual violence	Not yet well tested
Sexual Violence Risk-20 (SVR-20; Boer et al. 1997)	Easy to use Dynamic and static factors Moderate predictive validity	Not empirically derived
Risk Matrix 2000 Sexual (Hanson & Thornton 2000)	Moderate predictive validity Easy to score	Not yet well validated
Pyschopathy Checklist-Revised (PCL-R; Hare 1991) 20 items	Recognized psychological test Well validated	Requires training No dynamic factors

templates are provided by the courts as documents required for completion prior to a commitment hearing. In these cases, there may be little if any flexibility in what is included in the report and how the information is organized. In those regions or settings when a report is required but there are no set parameters for what to include, it is recommended that the report be structured similarly to other forensic reports.

Generally for civil commitment to proceed the court must find a nexus between mental illness and a risk of harm if the person is not committed. In some states mental illness is defined by DSM category (e.g., Nevada Revised Statutes 433.164), though this is unusual. Massachusetts is more typical in defining mental illness as a "substantial disorder of thought, mood, perception, orientation, or memory that grossly impairs judgment, behavior, capacity to recognize reality or meet the ordinary demands of life" (104 Code of Massachusetts Regulations 27.05).

Risk for the purpose of mental health commitment is generally a three-fold concept: risk of harm to self by virtue of suicidal behavior or intent, risk of physical harm to others, and inability to care for self, also referred to as "grave disability." Some jurisdictions make allowance for the commitment of an individual who is in need of treatment if other factors exist, who presents a risk to the rights of others or who lacks the capacity to make responsible treatment decisions (Ohio Revised Code s. 5122.01(B)(4); South Carolina Code 44-17-80(A)(1)). A small number of jurisdictions incorporate a standard that justifies commitment on the grounds of a risk of physical deterioration if not so committed (e.g., Kansas Statute 59-2946(f)(3)) and of people who present a risk of harm to property (e.g., Alaska Statutes 47.30.915(10)(B)).

Clinical and judicial decision-making around the legal standards have proven challenging at times (Lidz et al. 1989). Jurisdictions vary as to whether the risk must be based on a recent act (e.g., Pennsylvania Statutes s. 7310(b)) or whether there would have to be a substantial likelihood of serious risk of harm (e.g., Mass. General Laws, c. 123) if the person were not committed.

Finally, since *Lake* v. *Cameron* (1966) commitment criteria have increasingly included reference to the need to adopt the least restrictive alternative for treatment of the respondent. Though the exact meaning and ethical analysis of least restrictive alternative remains subject to debate (Lin 2003), in general the evaluator must explore whether other treatment settings (e.g., outpatient, day programming, residential placements) are available that would sufficiently mitigate the risk presented.

Sex-offender commitment

As with mental health commitments, in writing a report the evaluator needs to be aware of the sex-offender commitment statute in the particular jurisdiction, including whether it is institutional and/or outpatient-based. All sex-offender commitment statutes require the presence of some kind of mental abnormality, typically defined as a congenital or acquired condition that affects the emotional, cognitive, or volitional capacities of the individual and that predisposes the person to commit sexually violent acts.

The second general issue for reports in all jurisdictions is the risk for violence. The risk for violence must be tied to the mental illness or mental abnormality. Generally the statutes use the term "likely" as the standard required for commitment. Others may use "more likely than not." It may be helpful to discuss with counsel prior to the evaluation and to state explicitly in the report how those phrases are interpreted. If this is not done at the outset it may be a focus of a challenging cross-examination. A third issue, just as was reviewed in the section related to commitment of persons with mental illness, is the issue of "lesser restrictive alternative" in some jurisdictions. This is again an issue that needs to be discussed with counsel prior to the evaluation.

10.3 The report

The elements of the psychiatric report that were described in Chapter 7 and that warrant distinctive treatment in reports on civil and sex-offender commitment are shown in Box 10.1.

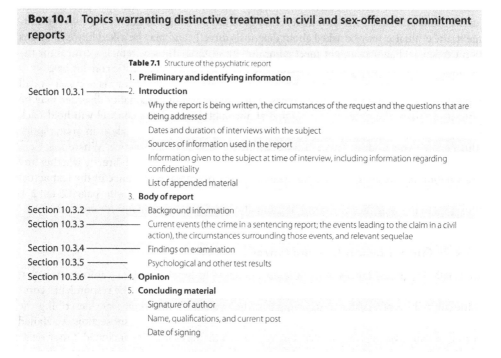

Box 10.1 Topics warranting distinctive treatment in civil and sex-offender commitment reports

Table 7.1 Structure of the psychiatric report

1. **Preliminary and identifying information**

Section 10.3.1 ——— 2. **Introduction**

Why the report is being written, the circumstances of the request and the questions that are being addressed

Dates and duration of interviews with the subject

Sources of information used in the report

Information given to the subject at time of interview, including information regarding confidentiality

List of appended material

3. **Body of report**

Section 10.3.2 ——— Background information

Section 10.3.3 ——— Current events (the crime in a sentencing report; the events leading to the claim in a civil action), the circumstances surrounding those events, and relevant sequelae

Section 10.3.4 ——— Findings on examination

Section 10.3.5 ——— Psychological and other test results

Section 10.3.6 ——— 4. **Opinion**

5. **Concluding material**

Signature of author

Name, qualifications, and current post

Date of signing

10.3.1 Introduction

For civil commitment, the introduction should contain the basic circumstances of admission, relevant dates, and facts (legal and clinical) that articulate the context. In sex-offender commitment, it is important to differentiate whether this is a pre-referral assessment or pre-commitment assessment. Many states in the Unites States require pre-referral assessments, which can inform prosecutors whether there is a reasonable prospect of success at a probable cause hearing. For both civil and sex-offender commitment, the question is whether the respondent fulfills the criteria in that jurisdiction. It can be helpful to quote directly at the outset the legal standard as defined by statute or case law, including whether the least restrictive alternative needs consideration.

The evaluator should list all pertinent information reviewed. For those being civilly committed following a short-term hospital stay, relevant documentation may include emergency detainment papers, emergency mental health assessments, and progress notes. Documentation identified in reports related to the longer-term patient will likely include a more extensive list of information obtained over the course of the hospitalization and the review may be less focused on the initiating documentation. Sex-offender commitment evaluations, more than traditional mental health civil commitment evaluations, are frequently very adversarial. This makes using a variety of collateral sources and listing those sources in the report particularly important.

10.3.2 Background

For civil commitment evaluations, the background content should contain traditional clinical historical information of relevance. More detailed information regarding the respondent's history of violence or public safety risk-taking behaviors, suicide attempts, and concerns related their ability to care for themselves historically will lend weight to the opinions. Although jurisdictions often use their own interpretation of mental illness to qualify for civil commitment, the evaluator may be asked about diagnosis directly and may be asked how symptoms of a particular diagnosis might meet commitment criteria. Thus, it remains critical for the evaluator to articulate in the background data the basis for any diagnostic conclusions.

In sex-offender commitment, a thorough personal and family history is necessary in all reports and particularly so where the issue of a diagnosis of personality disorder may be crucial to satisfy the criterion for mental abnormality. Sometimes counsel will hold back damaging information hoping that you will skip over it or not include it in your report. This exposes you to destructive cross-examination and is poor practice. Where there are concerns that this might be happening, retaining counsel can be asked directly whether any information has been held back. An evaluator should generally reference in the text actual file information referenced (e.g., "according to interview with subject's wife, page 12, tab 2"). This goes to the weight of the testimony and also prepares the evaluator for cross-examination, when they would have to cite the exact information.

10.3.3 Current events/circumstances

Especially in circumstances where there is an acute hospitalization, any information that relates to the more recent events that lead to the need to petition for the respondent's commitment will be of assistance in laying out the evaluator's thinking. Data describing the course of the current hospitalization should be presented as a separate subsection. A detailed review of daily events is not needed, but a review of themes should be included if they relate to the commitment question (e.g., episodes within the hospital of self-injurious behavior, medication non-adherence, and/or aggression).

In sex-offender commitment, it is important to discuss a detailed account of the circumstances leading to the convictions. In particular it is important to discover and report whether the subject fantasized about the behaviors prior to engaging in them. A DSM IV paraphilia diagnosis requires "recurrent, intense, sexually arousing fantasies, sexual urges, or behaviors generally involving ..." (American Psychiatric Association 2000) the specific anomalous object or activity. All convictions should be delineated in detail. It is also helpful to review whether the subject has a history of sexual acting out that did not lead to conviction. This does raise some ethical issues in that there could be various repercussions for the respondent from such an admission and its subsequent inclusion in a report. In the ongoing attention to the informed consent process during the assessment, this is perhaps one of the areas about which the individual may wish to consult with counsel.

10.3.4 Examination findings

For the purposes of civil commitment, mental status examination findings should be included, along with a description of the respondent's functioning and insight into their need for treatment and willingness to engage in treatment if not committed. The report should also reflect how the respondent views their own risk, again focusing on the standards for commitment in a particular jurisdiction. Reports for sex-offender commitment hearings should be set out in a manner corresponding to the order in which the basis of the opinion was set out at the beginning of the report (see Table 10.3), using headings and subheadings as necessary.

10.3.5 Psychological testing

Adjunctive testing is more commonly used in sex-offender evaluations than in civil commitment evaluations, though in either case certain tests may be helpful in examining diagnostic and risk-related issues. The interpretation of any adjunctive testing might include the strengths and limitations of each particular test as applied in the context of the report. For instance, in sex-offender evaluations, if penile plethysmography (PPG) testing is performed then a discussion of its reliability, validity, and application should be included (Bourget & Bradford 2008). This would also apply to the use of actuarial or other instruments aimed at predicting sexual violence (Vincent et al. 2009). The evaluator should be careful when interpreting actuarial tests to choose the precise language that the test is designed to establish, thereby not going beyond the limits of the test. For instance, the test may offer an estimate only of where an offender ranks in a certain population, that population being the development sample (Mossman 2006).

10.3.6 Conclusions and recommendations

Civil commitment

The civil commitment report should include an opinion of whether and how the respondent meets the jurisdictional requirements for mental illness. The opinion should then provide the nexus between the mental illness and the prongs related to risk of harm required by the local statute.

It is critical that report data related to civil commitment, and the opinions that follow, convey risk information in a meaningful way. Avoidance of conclusory statements (e.g., Mr. Jones has schizophrenia and has become agitated, and therefore meets criteria for commitment) should be avoided. Instead, statements are best when descriptive in nature (e.g., Mr. Jones carries a diagnosis of schizophrenia that is manifested by his talking to voices only he can hear, and most recently involved his yelling at perceived attackers, becoming more energized on the unit, screaming out loud and flailing his arms).

In terms of communicating risk issues, Heilbrun and colleagues (2002) propose a sample report that yields information relevant to risk factors, risk level, nature and imminence of harm, as well as protective factors that help lead the examiner to a reasoned prediction as to how likely it was that a particular patient, if not committed, would again try to kill themselves (Heilbrun et al 2002). They also articulate their consideration of whether the use of a formal risk assessment instrument would add to the report's opinion. In the case example they describe, where risk of harm was clear and imminence of risk was high, an actuarial tool was not viewed as a useful adjuvant. This example further highlights that these tools are not necessary for most evaluations related to civil commitment, particularly the obvious cases, but they may be helpful as a component of the evaluation in more ambiguous or complex situations.

Heilbrun and colleagues (2002) further note that clinicians who typically communicate risks by utilizing a risk assessment and management approach may need to use an approach that more specifically establishes whether an individual would meet the civil commitment criteria of a particular jurisdiction. The court must see the data as they relate to the dichotomous question at hand. The judge or finder of fact must determine, "Does this person meet the criteria for commitment or not at this time?" Thus, a report should not simply lay out a clinical formulation with risk management suggestions as one might do in a risk assessment consultation. Instead, the report should address the components of the commitment directly.

Sex-offender commitment

The Conclusion should include a summary of the main findings of the report and how these pertain to the psycho-legal issue outlined in the section on the purpose of the report. Psychiatric diagnosis should be laid out in the format of the current version of the DSM. The report should indicate whether there is a link between the psychiatric diagnosis and a predisposition to commit sexually violent offenses.

Doren (2002) outlines a very helpful template for the report. He advocates setting out conclusions as defined in the statute, and using the words of the statute. Whether or not to use the exact words of the statute may be discussed with counsel. Some forensicists are more comfortable using psychiatric rather than legal language in part because the legal language may appear too close to rendering the ultimate legal opinion at hand. The conclusions should explain the reasoning establishing or refuting the link between the psychiatric diagnosis or mental abnormality and the assessment of risk, if any.

In summarizing the issues of risk, it would be unfortunate if static factors ticked on a checklist were the only criteria for a comprehensive assessment (Glancy 2007). These factors may not assist the assessor in looking at unique relevant factors in an individual client such as one who may have a few past offenses who presents with overwhelming urges to molest in a new situation where a child relative has moved into his house temporarily.

The SONAR and the SVR-20 represent a development of previous tools in that they address dynamic factors. Current experts in the field argue (Sreenivasan et al. 2000; Norko & Baranoski 2005) that the responsibility of the clinician is to understand how the individual risk factors are represented in a specific patient. They have concluded that guided clinical judgment should be the norm. In this process clinical examination is guided by the various tests discussed above, thereby coming to a more fully informed opinion, applied to this particular case in this context.

Treatment recommendations, taking into account the fact that the subject may or may not be in a secure treatment facility, should be clearly enunciated. It may be important to make an estimate of whether the subject is motivated and has the characteristics of one who is likely to benefit from treatments and whether these treatments will attenuate risk. Treatment recommendations may include recommendations about a treatment should the court not find the subject a sexually violent predator (SVP) as well as possible suggestions regarding least restrictive alternatives.

10.4 Frequently asked questions in cross-examination

10.4.1 Civil commitment

Cross-examination in typical hospital proceedings may not be as rigorous as in sex-offender proceedings (see below). In fact, at times respondents may waive the hearing or attorneys may stipulate facts under consideration. In many situations, vigorous legal advocacy related to liberty interests of respondents is not seen. Nevertheless, there are commitment hearings that are contested through robust cross-examination, such that it would behove the individual expert to be well versed in testimony and common challenges in these proceedings.

Thatcher and Mossman (2009) identify several themes that clinicians are likely to encounter during testimony, including questions related to diagnosis and how its symptoms affect the respondent and lead to risk-related behavior, why hospitalization is the least restrictive alternative to provide for treatment for the individual, and the current medication regimen. They suggest that the testifying clinician be prepared to defend why their diagnosis of the respondent may differ from diagnoses given by other clinicians and to explain the respondent's view of the risk-related allegations in the chart.

There may also be challenges by either side toward allowing evidence into the record. The respondent's own statements may be excluded under certain circumstances. Although most state laws allow exceptions to privilege for the purpose of civil commitment (e.g., Texas Rules of Evidence S. 509(e)(6)), some jurisdictions have specific case law related to when a clinician needs to advise a patient of the limits of confidentiality and the potential that information they reveal may be used in certain commitment proceedings (e.g., *Commonwealth v. Lamb*, 1974). Without such a warning in those jurisdictions where this may apply, use of information taken from the interview can be objected to in court.

Issues of hearsay become of major significance in contested cases of civil commitment. Hearsay, which is a statement made out of court that is brought in as evidence, may include statements made by family and friends who witnessed behavior of the respondent that can be critical to the civil commitment evidence. Nonetheless, the expert should be prepared to deal with reframing testimony after hearsay challenges.

Inevitably in any cross-examination of a psychiatrist on forensic matters the issue of malingering arises. This may not be seen as frequently in mental health civil commitments, but it is still important to bear in mind as it does happen on occasion. Generally speaking, the evaluator needs to have a clear explanation of how malingering was addressed since conclusions may largely rely on the evaluee's self-report.

10.4.2 Sex-offender commitment

It is likely that anyone who appears in court as an expert in an SVP hearing will be cross-examined in a thorough manner. They may be subject to impeachment on published material (Mauet 2005). The more one has written the more fodder there is for cross-examination.

One of the most contentious areas of cross-examination is that of the diagnosis of a paraphilia (Frances et al. 2008). If a respondent has a stated criterion for a DSM-IV paraphilia, a careful cross-examination on the criterion can be stressful. In SVP cases this often becomes even more difficult, particularly when the expert relies upon a diagnosis of Paraphilia Not Otherwise Specified. This may particularly be the case if there is a preferential rape pattern or hebephilia, both of which may be difficult to establish using strict criteria. First and Halon (2008), in a thoughtful discussion, caution not to make the diagnosis of a paraphilia based solely on the sexual offenses themselves.

Similar comments can be made about the second diagnosis frequently used to meet the definition of mental abnormality in SVP cases, that of personality disorder. In court one can realize that at times DSM diagnoses that seem so complete in case conferences can be difficult to justify under searching cross-examination. The lack of thresholds and clarity in the criteria can be particularly difficult to defend. Sometimes it is helpful to have the support of psychological testing. Further refinement of practice relevant to diagnoses in sex-offender evaluations may be needed given the evolution of a new version of DSM on the horizon at the time of this writing.

Regardless, both sides may raise in cross-examination the large published literature comparing clinical and actuarial predictions. A skillful cross-examiner can establish that there is a significant amount of evidence suggesting that clinical impression alone is not adequate in predicting sexual violence. Counsel have attempted to point out that the best actuarial instruments likely have a ceiling of prediction represented by the area under the curve receiver operating characteristic (AUC-ROC) of 0.79 (personal observation, G. Glancy). Questions should be expected regarding this ceiling and regarding the fact that these measures are a comparison of the hits versus the misses in prediction.

For example, there may be questions on cross-examination if there are a significant number of misses as to why the individual does not fall in the miss group rather than the hit group. Additionally, scoring of these types of instruments is typically called into question. It is not uncommon for individual items on particular scales to be questioned in court such that the court deliberations yield scores that differ from those of the evaluator. It can be helpful at the time of finalizing these tests (even the tests that are most established such as the Psychopathy Checklist Revised; Hare 1991) and prior to a court appearance to consult a colleague and spend time going through each item, noting how scores for particular items were justified.

It is likely that handwritten notes or an electronic record of the interview will be in the hands of counsel, so interpretation of various answers may be called into question. The sufficiency and quality of collateral information is another issue that will likely be canvassed. Attorneys in these cases have devoted weeks of their time to the case and can uncover additional information. There is some debate about whether examiners should speak to victims, but in any event there is usually someone who has not been accessible for one reason or another and one should expect to be confronted with this.

In an ideal world counsel would have alerted the expert when some critical information has been ruled inadmissible earlier in the course of the hearing, but in the real world this omission is a possibility. Another situation arises when some of the material relied upon in the report has not been entered into evidence at trial such as knowledge about charges that were previously dismissed. Along these lines some of the actuarial tools actually use charges that did not lead to convictions as one of their criteria. Prior experience has shown this can gravely concern lawyers and exposes one to serious potential damage in cross-examination. Such evidence should be discussed with counsel prior to testimony.

10.5 Conclusions

Commitment hearings for persons with mental illness are often done at a local facility, with the treating psychiatrist acting as the expert witness, though independent examinations may also be conducted in these contexts. Hearings can be contested, but often they are not. Reports can range from brief affidavits to more formal forensic reports. Sex-offender commitment evaluations, in contrast, have evolved to include a complex menu of options for formal assessments, and the cases tend to draw much more rigorous cross-examination, requiring a more detailed report. The mental health professional engaging in civil commitment assessments for mental illness or sexual offenders should be familiar with existing practices and legal standards and apply known risk factors to an individual in the context of the individual's current state and unique circumstances. In approaching civil commitment evaluations, it is critical for the mental health practitioner to recognize the loss of liberty involved in the confinement for treatment, and the need to balance this interest with the interests of the public at large as a necessary component of these forensic clinical endeavors.

References

104 Code of Massachusetts Regulations 27.05.

Abel, G. & Wiegel, M. (2009) Visual reaction time: development, theory, empirical evidence, and beyond. In *Sex Offenders, Identification, Risk Assessment, Treatment, and Legal Issues*, vol. 8, ed. F. M. Saleh, A. J. Grudzinskas, Jr., J. M. Bradford, & D. J. Brodsky. New York: Oxford University Press, pp. 101–118.

Abel, G., Becker, J., Cunningham-Rathner, J., et al. (1984) *Treatment of Child Molesters*. Atlanta, GA: Emory University School of Medicine.

Abel, G., Huffman, J., Warberg, B., & Holland, C. l. (1998) Visual reaction time and plethysmography as measures of sexual interest in child molesters. *Sexual Abuse: A Journal of Research and Treatment* 10(2): 81–95.

Addington v. Texas, 441 US 418, 99 S.Ct. 1804 (1979).

Alaska Statutes 47.30.915(10)(B).

Allen v. Illinois, 478 US 364 (1986).

American Academy of Psychiatry and the Law (2005) Ethics guidelines for the practice of forensic psychiatry. Available at http://www.aapl.org/ethics.htm, accessed November 6, 2009.

American Psychiatric Association (2000) *Diagnostic and Statistical Manual of Mental Disorders, Fourth Edition, Text Revision*. Washington, DC: American Psychiatric Press, Inc.

American Psychiatric Association (2003) *Practice Guideline for the Assessment and Treatment of Patients with Suicidal Behaviors*. Washington, DC: American Psychiatric Press, Inc.

Appelbaum, P. S. (1994) *Almost a Revolution: Mental Health Law and the Limits of Change*. New York: Oxford University Press.

Beck, A. T., Kovacs, M. & Weissman, A. (1979) Assessment of suicidal intention: the Scale for Suicide Ideation. *Journal of Consulting and Clinical Psychology* 47: 343–352.

Boer, D. (2006) Sexual offender risk assessment strategies: is there a convergence of opinion yet? *Sex Offender Treatment* 1: 1–4.

Boer, D., Hart, S., Kropp, P., & Webster C. (1997) *Manual for Sexual Violence Risk – 20 (SVR20): Professional Guidelines for Assessing Risk of Sexual Violence*. Vancouver, BC, Canada: British Columbia Institute Against Family Violence.

Bourget, D. & Bradford, J. M. W. (2008) Evidential basis for the assessment and treatment of sex offenders. *Brief Treatment and Crisis Intervention* 8: 130–146.

Burt, M. (1980) Cultural myths and supports for rape. *Journal of Personality and Social Psychology* 38: 217–230.

Check, J. (1988) Hostility toward women: some theoretical considerations. In *Violence in Intimate Relationships*, ed. G. Russell. Great Neck, NY: PMA Publishing, pp. 29–42.

Commonwealth v. Lamb, 311 N. E.2d 47 (1974).

Deutsch, A. (1945) *The Mentally Ill in America: A History of Their Care and Treatment from Colonial Times*. New York: Columbia University Press (first published in 1937).

Doren, D. M. (2002) *Evaluating Sex Offenders: A Manual for Civil Commitments and Beyond*. Thousand Oaks, CA: Sage Publications, Inc.

Douglas, K. S., Webster, C. D., Eaves, D., Hart, S. D. & Ogloff, J. R. P. (eds.) (2001) *HCR-20 Violence Risk Management Companion Guide*. Burnaby, BC, Canada: Mental Health Law and Policy Institute, Simon Fraser University and Louis de la Parte Florida Mental Health Institute, University of South Florida.

Epperson, D., Kaul, J., & Hesselton, D. (1998) Final report of the development of the Minnesota Sex Offender Screening Tool – Revised. Presentation at the 17th Annual Research and Treatment Conference of the Association for the Treatment of Sexual Abusers, Vancouver, BC, Canada.

Federoff, J. P., Kuban, M., & Bradford, J. M. W. (2009) In: *Sex Offenders: Identification, Risk Assessment, Treatment, and Legal Issues*, vol. 7, ed. F. M. Saleh, A. J. Grudzinskas, Jr., J. M. W. Bradford, & D. Brodsky. New York: Oxford University Press, pp. 89–100.

First M. B. & Halon R. L. (2008) Use of DSM paraphilia diagnoses in sexually violent predator commitment cases. *Journal of the American Academy of Psychiatry and the Law* **36**(4): 443–454.

Foucha v. *Louisiana*, 504 US 71 (1992).

Frances, A., Sreenivasan, S., & Weinberger L. E. (2008) Defining mental disorder when it really counts: DSM-IV-TR and SVP/SDP Statutes. *Journal of the American Academy of Psychiatry and the Law* **36**(3): 375–384.

Glancy, G. (2007) Caveat usare: actuarial schemes in real life. *Journal of the American Academy of Psychiatry and the Law* **34**: 272–275.

Glancy, G. & Bradford, J. (2007) The admissibility of expert evidence in Canada. *Journal of the American Academy of Psychiatry and the Law* **35**: 350–356.

Glancy, G. & Regehr, C. (2004) Assessment measures for sexual predators. In *Evidence Based Practice Manual: Research and Outcome Measures in Health and Human Sciences*, ed. A. Roberts & K. Yeager. New York: Oxford University Press.

Grove, W. & Meehl, P. (1996) Comparative efficiency of informal (subjective impressionistic) and formal (mechanical, algorithmic) prediction procedures: the clinical statistical controversy. *Psychology, Public Policy and Law* **2**: 293–323.

Hanson, R. (1997) *The Development of a Brief Actuarial Risk Scale for Sexual Offense Recidivism. (user report)* Ottawa: Department of the Solicitor General.

Hanson, R. & Harris, A. (1998) *Dynamic Predictors of Sexual Recidivism. (user report).* Ottawa: Department of the Solicitor General.

Hanson, R. & Thornton D. (2000) Improving risk assessments for sex offenders: a comparison of three actuarial scales. *Law and Human Behaviour* **24**: 119–136.

Hanson, R. K. & Thornton, D. (2003) Notes on the development of Static-2002. (Corrections Research User Report No. 2003–01.) Ottawa: Department of the Solicitor General of Canada.

Hare, R. (1991) *Manual for the Revised Psychopathy Checklist.* Toronto: Multihealth Systems.

Heilbrun, K., Marczyk, G. R., & DeMatteo, D. (2002) *Forensic Mental Health Assessment.* New York: Oxford University Press.

Johnson S. & Listiak, A. (1999) The measurement of sexual preference-a preliminary comparison of phallometry and the Abel assessment. *The Sex Offender* **3**(26): 1–19.

Kansas v. *Crane*, 534 US 407 (2002).

Kansas v. *Hendricks*, 521 US 346 (1997).

Kansas Statute 59–2946(f)(3).

Krueger, R., Bradford, J., & Glancy, G. (1998) Report from the Committee on Sex Offenders: The Abel Assessment for Sexual Interest – a brief description. *Journal of the American Academy of Psychiatry and the Law* **26**(2): 277–280.

Lake v. *Cameron*, 364 F.2d 657 (1966).

Langevin, R. & Paitich, D. (2005) *The Clarke Sexual History Questionnaire for Males – Revised.* Toronto: Multihealth Systems.

Langevin, R. & Watson, R. (1996) Major factors in the assessment of paraphilias and sex offenders. *Journal of Offender Rehabilitation* **23**: 39–70.

Lessard v. *Schmidt*, 349 F. Supp. 1078 (ED Wis. 1972).

Letourneau, E. J. (2002) A comparison of objective measures of sexual arousal and interest: visual reaction time and penile plethysmography. *Sexual Abuse: A Journal of Research and Treatment* **14**(3): 207–223.

Lidz, C. W., Mulvey, E. P., Appelbaum, P. S., & Cleveland, S. (1989) Commitment: the consistency of clinicians and the use of legal standards. *American Journal of Psychiatry* **146**: 176–181.

Lin, C. Y. (2003) Ethical Exploration of the least restrictive alternative. *Psychiatric Services* **54**: 866–870.

Massachusetts General Laws, Chapter 123.

Mauet, T. A. (2005) *Trials, Strategy, Skills, and the New Power of Persuasion.* New York: Aspen Publishers.

Miller, F. G. & Lazowski, L. E. (1999) *The Adult SASSI-3 Manual.* Springville, IN. The SASSI Institute.

Monahan, J, Steadman, H., Appelbaum, P. S., et al. (2005) *Classification of Violence Risk™ (COVR™).* Lutz, FL: Psychological Assessment Resources.

Mossman, D. (2006) Another look at interpreting risk categories. *Sexual Abuse: A Journal of Research and Treatment* **19**: 41–63.

Nevada Revised Statutes 433.164.

Norko, M. & Baranoski, M. (2005) The state of contemporary risk assessment. *Canadian Journal of Psychiatry* **50**: 18–26.

O'Connor v. *Donaldson*, 422 US 563 (1975).

Ohio Revised Code s. 5122.01(B)(4).

Pennsylvania Statutes s. 7310(b).

Pinals, D. A., Tillbrook, C. E., & Mumley, D. (2009) Violence risk assessment. In *Sex Offenders, Identification, Risk Assessment, Treatment, and Legal Issues*, ed. F. M. Saleh, A. J. Grudzinskas, Jr., J. M. Bradford, & D. J. Brodsky. New York: Oxford University Press.

Quinsey, V., Harris, G., Rice, M., & Cormier, C. (1998a)) *Violent Offenders: Appraising and Managing Risk.* Washington, DC: American Psychological Association.

Quinsey, V., Khanna, A., & Malcolm, P. (1998b) A retrospective evaluation of the regional treatment sex offender treatment program. *Journal of Interpersonal Violence* **13**: 621–624.

Scott, L. (1994) Sex offenders. In *Critical Issues in Crime and Justice*, ed. A. Roberts. Thousand Oaks, CA: Sage Publications, pp. 61–76.

Selzer, M. (1971) The Michigan Alcohol Screening Test: The quest for a new diagnostic instrument. *American Journal of Psychiatry* **127**: 1653–1658.

Skinner, M. (1982) *Drug Abuse Screening Test (DAST-20).* Toronto, ON: CAMPH Publications.

South Carolina Code 44–17–580(A)(1).

Specht v. *Patterson*, 386 US 605 (1967).

Sreenivasan, H., Kirkish, P., Garrick, T., Wineberger, L., & Phenix, A. (2000) Actuarial risk assessment models: a review of critical issues related to violence and sex offender recidivism assessments. *Journal of the American Academy of Psychiatry and the Law* **28**: 438–448.

Stone, A. A. (1984) *Law, Psychiatry, and Morality.* Washington, DC: American Psychiatric Press, Inc.

Strasburger, L. H., Gutheil, T. G., & Brodsky, A. (1997) On wearing two hats: role conflict in serving as both psychotherapist and expert witness. *American Journal of Psychiatry* **154**: 448–456.

Texas Rules of Evidence S. 509(e) (6).

Thatcher, B. T. & Mossman, D. (2009) Testifying for civil commitment: helping unwilling patients get treatment they need. *Current Psychiatry* **8**: 51–55.

Vincent, G. M., Maney, S. M., & Hart, S. D. (2009) The use of actuarial risk assessment instruments in sex offenders. In *Sex Offenders, Identification, Risk Assessment, Treatment, and Legal Issues* ed. F. M. Saleh, A. J. Grudzinskas, Jr., J. M. Bradford, & D. J. Brodsky. New York: Oxford University Press, pp. 70–89.

Washington Code 71.09.010 et seq. (1990).

Webster, C. D., Douglas, K. S., Eaves, D., & Hart, S. D. (1997) *HCR-20: Assessing Risk for Violence (Version 2).* Burnaby, BC, Canada: Mental Health, Law, and Policy Institute, Simon Fraser University.

In re Young & Cunningham, 857 P.2d 989 (1993).

Zonana, H. (1999) Dangerous Sex Offenders. A Task Force Report of the American Psychiatric Association. Washington DC: American Psychiatric Association.

Zonana, H. (2000) Sex offender testimony: Junk science of unethical testimony. *Journal American Academy Psychiatry and the Law* **28**: 386–388.

Competency to practice and licensing

Jeffrey S. Janofsky

11.1 Introduction

A physician's ability to practice medicine in the United States is regulated by each state's Medical Practice Act. The Act establishes a State Medical Board to implement the Act's requirements. All Boards have physician and lay members. The Federation of State Medical Boards published *A Guide to the Essentials of a Modern Medical and Osteopathic Practice Act* (henceforth, the *Guide*) in 2009. This includes requirements for licensure (including training, examinations, and continuing education), grounds and procedures for professional discipline and measures for dealing with incompetent physicians.

The *Guide* defines competence as, "possessing the requisite abilities and qualities (cognitive, non-cognitive and communicative) to perform effectively within the scope of the physician's practice while adhering to professional ethical standards (2009, p. 5)." Physicians may become incompetent to practice because of impairment or "dyscompetence." Impairment in this context means the inability to practice medicine with reasonable skill and safety due to:

1. mental, psychological or psychiatric illness, disease or deficit;
2. physical illness or condition, including, but not limited to, those illnesses or conditions that would adversely affect cognitive, motor or perceptive skills; or
3. habitual, excessive or illegal use or abuse of drugs defined by law as controlled substances, illegal drugs or alcohol or of other impairing substances (2009, p. 5).

Dyscompetence means, "failing to maintain acceptable standards of one or more areas of the physician's practice."

Physician sexual misconduct with patients is regarded as a special case of physician incompetence. Prior to publishing the *Guide*, the Federation of State Medical Boards had issued separate guidelines to help state Medical Boards deal with sexual misconduct cases (2006). These define sexual misconduct as, "behavior that exploits the physician–patient relationship in a sexual way," and subdivide physician sexual misconduct into sexual impropriety and sexual violations. Sexual impropriety is comprised of physician "behavior, gestures, or expressions that are seductive, sexually disrespectful of patient privacy, or sexually demeaning to a patient" (2006, p. 2). Sexual violations include "physical sexual contact between a physician and patient, whether or not initiated by the patient, and engaging in any conduct with a patient that is sexual or may be reasonably interpreted as sexual" (2006,

The Psychiatric Report, ed. Alec Buchanan and Michael A. Norko. Published by Cambridge University Press. © Cambridge University Press 2011.

p. 3). Both may be the basis for disciplinary action by a State Medical Board if the Board, "determines that the behavior exploited the physician–patient relationship."

The Council of the Ethical and Judicial Affairs (CEJA) of the American Medical Association prohibits sexual contact with current patients and notes that, "sexual or romantic relationships with former patients are unethical if the physician uses or exploits trust, knowledge, emotions, or influence derived from the previous professional relationship" (2009). The current American Psychiatric Association ethics code explicitly prohibits psychiatrist "sexual activity with a current or former patient" (2009, Section 2.1).

The *Guide* lists 53 potential grounds for disciplinary action (2009, pp. 16–19). Most do not require the participation of a psychiatrist. Disciplinary grounds that might require a psychiatric report include:

1. failure to meet appropriate standards of quality medical and surgical care or failure to keep adequate medical records;
2. giving false or fraudulent testimony in the practice of medicine;
3. being found mentally incompetent by a court of competent jurisdiction;
4. being physically or mentally unable to engage in the practice of medicine;
5. commission of an act of sexual misconduct or other conduct which violates a patient's trust or professional boundaries;
6. habitual or excessive use of drugs or alcohol that impair ability;
7. disruptive behavior that interferes with patient care; and
8. failure to cooperate with a lawful investigation conducted by the Board.

Psychiatrists may be asked to provide treatment for physicians as a condition of continued practice after a finding of impairment or after referral from an impaired physician program (Federation of State Medical Boards of the United States, Inc 1995).

Physicians who practice in hospitals and other health care organizations are further regulated by medical staff bylaws that are, in turn, governed in part by Joint Commission and other oversight body requirements (Joint Commission 2008, Sec. MS.09.01.01). The Joint Commission is an independent standards setting organization that evaluates and accredits health care organizations (Joint Commission 2010). Like Medical Practice Acts, medical staff bylaws require that physicians practice competently. Medical Practice Acts and Medical Staff Bylaws require that physicians who are suspected of impairment submit to professional evaluation as a condition of continued practice, and physicians who are suspected of dyscompetence undergo practice reviews. This chapter discusses the writing of reports subsequent to a psychiatric evaluation or review.

11.2 Special considerations in conducting the evaluation and writing the report on competency to practice and licensing

11.2.1 Agency

Evaluating psychiatrists may be retained by the Board of Medicine, a Health Care Organization (HCO), or the respondent physician's attorney. Sometimes physicians responding to a complaint attempt to retain the psychiatrist evaluator directly. Such direct retention should usually be avoided. Attorneys can help to clarify with the retained psychiatrist what questions are to be answered and can be useful intermediaries if the evaluating psychiatrist's findings are not helpful to the physician (Johnston 1996; Brent 2002).

Before beginning the evaluation, the evaluating psychiatrist must know to whom a duty is owed and the limits of confidentiality. The duties of psychiatrists retained by a Board to conduct an evaluation are usually contained in the state's Medical Practice Act, and may include duties to maintain confidentiality and qualified immunity if acting in good faith. Some Boards of Medicine require the physician respondent to pay for the cost of the evaluation. Other Boards pay the psychiatrist evaluator directly. Such issues should be clearly delineated in the retention letter between the evaluating psychiatrist and the Board, and should be explained to the physician evaluee prior to the start of the evaluation.

Rules surrounding evaluation of physicians for HCOs are generally less clear. Psychiatrist evaluators should ideally be retained by an attorney representing the HCO, rather than directly by the organization. The attorney is usually in a better position to ensure that all confidentiality- and employment-related rules are followed. Restrictions on the amount of time that may be spent in an evaluation, the number and kind of collaterals contacted, and additional psychological testing may all have been negotiated between the HCO and the responding physician's attorney prior to the evaluating psychiatrist's retention. It should also be clarified to whom the report will be released. Such restrictions should be carefully reviewed by the evaluating psychiatrist and agreed to or modified before the psychiatrist accepts to undertake the evaluation. Any restrictions should be clearly delineated in the report.

Psychiatrists hired by the physician's attorney owe a duty to communicate data and opinions completely and honestly to the attorney. In some jurisdictions, the opinions of defense experts in civil cases are covered under the attorney–client privilege (*Sowders* v. *Lewis*). This means that if the psychiatrist's opinions are not used by the defense, they are not discoverable. In such situations the defense attorney may ask the evaluating psychiatrist not to write a report and the findings will not be discoverable by the Board of Medicine. In other jurisdictions, no attorney–client privilege applies to information or facts acquired by attorneys from non-client sources in civil matters (*Granger* v. *Wisner*). Furthermore, the *Guide* requires every physician with evidence that another physician is incompetent or unfit to practice to report the evidence to the Board (2009, Sec. IX, 31). The evaluating psychiatrist should clarify whether privilege protects the information obtained during the evaluation and whether the attorney has clarified this with the physician being evaluated.

11.2.2 Physician impairment

The American Medical Association's ethics opinions note that physicians have a responsibility to maintain their own health and that, "when failing physical or mental health reaches the point of interfering with a physician's ability to engage safely in professional activities, the physician is said to be impaired" (2009, p. 597). Physician impairment evaluations are a subset of fitness for duty evaluations. The American Academy of Psychiatry and the Law has published a Practice Guideline (Gold et al. 2008, S40–S45) and the American Psychiatric Association has published a Resource Document (Anfang et al. 2005). Both contain recommendations for performing physician impairment evaluations.

Impairment evaluations requested by HCOs generally occur when there is suspicion that a psychiatric or medical disorder has affected a staff physician's behavior or performance, and that suspicion is not clear enough to warrant an immediate suspension of hospital privileges. Such a suspension of privileges would trigger an automatic referral to the Board of Medicine. The HCO should provide the evaluating psychiatrist with all quality assurance and risk management data regarding the alleged impaired physician, not just data surrounding the most recent event. The database the HCO can provide the evaluating psychiatrist may be relatively limited compared with a Board of Medicine, as the HCO lacks subpoena power and cannot compel participation of anyone outside of hospital employees or medical staff.

The psychiatrist evaluator should consider directly contacting any hospital staff members who witnessed any problematic behaviors. Care should be taken before contacting any of the physician's economic competitors, as the data that they provide may be biased, and they may misuse the knowledge that their colleague is being investigated. Patients who may have witnessed problematic behaviors should not be contacted. Instead, any written patient complaints made to the HCO about the physician should be considered.

Board of Medicine physician impairment evaluations may be triggered after a patient complaint, a suspension or revocation of hospital privileges, a referral by another physician, an arrest, or the physician's own disclosure on a licensing application or renewal of a physical or mental condition that might impair the ability to practice medicine. The physician's own atypical behavior towards Board of Medicine investigators after being notified of a Board complaint might also result in an impairment evaluation request. Board of Medicine investigators may have interviewed the physician and may have their own direct concerns regarding the physician's medical or psychiatric condition.

Some states refer cases of alleged physician impairment to a Committee on Physician Impairment, usually run in cooperation with the state's Medical Society. The Committee evaluates the physician, makes recommendation for management including a treatment contract, and monitors the physician (Bloom et al. 1991; McIntyre & Hamolsky 1994). Other states retain independent physician evaluators.

Some states divert from discipline respondent physicians who are impaired, who cooperate with the Board contract and treatment plan, and for whom there is no corresponding standard of care complaint. If the respondent physician follows the contract and recovers, the disciplinary file is closed without a sanction. Other State Boards of Physicians suspend the impaired physician's license and then either immediately stay the order and place the impaired physician on probation with conditions or suspend the physician without a stay (Dorsey & Scheer 1987). The burden is then placed on the physician to obtain treatment and show recovery before the sanction is lifted, sometimes with the help of an impaired physician's program sponsored by the State Medical Society (Krebs-Markrich & Perrine 1996).

Before meeting with the alleged impaired physician, psychiatrist evaluators should familiarize themselves with all background material including, in Board cases, material collected by Board of Medicine staff. Summaries or transcripts of interviews with collateral informants should be reviewed prior to any evaluation. Medical and psychiatric treatment records should be reviewed as well. Respondent physicians will be ordered by the Medical Board to comply with the psychiatric impairment evaluation. Although an authorization for the release of independent medical evaluation in connection with legal proceedings is only required for covered entities under HIPAA, the authorization is a useful tool for clarifying agency and confidentiality for all impairment evaluators. A sample authorization form is provided in Figure 11.1.

Physicians forced to undergo psychiatric evaluations may find such evaluations "particularly upsetting and threatening acts" (Murray 1993). Physicians may also be under financial stress as most malpractice policies do not cover costs for defending against Board of

AUTHORIZATION FOR RELEASE OF HEALTH INFORMATION AND INDEPENDENT MEDICAL EVALUATION IN CONNECTION WITH LEGAL PROCEEDINGS

All items on this authorization must be completed or the request will not be honored. Use "N/A" if not applicable.

Name: _____
           (first)   (m. initial)   (last)

Address: _____
                              (street address)

_____
        (city)   (state)   (zip code)

Phone #: _____ Birth Date: _____

I understand that certain health information about me is to be provided to, or I am to be evaluated by:

_____

(insert name of physician evaluator)

for the purpose of conducting a medical evaluation in connection with a legal matter in which I am involved. (Such a medical evaluation is sometimes called an "independent medical evaluation," or a "defense medical evaluation" or a "plaintiff's medical evaluation," depending upon who has requested that it be done. Such a medical evaluation does not establish a doctor-patient relationship.)

For this authorization, "My Health Information" means information obtained during the evaluation of me or of the health information provided, including but not limited to, neuropsychological test results; physical examinations; history learned from records, questionnaires, and interviews (including any transcript of the interview); and _____

_____;

and includes any analyses and evaluations related to those items.

My Health Information includes the following, if initialed by me:

_____ audio recording of the evaluation   _____ video recording of the evaluation.

I authorize the physician named above. to provide My Health Information to: _____
                                                             (name)

_____ ("Recipient") upon completion of the evaluation.
                    (address)

This authorization may be revoked until My Health Information is provided by the physician named above, or until my evaluation has begun. Once that physician receives My Health Information or my evaluation has begun, the physician is authorized to provide the analyses and evaluation to Recipient.

I understand that once My Health Information is disclosed as requested in this authorization My Health Information may no longer be protected by federal and state privacy laws and potentially may be re-disclosed by the person who is receiving my information.

I understand that the independent medical evaluation may not be performed unless I sign this authorization.

I am entitled to receive a copy of this authorization from the person who asks me to sign it.

By signing this authorization, I understand that medical records released may contain information related to HIV status, AIDS, sexually transmitted diseases, mental health, and drug and alcohol abuse.

Signature of Patient only:	_____	Date:	_____

Modified from a form used at the Johns Hopkins Hospital. (used with permission)

Figure 11.1 Authorization for release of health information.

Medicine Actions. The psychiatric evaluator should take such situational stressors into consideration when performing the impairment evaluation.

11.2.3 Physician dyscompetence

Medical Boards are authorized to discipline physicians who fail to meet appropriate standards of medical care or who fail to keep appropriate medical records. Questions about standard of care violations usually arise after a patient complains to the Board and the Board has completed a preliminary investigation. Board investigators may speak to the complainant, ask the physician for a response, and review treatment records. Many complaints are resolved at this stage.

Medical Boards may hire physician peer reviewers in order to establish a standard of care violation. Some Boards of Medicine contract with state medical societies or independent peer review agencies. Others contract with physicians independently. Peer reviewers must be in the same specialty or subspecialty as the physician. Before agreeing to perform a peer review, the potential peer reviewer should be sure they are licensed in the same state as the respondent physician, and have experience treating patients in similar age groups as the complainant, with similar diagnoses and with similar treatment modalities.

Peer reviewers should avoid conflicts of interest before agreeing to perform a review. Peer reviewers should not have personal or professional relationships with the physician under review, the patients whose cases are reviewed, or the complainant. Particular attention should be paid to avoiding reviewing the medical care provided by or to friends, family members, economic partners, or competitors.

Peer reviewers should review all of the relevant medical records, the complaint, the response to the complaint, and if available, investigative reports and depositions. Some Medical Practice Acts allow peer reviewers to directly contact the complainant/patient or the physician being reviewed. The peer reviewer should clarify with the referring Board whether such direct contact is permissible. Peer reviewers act as agents of the Medical Board. They must hold all records reviewed and data collected in the strictest confidence, and maintain all confidentiality provisions of their peer review contract. Failure to maintain confidentiality may cause the peer reviewer to lose qualified immunity or indemnification provided by the state's Medical Practice Act or peer review contract.

A Medical Board may ask a peer reviewer to also perform a practice review. In these cases the peer reviewer is asked to review either a random sample of the physician's charts, charts from a particular time period, or charts with specific diagnoses or treatment regimes. The practice review initially focuses on potential problems generated by the initial complaint. The practice review may discover additional standard of care violations. Because the patients in a practice review are not aware that their charts are being reviewed, they should not be contacted by the reviewing physician.

11.2.4 Assessment of physician accused of sexual misconduct

The role of the psychiatrist evaluator in Board of Medicine sexual misconduct cases is usually limited to providing insight into psychological factors that led to the sexual misconduct and for opining on a respondent physician's rehabilitation potential. Future risk to the public and ways of minimizing those risk factors should also be assessed by the psychiatric evaluator.

Forty-four percent of physicians disciplined for sex-related offenses will surrender their medical licenses or have them revoked. The remainder will have their licenses suspended or be placed on probation or a less serious action (Dehlendorf & Wolfe 1998). Besides the usual psychiatric history and mental status evaluation, the psychiatric report for a physician accused of sexual misconduct should include a detailed sexual history, including considering the presence of paraphilias. Interviews with the respondent physician's prior sexual partners may be indicated. Assessment of the presence of narcissistic and antisocial personality traits or disorder, thorough history taking, and psychological testing is essential.

Gabbard (1994) found that most therapists who transgress sexual boundaries suffer from either a psychotic disorder or major mood disorder; predatory psychopathy and paraphilia; lovesickness; or masochistic surrender. Such a typology is useful for categorizing non-psychiatrist physicians as well. Therapists suffering from psychotic or major mood disorders become sexually involved with patients as a direct result of their symptomatology. These therapists' potential for rehabilitation and risk factors for recurrence turn directly on the treatability of the underlying illness.

Gabbard's predatory psychopaths usually demonstrate other signs of antisocial or narcissistic personality disorders. He includes in this category therapists with paraphilia "who act on their paraphilic impulses with patients under their care (1994, p. 126)." They are master manipulators who may pretend to be remorseful, regard patients as mere objects, and are refractory to treatment.

Therapists who suffer from lovesickness believe they are actually in love with their patients. Some of these therapists are not suffering from a diagnosable mental disorder but are suffering from psychosocial stressors caused by relationship difficulties. Others may be suffering from less severe narcissistic or borderline personality disorders. Gabbard believes these therapists are difficult to treat until their infatuation with their patient dissipates. At that point they may be amenable to insight-oriented psychotherapy.

Some therapists allow themselves to be tormented, intimidated, and controlled by their patient. The therapist becomes involved in ever worsening boundary violations with the patient as a way to prevent the patient from self-harming. Therapists suffering from such masochistic surrender "attempt to accommodate these demands, even though they know better" (Gabbard 1994, p. 132). Gabbard believes these therapists are remorseful and eager to receive therapy so that they will likely not repeat the boundary violation.

11.2.5 Treatment

A physician may accept ongoing psychiatric treatment and monitoring of that treatment as a condition of continued licensure or hospital staff membership. Aside from the usual purposes of psychiatric treatment, ongoing treatment allows for monitoring of psychiatric symptoms that may cause impairment. When a psychiatrist agrees to treat a physician patient under such circumstances the combined treatment and monitoring roles can complicate effective treatment and interfere with the usual psychiatrist–patient relationship (Strasburger et al. 1997).

In order to minimize treatment disruption the psychiatrist and physician-patient should agree in advance how many data about treatment should be routinely shared with the supervising agency (see Boxes 11.1 and 11.2).

Box 11.1 Sample letter for a physician who is doing well in treatment

Doctor Martin requested that I send you another letter regarding his psychiatric treatment with me.

Doctor Martin remains in treatment with me. He has been in treatment continuously from January 2006 to the present. His most recent visit was today, September 12, 2009. He now sees me every three months. His symptoms have remained in remission and he reports that he continues to do well in his practice.

Based on the data I have available, I see no current psychiatric impairment in Doctor Martin's ability to function as a physician. He continues to respond appropriately to psychotherapy and medications. He has no impairment in his ability to focus and render care to patients. He continues to do well.

Box 11.2 Sample letter for a physician who is having difficulty in treatment

I am writing to provide new information regarding Doctor Jones.

Doctor Jones remains in treatment with me. He has been in treatment continuously from March 2004 to the present. His most recent visit was today, after Doctor Jones had requested an emergency visit. Doctor Jones reported that he has had a recurrence of his symptoms of depression, similar in severity to the prior episode of depression that had occurred around the time he had first been brought to the attention of the Board. Doctor Jones agreed to be voluntarily admitted to a psychiatric hospital today. He notified his business partner of the hospitalization, and his partner agreed to cover his practice. I will see Doctor Jones once he is discharged from the hospital. At that time I will reassess whether Doctor Jones might be suffering from a psychiatric impairment that would affect his ability to function as a physician. Doctor Jones is aware of the contents of this letter.

The physician-patient must also be informed of the treating psychiatrist's responsibilities to inform the Board of Medicine if the physician is not compliant with treatment, or is exhibiting symptoms that could cause impairment in the ability to practice medicine. The physician or his attorney may have negotiated with the Board what and under what circumstances treatment data will be revealed to the Board. Agreed limits on what must be shared with the Board of Medicine should be confirmed with the Board prior to beginning treatment. Of course, if not comfortable with prior negotiated limits, the treating psychiatrist should feel free to not initiate a treatment relationship with the physician.

11.3 The report

The elements of the psychiatric report that were described in Chapter 7 and that warrant distinctive treatment in reports on physician impairment are shown in Box 11.3.

11.3.1 Impairment

(a) Introduction to the report

This section should contain, at a minimum, details of who requested the evaluation and what the evaluator was requested to do. Questions that psychiatrists may be asked to answer include:

Box 11.3 Topics warranting distinctive treatment in physician impairment reports

Table 7.1 Structure of the psychiatric report

1. **Preliminary and identifying information**

Section 11.3.1a ——————2. **Introduction**

Why the report is being written, the circumstances of the request and the questions that are being addressed

Dates and duration of interviews with the subject

Section 11.3.1c —————— Sources of information used in the report

Section 11.3.1b ————— Information given to the subject at time of interview, including information regarding confidentiality

List of appended material

3. **Body of report**

Section 11.3.1d ————— Background information

Section 11.3.1e ————— Current events (the crime in a sentencing report; the events leading to the claim in a civil action), the circumstances surrounding those events, and relevant sequelae

Section 11.3.1f ————— Findings on examination

Psychological and other test results

Section 11.3.1g —————4. **Opinion**

5. **Concluding material**

Signature of author

Name, qualifications, and current post

Date of signing

(1) whether another psychiatrist's treatment met the standard of care; or
(2) whether another physician is so impaired by a mental disorder that person cannot function competently as a physician.

The psychiatrist evaluators should clarify the question in consultation with the referrer, usually a State Medical Board, hospital, or doctor's attorney.

(b) Description of warning regarding confidentiality

The reporter should provide a description of informed consent and limits of confidentiality. An example is provided in Box 11.4.

Box 11.4 Sample description of warning regarding confidentiality

Prior to my evaluation of Doctor Jones, I informed him that I had been formally designated by the Board of Medicine as his evaluator. I also informed him that we were not forming a physician–patient relationship, that I was not undertaking to treat him and that anything he told me could be revealed in a report or in Court, as per the Board of Medicine regulations. Doctor Jones understood and agreed to proceed with the interview.

(c) Sources of information

The report author should list all data considered. Include the dates and total interview time spent with the physician. Summarize data collected by Board or HCO investigators through their direct interviews or depositions. Include other written data provided by the retaining attorney or agency, any written material provided by the physician, and any material that you obtained through medical records request or other means.

For interviews with collateral sources, the report should list all sources contacted and the time spent speaking with them. Record the relationships to the physician of the persons interviewed and indicate whether they are a colleague, supervisor, or economic competitor. For record reviews, if there are extensive medical, psychiatric or other data, it may be useful to record by date, source, and legal document pagination (or by Bates numbering) and then sort the data by date.

In contrast to impairment evaluations done for Boards of Medicine, evaluations done for HCOs may omit or summarize personal information not directly relevant to the impairment question. This is because a physician's colleagues or competitors on the medical staff may have eventual access to the report. If personal information is omitted or summarized, that fact should be clearly stated in the report (Anfang et al. 2005 p. 87).

(d) Background

In impairment reports, particular focus should be placed on educational, occupational, and past psychiatric and medical history. Family history can generally be brief. Be sure to include whether there is any family history of psychiatric illness. Consider including information regarding any family history of criminal behavior, substance abuse, or physical illness if relevant to the inquiry. Include any childhood developmental or behavioral difficulties, if relevant to the inquiry.

Educational history should be taken in detail, especially medical school, residency, and fellowship training. Document any academic difficulties, or academic awards and achievements. Ask the physician to account for all periods of time from college through fellowship. If education occurred outside the United States, ask the physician to explain training differences from the typical US training regime. If education was not continuous, ask for an explanation. Consider comparing what the physician reports to what they reported to the Board of Medicine when applying for licensure. If there were personal or academic difficulties during training, ask the physician for an explanation.

Describe pre-medical school employment and any outside employment during medical education. Describe all medically related employment post residency, including hospital practice, private practice, and research. Document any non-medically related employment. Document why the physician changed jobs, and whether there were employment difficulties. Contrast what the physician tells you with what other data sources reveal. Document number of marriages and children and whether the stress of a divorce or child custody proceeding is problematic and may be causing symptoms. Document all past criminal and civil actions, including past Board of Medicine and malpractice actions.

Document longitudinal and current use of alcohol, prescribed addictive drugs, and illicit drugs. Record signs and symptoms of dependence and impairment, as well as past treatment attempts. Ask the physician whether intoxication on any substance has ever affected their performance as a physician.

Document what the physician tells you about the presence of any acute or chronic medical conditions. If the physician is on medications, document who prescribes them. Ask whether the physician has a primary care physician, and when the last primary care visit occurred. Ask if the physician is self-prescribing, or whether the physician's group is prescribing medications for him or her. If there are only a few collateral medical treatment records they may be reviewed here. Otherwise they should be placed in a separate record review section below.

Document what the physician tells you about any past inpatient or outpatient psychiatric treatment history or history of prior impairment evaluations. Ask for the physician's understanding of the psychiatric diagnosis, psychotherapeutic and pharmacological treatment, and goals for treatment. Review collateral psychiatric treatment records here, or in a separate record review section.

(e) Current events/circumstances

Summarize allegations contained in the Board of Medicine or HCO referral. Describe in detail the physician's response to the allegations that generated the current Board or HCO action. Include both open-ended responses and responses to specific allegations of problematic behaviors.

(f) Examination findings

The usual elements should be included. Screens for cognitive impairment such as the Mini-Mental Status Examination (Folstein et al. 1975) should be recorded here, as well as any screening tests for executive functioning.

Some evaluators administer a personality inventory such as the MMPI, PAI, or MCMI and rely on the results to complement the data collected from collaterals or direct interview (Meyer & Price 2006). If possible cognitive impairment is a major issue in the case, the physician respondent should be referred to a neuropsychologist for neuropsychological testing, unless the evaluating psychiatrist is also trained to complete such testing. Data from such sources should be summarized.

(g) Conclusions and recommendations

The Opinion section should provide a summary of the database and a psychiatric diagnosis. Past and current episodes of impairment should be documented. Risk of future impairment should be addressed. If possible, how psychiatric impairments affected competency to practice medicine in the past and how the impairments might affect the evaluee's competency to practice medicine in the future should be addressed. Recommendations for treatment, if indicated, and how treatment might mitigate impairment should also be provided.

11.3.2 Dyscompetence

In dyscompetence assessments, the report generated by the peer reviewer should show that the reviewer understands the background of the complaint and of the medical treatment at issue. The reviewer should state what standard of care is required in the matter at hand, and whether the care actually rendered by the physician under review met that standard. The peer reviewer should outline the basis for the reviewer's opinion as to why the standard of care was met or not met in each case. The peer reviewer should also detail whether the physician's documentation was adequate, and if not, why not. These considerations also apply to a report on the cases covered by a practice review.

11.4 Conclusions

Boards of Medicine are charged with attempting to insure that physicians practicing in their state have the necessary knowledge base to practice competently, and are not suffering from psychiatric or medical disorders that might impair their ability to practice. Psychiatrists retained by the Board of Medicine to act as peer reviewer are asked to assess whether a psychiatrist is practicing at or below the standard of care. Forensic psychiatrist evaluators may be asked to perform an independent medical evaluation about a physician to assess whether this physician is impaired by any mental disorder that might affect their ability to practice medicine competently. Psychiatrists may also be asked to treat physicians with psychiatric impairments and make periodic reports to the Boards of Medicine regarding the physician's continued competency to practice. Finally forensic psychiatrist to evaluators may be asked to assess a physician who has been accused of sexual misconduct, to look at potential mitigating or aggravating factors.

All such evaluations may be particularly difficult for the physician respondent, who may be defensive about possible impairment and embarrassed to be accused of incompetence to practice medicine. Physician respondents may feel particularly intimidated because unlike usual fitness for duty evaluations, Board of Medicine competency evaluations are initiated by state agencies with large budgets and the ability to compel testimony and record releases. Psychiatrists performing such evaluations must be particularly careful to clarify agency relationships with the physician being evaluated, particularly if the physician is asked to fund the costs of the evaluation and the evaluating psychiatrist is actually working for the Board of Medicine or HCO and not for the physician. Psychiatrists performing physician evaluations do a public service both by protecting the public from dyscompetent and impaired physicians, but also by protecting falsely accused physicians.

References

American Medical Association (2009) *Principles of Medical Ethics: E-9.0305 Physician Health and Wellness*. Available: http://www.ama-assn.org/ad-com/polfind/Hlth-Ethics.pdf [Accessed August 2, 2009].

American Psychiatric Association (2009) *The Principles of Medical Ethics With Annotations Especially Applicable to Psychiatry*. Available: http://www.psych. org/MainMenu/PsychiatricPractice/ Ethics/ResourcesStandards/ PrinciplesofMedicalEthics.aspx [Accessed August 13, 2009].

Anfang, S. A., Faulkner, L. R., Fromson, J. A., & Gendel, M. H. (2005) The American Psychiatric Association's Resource Document on Guidelines for Psychiatric Fitness-for-Duty Evaluations of Physicians. *Journal of the American Academy of Psychiatry and the Law* **33**(1): 85–88.

Bloom, J. D., Resnick, M., Ulwelling, J. J., et al. (1991) Psychiatric consultation to a state board of medical examiners. *American Journal of Psychiatry* **148**(10): 1366–1370.

Brent, N. J. (2002) Protecting physicians' rights in disciplinary actions by a medical board: A brief primer. *Journal of Medical Practice Management: MPM* **18**(2): 97–100.

Council on Ethical and Judicial Affairs (2009) *E-8.14 Sexual Misconduct in the Practice of Medicine*. Chicago, IL: American Medical Association.

Dehlendorf, C. E. & Wolfe, S. M. (1998) Physicians disciplined for sex-related offenses. *JAMA: The Journal of the American Medical Association* **279**(23): 1883–1888.

Dorsey, D. M. & Scheer, R. (1987) Licensing boards and impaired professionals. *Maryland Medical Journal* **36**(3): 238–240.

Federation of State Medical Boards of the United States, Inc (1995) Report of the Ad Hoc Committee on Physician Impairment. Available: http://www.fsmb.org/pdf/1995_ grpol_Physician_Impairment.pdf [Accessed August 23, 2009].

Federation of State Medical Boards of the United States, Inc (2006) Addressing Sexual Boundaries: Guidelines for State Medical Boards. Available: http://www.fsmb.org/pdf/ GRPOL_Sexual%20Boundaries.pdf [Accessed August 13, 2009].

Federation of State Medical Boards of the United States, Inc (2009) A Guide to the Essentials of a Modern Medical and Osteopathic Practice Act. Available: http://www.fsmb.org/pdf/GRPOL_essentials.pdf [Accessed August 23, 2009].

Folstein, M. F., Folstein, S. E., & McHugh, P. R. (1975) "Mini-mental state". a practical method for grading the cognitive state of patients for the clinician. *Journal of Psychiatric Research* **12**(3): 189–198.

Gabbard, G. O. (1994) Psychotherapists who transgress sexual boundaries with patients. *Bulletin of the Menninger Clinic* **58**(1): 124–135.

Gold, L. H., Anfang, S. A., Drukteinis, A. M., et al. (2008) AAPL Practice Guideline for the Forensic Evaluation of Psychiatric Disability. *Journal of the American Academy of Psychiatry and the Law* **36** (Suppl.): S3–50.

Granger v. *Wisner*, 134 Ariz. 377, 656 P.2d 1238 (Ariz. 1982).

Johnston, M. E. (1996) "When the board comes a'callin". *Journal of the Tennessee Medical Association* **89**(2) 54–55.

Joint Commission (2008) 2009 Comprehensive Accreditation Manual for Hospitals: The Official Handbook (CAMH). Joint Commission Resources.

Joint Commission (2010) *Accreditation Process Overview*. Available: http://www.jointcommission.org/assets/1/6/Accreditation%20Process%20Overview%2012%20091.PDF [Accessed February 2, 2011].

Krebs-Markrich, J. & Perrine, K. W. (1996) Defending the impaired physician. *Virginia Medical Quarterly: VMQ* **123**(4 Suppl.): 14–16.

McIntyre, B. W. & Hamolsky, M. W. (1994) The impaired physician and the role of the Board of Medical Licensure and Discipline. *Rhode Island Medicine* **77**(10): 357–358.

Meyer, D. J. & Price, M. (2006) Forensic psychiatric assessments of behaviorally disruptive physicians. *Journal of the American Academy of Psychiatry and the Law* **34**(1): 72–81.

Murray, M. J. (1993) Are you ready for an encounter with the board of medical practice? *Minnesota Medicine* **76**(5): 11–12.

Sowders v. *Lewis*, 241 S.W.3d 319 (Ken. 2007).

Strasburger, L. H., Gutheil, T. G., & Brodsky, A. (1997) On wearing two hats: role conflict in serving as both psychotherapist and expert witness. *American Journal of Psychiatry* **154**(4): 448–456.

Chapter

12

Child custody

Peter Ash

12.1 Introduction

Child custody evaluations are more complex than almost all other forensic evaluations. Most forensic evaluations focus on one person. An evaluator in a child custody case needs to typically assess each parent, each child, and potentially other caretakers such as new spouses. Not only does each of those people need to be assessed as an individual, the interactions among all of those people also need to be assessed. Such evaluations garner a great amount of data: a relatively straightforward pre-divorce custody evaluation involving only two parents and one child is likely to involve a minimum of 9 hours of interviews, several additional hours of document review and telephone calls with collateral sources, and time devoted to psychological testing. Cases that involve step-parents, many children, allegations of sexual abuse, or other complicating factors can easily double those numbers. Synthesizing all the relevant information obtained into a report that contains conclusions and recommendations that will appear reasonable to the parties involved, their lawyers, and the judge, is a major task.

This chapter will focus primarily on reports on child custody evaluations in the context of divorce. Child custody may arise in abuse/neglect cases, and reports for such cases will be treated as a variation of the custody report near the end of this chapter. Evaluations of visitation or access will likewise be treated as a variation. The chapter will focus on the report, and is not a manual on how to conduct a child custody evaluation. The reader interested in custody evaluation techniques may wish to read some of the professional organizations' published standards for such evaluations (see American Academy of Child & Adolescent Psychiatry [Herman S. P. principal author] 1997; American Psychological Association Committee on Professional Practice and Standards (COPPS) 1994; Association of Family and Conciliation Courts Task Force 2007) or explore the extensive literature on conducting such evaluations (see, for example, Bow & Quinnell 2001; Bernet 2002; Galatzer-Levy & Kraus 2009; Ludolph 2009).

12.2 Special considerations in the conduct of the evaluation

12.2.1 The legal test: best interests of the child

Public policy is oriented towards encouraging divorcing parents to develop their own parenting plans for their children. Policies such as mandatory parent education when parents file for divorce or mediation of divorce disputes have this goal in mind. Custody evaluations are

The Psychiatric Report, ed. Alec Buchanan and Michael A. Norko. Published by Cambridge University Press. © Cambridge University Press 2011.

referred to mental health professionals after parents fail to make their own plan. The "best interests of the child" is the general test utilized in child custody decisions. However, the way that test is applied varies widely depending on the laws and precedents of the jurisdiction and the nature of the case.

"Best interests of the child," by itself, is a vague test. While some state statutes simply say that custody is to be decided in the best interests of the child, many state statutes give some guidance as to how that term is to be interpreted. Michigan was the first state to adopt a statute that explicitly listed factors, originally 11 of them, that comprised the child's best interests (for current law, see Michigan Child Custody Act 1993). Michigan judges need to make findings under each of the enumerated factors when they issue a custody decision. The Uniform Marriage and Divorce Act (1987), which has been adopted by many states, lists five broad factors: (1) the wishes of the parents; (2) the wishes of the child; (3) "the interaction and interrelationship of the child with his parent or parents, his siblings, and any other person who may significantly affect the child's best interest"; (4) "the child's adjustment to his home, school and community"; and (5) "the mental and physical health of all individuals involved."

In states that do provide some statutory guidance, it is useful for the report to address each of the statutory factors (see Opinions section, below), although courts are also allowed to consider other factors they deem important. Jurisdictions also vary in their definitions of terms (such as shared or joint custody), legal presumptions regarding standard of proof (e.g., in some states an "established custodial environment" may only be changed if there is clear and convincing evidence), presumptions regarding joint custody or grandparent visitation, and the weight to be given to a child's or adolescent's preference. The United States Commission on Child and Family Welfare (1996) recommended that courts focus on "parenting plans" rather than "joint custody," and some states have changed their statutes in accord with this principle. Evaluators need to be aware of the details of the applicable custody law and appropriate legal terms when formulating their opinions.

12.2.2 Nature of the case

The most straightforward situation is a pre-divorce case involving two parents who are contesting custody and visitation in which both parents start on legally equal footing. In some cases, non-parents may be involved, such as grandparents or foster parents, whose standing is typically less than that of a natural parent. Post-divorce disputes may raise different legal standards, depending on the weight given to an already established custodial environment. Some states have statutes that give grandparents specific rights to visitation. Cases involving allegations of sexual abuse may implicate child abuse law or criminal statutes. Such complicating factors affect both the nature of the evaluative process and the reasoning utilized in formulating opinions, and so shape the nature of the report.

12.2.3 Evaluator status and evaluator approach

There is a general consensus that the best position for an evaluator in a custody case is to be either appointed by the court or stipulated to by the attorneys or parties, rather than working solely for one side. Such a position defines the evaluator as not beholden to one side, and so reduces bias and, in principle, allows the evaluator to focus impartially on the children's best interests. In addition to reducing evaluator bias, a position of neutrality between the parents decreases the likelihood that the competing parties will see the evaluator as biased for or against them. A perception of bias by one party is likely to affect that party's cooperation with the evaluation and the way in which the party presents data. Finally, being the evaluator by court order will give the evaluator quasi-judicial immunity in many jurisdictions, which may protect the evaluator in the event of a later complaint by one party about how the evaluation was conducted.

However, there are times when an evaluator does enter a case at the request of only one party. Such a role generally calls for explicit discussion in the report, and, if the role also restricts who is interviewed, necessitates discussing the resulting limitations in the opinion. This chapter will generally assume that the evaluation is court-ordered, and indicate some of the places where the report needs to be modified if the evaluator's status is not court-ordered.

In addition to their explicit role in the process described above, evaluators vary in how they conceptualize their function. For example, some evaluators see their role as simply providing data and recommendations for the court to consider in reaching a decision. Since most custody cases settle prior to trial, others see the evaluation as part of a bargaining process that may result in a court imposing a decision, but more often provides information that affects the bargaining between the parties and their attorneys (Ash & Guyer 1986), and so the functional audience for the report becomes the attorneys. Some see the evaluation as overlapping with mediation and arbitration, and some take this so far as to see their role as actively negotiating a settlement and rarely even write a report. All of these variations affect the style of the report.

Finally, there are stylistic variations, both in how evaluators conduct evaluations (such as the extent to which they utilize psychological testing) and how they write about what they do. Many evaluators adopt an educational tone in their report in those sections where they are discussing how concepts of child development affect the case. Given the number of people evaluated and the multiplicity of relationships involved, one would expect considerable variation. In preparation for writing this chapter, a number of experts from diverse training backgrounds provided sample reports (see Acknowledgements at the end of the chapter), and the commonalities among reports were impressive. Bow and Quinnell (2002), in a study of psychologists' custody reports, also found many commonalities.

12.3 The report

The elements of the psychiatric report that were described in Chapter 7 and that warrant distinctive treatment in reports on child custody are shown in Box 12.1.

12.3.1 Introduction to report

As with most forensic reports, the introduction sets forth the circumstances of the referral, referencing the court order, if one was issued, and the general nature of the case, along the lines of:

> This child custody evaluation was conducted pursuant to an *Order for Evaluation* issued by the Honorable ＿＿ of the ＿＿ County Court on ＿＿, and arises out of an action for divorce between [parent or other party name] and [other party name]. The custody issue involves the parties' minor children: ＿＿ (d.o.b. ＿＿) and ＿＿＿ (d.o.b.＿＿). The court order specified that the issues to be addressed are … The children are currently [list current legal and actual arrangements] …

Box 12.1 Topics warranting distinctive treatment in child custody reports

Table 7.1 Structure of the psychiatric report

1. **Preliminary and identifying information**

Section 12.3.1 ——— 2. **Introduction**

Why the report is being written, the circumstances of the request and the questions that are being addressed

Dates and duration of interviews with the subject

Section 12.3.2 ——— Sources of information used in the report

Section 12.3.3 ——— Information given to the subject at time of interview, including information regarding confidentiality

List of appended material

3. **Body of report**

Section 12.3.4 ——— Background information

Current events (the crime in a sentencing report; the events leading to the claim in a civil action), the circumstances surrounding those events, and relevant sequelae

Section 12.3.5 ——— Findings on examination

Psychological and other test results

Section 12.3.6 ——— 4. **Opinion**

5. **Concluding material**

Signature of author

Name, qualifications, and current post

Date of signing

12.3.2 Description of warnings regarding confidentiality

As with all forensic evaluations, it is important to document what the parents and children were told about the nature of the evaluation, the role of the evaluator (including that the evaluator is not providing treatment), to whom the report is being sent, and limitations on confidentiality. It is recommended that parents and children be told that they have the right to refuse to answer any question and the right to refuse to give consent to see outside records. The parties' consent to participate in the evaluation should be noted. While children are usually not deemed competent to give legal consent, it is important for the evaluator to discuss the nature of the evaluation with them in a manner appropriate to their development and to pay special attention to not coercing them to provide information they are not comfortable providing.

12.3.3 Sources of information

The report should list all sources of information. Each type of interview should be itemized, noting who conducted the interview, where and when the interview took place, who (including what combination of people) was interviewed, and the duration of each interview. Other sources should also be listed, including records reviewed (clinical, legal, and school), questionnaires or psychological tests given, telephone interviews of collateral sources, etc.

If there are important limitations to the sources of information, they should be explicitly stated. For example, if one party was not interviewed because of a refusal to cooperate or for other reasons, the lack of that information should be made explicit and some statement made about how that limits the conclusions that can be made from the available data. Many of the published standards for custody evaluations and some ethics codes specify that a custody evaluator should not make comparisons about whom the child would do better with if one of the parties has not been evaluated.

Because custody evaluations related to divorce involve multiple people, a great deal of information is obtained. Not all of that information is put into the report. The information may not be relevant to the issue at hand. Custody reports tend to be long as it is, and mammoth reports run the risk of boring the reader with irrelevant facts. Since parties to the case generally see the report, often some care will also be taken to protect the children. For example, providing extensive quotations of what a child said that is negative about one parent may adversely affect that parent's feelings towards the child and so damage the future parent–child relationship. Therefore, the author generally includes the following statement at the end of the sources section:

> While a considerable amount of information was gathered during the course of this evaluation, only that specifically relevant and necessary for formulating my recommendations will be presented here.

This statement heads off later attacks on the expert who might otherwise later be painted in a bad light for not including some information an attorney thinks is important.

12.3.4 Background

The data section of the report begins with material about the background of the case. There is no established standard for how to organize the data, although what follows is one typical approach where the material is organized by person. This outline is given in Table 12.1.

Some evaluators prefer to organize the material by source (separate sections for interviews, records, collateral information, psychological testing, etc.).

It is generally advisable to separate sections containing data from sections containing opinions. If the significance of some item of data is not likely to be understood by an intelligent lay person, it may be appropriate to comment rather than expect the reader to remember the finding (e.g., "Fifteen-year-old Johnnie drew his family as all stick figures, which was an immature drawing for a mid-adolescent.")

Brief history of the current difficulties

This section is aimed to give the reader an overview of the major issues and disputes in the case. It begins with a brief history of the marriage and of the child care arrangements up to the present. Often the parties will dispute aspects of the history. In this section, it is best to focus on those items of the history on which the parties and children agree, and simply note important areas in which the histories differ. The section then includes a description of the parenting plan each parent is seeking, and their views as to why they have not been able to resolve the issues themselves without court involvement.

12.3.5 Examination findings

Each parent (or party)

Relevant information about each contesting adult is presented in a separate section. This will typically include relevant personal history, the parent's views on the important issues in dispute, mental health assessment, and history of relationship with the child. The emphasis in the data presented should be on those aspects that are directly relevant to parenting. Some evaluators like to organize information under "Parenting Strengths" and "Parenting Weaknesses."

Table 12.1 Data section of a typical custody report

History of marriage, overview of issues and concerns

Each parent or adult party

   History

   Parenting – strengths and weaknesses

   Psychiatric status

   Collateral information (from documents, therapists, others)

   Psychological testing

   Observation of interaction with child(ren)

Each child

   Interview data

   Psychiatric status

   Collateral information

   Psychological testing (if done)

   Observation of interaction with parents and siblings

Other persons as appropriate (e.g., step-parents, step-children, grandparents)

Child custody disputes often raise disputes about historical facts (e.g., who did most of the childcare previously, how much one parent drinks, whether spouse abuse took place, etc.). A determination of these facts may prove to be critical for the resolution of the case. Nevertheless, while it is appropriate for the evaluator to cite the relevant evidence, unless the weight of the evidence is clear, it is generally inappropriate for the evaluator to make a determination as to what actually happened. Therefore, the evaluator should eschew the role of a detective who seeks more and more evidence about past happenings. In that minority of cases in which the custody determination turns on one or two main findings of historical fact, it is better to point out the implications of the determination, but leave the contested fact-finding to the legally authorized finder of fact.

Some evaluators have separate sections for collateral data, but to the extent that such data bears directly on the parent–child relationship, the author finds it more useful to include it here. One source of collateral data frequently obtained is information from current or past therapists. That the parent is a patient, and the duration and type of treatment, can generally be put into the report. Records of medication treatment and inpatient treatment may also be useful. However, putting in details obtained in psychotherapy sessions, such as the nature of the patient's conflicts as reported by the therapist, invades the confidentiality of that treatment and undermines it. This is especially problematic because the other (ex-) spouse may be furious at the patient and all too ready to use such otherwise confidential material in a hurtful manner.

If the evaluator obtains written records from an outpatient psychotherapist, those records become discoverable at deposition or trial because they are part of the basis for the evaluator's opinions. Such written outpatient records are usually not very helpful: unless the evaluator is very familiar with the therapist's work, he or she has no solid basis for relying on the judgments of the therapist, and psychotherapy records typically do not contain much factual information that is useful in determining custody. For these reasons, it is generally better not to obtain written records of outpatient psychotherapy. A telephone call to the therapist (after obtaining an appropriate release) avoids most of the discovery problem and is likely to yield more useful information. It is better to use the therapist's information to guide the evaluator as to what issues may be significant, and the evaluator can then conduct his or her own assessment of those issues and their impact on parenting in further interviews with the patient-evaluee. If this is done, then the evaluator is relying on information obtained from his or her own interviews, and so does not need to cite details of the parent-patient's psychotherapy in the report. This somewhat protects the confidentiality of the treatment, avoids hearsay problems of relying on a statement one does not know to be accurate, and provides a clear basis for the evaluator's opinions.

Information from psychological testing, if conducted, is given in a subsection. Psychologists typically conduct their own testing as part of a custody evaluation. Many psychiatrists administer MMPIs or other personality tests to parents as well. Observational data about the parent–child interaction may be discussed here or may be discussed in a separate subsection (see below).

Because custody reports are fairly long and, unlike most other forensic reports, present a great deal of information about multiple people, some evaluators summarize the major findings and issues regarding each parent at the end of the section on that person so that the reader will not have to recall what detail went with which person when reading the evaluator's opinions at the end of the report.

Each child

Each child is typically interviewed. For very young children (under age 4), individual interviews may not be conducted, but the child will be assessed as part of family group interviews and through observations of parent–child interactions. The interview will include discussing the childrens' views of their family. In deciding the amount of such data that should be put in the report, the evaluator needs to consider how the information presented may affect the future parent–child relationship. This dilemma is clearest when discussing the child's preference. Leaving aside the technical questions of how and whether the child's preference should be ascertained in the interview, if the child's preference is known, there is the problem of addressing it in the report. State statutes vary widely in the legal weight given to a child's preference: some are silent on the subject, some consider it a factor, some consider it a factor only if the preference is "reasonable," and some, if the child is over a certain age (such as 13), find the preference determinative. Even if the child's preference is not a legal factor, it is often important evidence of the nature of the child's attachments. The problem is that if a parent doesn't know the child's preference, or if a parent erroneously thinks the child prefers to live with him or her the parent may feel rejected or betrayed by the child when reading the report. There are cases in which the evaluator is reasonably concerned that the parent's feelings of rejection would adversely affect the parent–child relationship, and thus do harm to the child. Evaluators are thus caught in the ethical problem that if full information is provided to the finder of fact, this will harm the child.

There is no simple resolution to this dilemma. The evaluator needs to weigh the need to fully discuss the child's feelings about each parent with the potential harm such a written discussion might bring. The evaluator should ascertain what each parent thinks the child prefers; it often turns out that the parents know, in which case discussing it in the report is seldom problematic. In many cases, the emphasis can be put on the reasons for the preference, rather than the action of choosing. In some cases the evidence for the recommendations is sufficiently clear on other grounds that the child's preference need not be discussed in detail, and the evaluator can comment on the child's loyalty conflict and the evaluator's concern about repercussions to the child. The crucial point is to write the report, particularly that part which contains information from the child, keeping in mind that the disappointed parent is likely to read it, and consider how that may affect the child.

Observations of parent–child interactions

Observations of parent–child interactions may be put in sections about the parent, the child, or contained in a separate section, depending on the stylistic preferences of the evaluator. The evaluator should specify the circumstances under which the observations took place (home or office, what instructions were given to the family, whether the evaluator was present or the session was observed through a one-way mirror, etc.), as well as the observations themselves. When parents know they are being observed, they will strive to put themselves forward in as favorable a light as possible, so the evaluator should think about how typical the observed interaction was. This assessment will include the parents' and children's responses to the question, "I know that being observed as part of an evaluation is an unusual and probably stressful situation. How typical do you think the interaction I saw was, compared to regular day-to-day life?"

12.3.6 Conclusions and recommendations

While the evaluator may have made some brief summary comments that contain opinions in the data section of the report, the bulk of the findings and recommendations should be placed in a separate section. It is useful to separate opinions about custody factors from the recommendations.

Opinions about custody factors

The structure of this section will vary depending on the specific test in the jurisdiction and the nature of the question being asked. It is useful to introduce opinions with the statement that the opinions are held with a "reasonable degree of medical certainty."

In states that have statutes or court rulings that define factors of the best interests test, it is best to organize opinions around those factors. The evaluator should list each factor, discuss opinions relevant to it, and whether that factor favors one parent or the other. In states where factors of the best interests test are not clearly defined, evaluators should strongly consider developing their own lists to provide a comprehensive approach to defining best interests. If evaluators create their own factors, they should introduce them with a statement that indicates that this is how the evaluator is breaking down a complex concept into more manageable components, something along the lines of, "In order to more clearly address the best interests of the child, those interests will be discussed under the various factors listed below." A list of factors to consider is given in Table 12.2.

In addition to best interests, the case may present special factors, such as whether sexual abuse took place, which should be addressed. The relevant jurisdiction may have special terms that are relevant to determinations in that state, such as whether an "established custodial environment" exists, or factors that trigger a presumption in favor of joint custody, which call for explicit opinions on those issues.

In most cases, not all factors tilt in the same direction, and the evaluator must weigh some factors against others. There is relatively little research and relatively little in the literature to guide evaluators in how to conduct this weighing, but it is important for them to lay out their reasoning process in evaluating the relative importance of various factors. The

Table 12.2 A listing of possible factors to consider as comprising the "best interests of the child" (adapted from Georgia statute OCGA 19–9-3(3))

(A) The love, affection, bonding, and emotional ties existing between each parent and the child

(B) The love, affection, bonding, and emotional ties existing between the child and his or her siblings, half siblings, and stepsiblings and the residence of such other children

(C) The capacity and disposition of each parent to give the child love, affection, and guidance and to continue the education and rearing of the child

(D) Each parent's knowledge of and familiarity with the child and the child's needs

(E) The capacity and disposition of each parent to provide the child with food, clothing, medical care, day-to-day needs, and other necessary basic care, with consideration made for the potential payment of child support by the other parent

(F) The home environment of each parent considering the promotion of nurturance and safety of the child rather than superficial or material factors

(G) The importance of continuity in the child's life and the length of time the child has lived in a stable, satisfactory environment and the desirability of maintaining continuity

(H) The stability of the family unit of each of the parents and the presence or absence of each parent's support systems within the community to benefit the child

(I) The mental and physical health of each parent

(J) Each parent's involvement, or lack thereof, in the child's educational, social, and extracurricular activities

(K) Each parent's employment schedule and the related flexibility or limitations, if any, of a parent to care for the child

(L) The home, school, and community record and history of the child, as well as any health or educational special needs of the child

(M) Each parent's past performance and relative abilities for future performance of parenting responsibilities

(N) The willingness and ability of each of the parents to facilitate and encourage a close and continuing parent–child relationship between the child and the other parent, consistent with the best interest of the child

(O) Any recommendation by a court-appointed custody evaluator or guardian *ad litem*

(P) Any evidence of family violence or sexual, mental, or physical child abuse or criminal history of either parent

(Q) Any evidence of substance abuse by either parent

(R) Any other factor that appears relevant

evaluator may also want to educate the reader as to why certain factors are especially important (e.g., with a discussion of developmental concepts regarding how very young children react to separations of varying lengths). In some cases, the reasoning process may be better suited to the recommendations section.

Recommendations

There is some controversy regarding whether an evaluator should make recommendations about custody and visitation at all (Tippins & Wittmann 2005), but most evaluators do make recommendations. Parties, or the court, may be required to formulate a parenting plan, and evaluators should formulate their recommendations along those lines. Some statutes specify the elements of a parenting plan. In the absence of specific guidelines, the evaluator would usually address the time the child should spend with each parent (physical custody or visitation and access), how legal decision-making authority should be apportioned between the parents, and recommendations for therapy. Specific recommendations are more helpful than vague ones. In many cases, it is also appropriate to address how to resolve future disputes (e.g., if parents share decision-making authority, in the event they disagree, how should the dispute be resolved? One parent gets more weight? Mediation? Third party arbitration?). In some cases, it is appropriate to anticipate the arrangement is likely to change in the future and may call for re-evaluation. For example, in cases involving preschool children, it may be appropriate to think of the proposed recommendations as good for the next 2 years, to be re-evaluated later in light of the family's experience. Finally, the evaluator may make a recommendation as to what legal term the proposed arrangement should be called (e.g., sole custody with visitation, joint legal custody, joint custody, shared parenting, or other terms used in the jurisdiction).

The rationale for the recommendations should be made explicit. While there is considerable research about children of divorce and joint custody, there is much less regarding children of high-conflict parents who contest custody, and that research is usually too non-specific to allow easy applicability to an individual case. Disputed custody cases present a wide array of fact situations, and parenting plans cover a large variety of options. Thus, providing a compelling rationale for a particular recommendation is often one of the most difficult parts of the report to write. Nevertheless, parents, their attorneys, and the court find it very useful to understand how the evaluator reached the specific recommendations.

Interpretive sessions

After a draft of the report has been prepared, many evaluators conduct feedback sessions with each parent separately and/or with attorneys to explain their thinking, give the parent or party the opportunity to comment, bring some closure to the process, or to enlist the attorneys in an effort to reach a settlement. If such feedback sessions are conducted, it is important to document what occurred in those sessions in the report. Such documentation is often included as a separate section at the end of the report. While placement at the end goes against the usual practice of not including new data in the Opinion section of the report, the data being presented focuses on the parents' reactions to the evaluator's conclusions and recommendations, so logical flow is best preserved by placing this section after those opinions are spelled out.

12.3.7 Variations

The above discussion focused on pre-divorce custody reports. Some variations on this basic model are called for in other situations.

Post-divorce custody evaluations

Post-divorce custody evaluations are often conducted slightly differently: evaluators are less likely to conduct an initial joint session with parents, other persons in the proposed custodial environment such as step-parents and step-siblings need to be considered, and the jurisdiction may have specific legal thresholds for considering a change of custody (e.g., in

Michigan an established custodial environment can only be changed if there is a showing that it is in the child's best interest by clear and convincing evidence). All of those issues then need to be addressed in the report, although the general report structure remains the same.

Cases involving allegations of sexual or physical abuse

Cases involving allegations of sexual abuse tend to be quite heated, and the stakes may go beyond custody and involve termination of parental rights and criminal penalties if a parent is found to have abused a child. The frequency of false allegations of sexual abuse is considerably higher in contested custody cases than in allegations arising in other contexts, reflecting the fact that one parent often has something to gain if the allegation is found to be true. The evaluation of abuse allegations, particularly of preschool children, is complicated in custody cases by the heightened possibility of contamination of the child's memory by suggestive comments from one or both of the parents.

The report in a case involving sexual abuse allegations will generally need to address the question of whether abuse took place. Evaluators will need to be clear about their methods of evaluation, reasoning process, and level of confidence in their findings. In many cases, the question of whether abuse took place will be adjudicated either in an abuse/neglect hearing in juvenile court or a criminal trial. The evaluator should keep in mind that the report may be used in those proceedings. In sum, the report will combine the structure of a custody evaluation report and the report of a sexual abuse assessment.

Visitation/access evaluations

Custody evaluations generally address visitation or access issues, so evaluations that address only visitation follow much the same structure as custody evaluations but are more limited in scope. Visitation evaluations emphasize the assessment of the child(ren)'s relationship with the visiting party (usually a parent or grandparent) and the child's best interest in fostering that relationship. Therefore the report format is similar, but some sections (such as the assessment of the custodial parent) will be more abbreviated. Care needs to be taken to use the language appropriate to the jurisdiction (visitation, access, alternating custody, shared parenting time, etc.).

Parenting evaluations in the context of established prior neglect or abuse

The prototypical evaluation involves a child who has been removed from a parent's custody, the parent has undergone some intervention and potentially improved his or her parenting, and child protective services (CPS) or the juvenile court are considering returning custody of the child(ren) to the parent. Such evaluations differ from divorce-custody evaluations in that the standards utilized in abuse/neglect proceedings differ from standards used in divorce. Public policy supports the reunification of families subject to the conditions of parental fitness and promotion of the child's best interest. The central question tends to be the risk of the abuse or neglect recurring. As with all evaluations, the evaluator needs to be conversant with the operative test in the jurisdiction.

The general structure of the custody issue in a divorce report can be used in the assessment of parenting, although typically only one parent is considered and the opinions focus on a different test. Many evaluations of parenting do not include the child in the assessment, and parent–child interaction is not observed directly, in which case the evaluator should not make a formal recommendation that the child be returned. The evaluator may have sufficient grounds to determine that the child should *not* be returned, based solely on the parent's limitations. If the evaluee's parenting appears acceptable, then the opinion may include statements to the effect that no contraindications to returning the child were found, but that since the parent–child interaction and the particular child's parenting needs were not assessed directly, the evaluator cannot form an opinion regarding whether a particular child should be returned.

12.4 Frequently asked questions in cross-examination

Most custody cases settle without going to trial. Attorneys of the parents who gain the least from evaluation reports will be assessing whether they can successfully attack the report's recommendations. If they do not think they can, they will typically encourage the client to trade not going to trial for a somewhat better resolution than the report suggests. Trials are very expensive, and to go into one when it is fairly certain one will lose is not an appealing prospect to most parties. To the extent the report reduces uncertainty of the trial's outcome, it reduces the likelihood of trial. Since most custody evaluations are conducted on court order or by stipulation, battles of the experts are rare and it is difficult to show in court that the evaluator was biased. Occasionally cases go to trial because of parents' wishes to continue the fight to the bitter end, but more commonly they go to trial when one of the attorneys thinks there is a chance of persuading the finder of fact (a judge in most jurisdictions) to ignore crucial aspects of the recommendations. These situations fall into several areas.

12.4.1 The attorney thinks the facts have changed

Unlike most forensic cases where the time period under scrutiny is demarcated in time, such as the time of the crime or when malpractice allegedly took place, custody determinations focus on relationships that are ongoing. A trial frequently takes place a considerable time after the evaluation, and during this time, new allegations may develop (e.g., the child now says he doesn't want to visit, one spouse has resumed drinking, etc.). Cross-examination in such instances will typically be a hypothetical of the sort, "Doctor, assuming [allegation about new facts] is true, how would that affect your conclusion about ...?" There are certainly instances in which such facts might lead evaluators to change their opinions.

Prior to trial, it is useful for the evaluator to find out from the attorneys whether substantial new facts have developed. If they have, the evaluator can consider proposing to the attorneys that the evaluator see the parties to update the information. If that proposal is turned down, the evaluator on the stand can make clear that he or she suggested looking into the matter, which tends to bolster the evaluator's testimony as open-minded and non-biased.

12.4.2 The attorney thinks the evaluator got the facts wrong or missed crucial facts

As discussed above, custody evaluators frequently encounter conflicting stories of what happened previously, and evaluators have limited expertise in playing detective and getting to the truth of such allegations. In the event the evaluator does make such a determination, an attorney may think there are good grounds to show that the evaluator simply got it wrong, especially if compelling testimony has been provided earlier in the trial that would lead to a different conclusion.

There are many situations in which evaluators do not make a determination of conflicting allegations and base their recommendations on data that are more verifiable. For example, suppose the mother asserts that the father is a heavy drinker, but the father denies drinking. The evaluator finds no evidence of heavy drinking (including eliciting a history from the child that suggests the child does not see the father drunk). The evaluator might conclude that there is no evidence that the father's drinking, if present, significantly impairs his parenting, and so not weigh the allegation as important. If mother's attorney has compelling evidence that father is frequently drunk, the attorney may confront the evaluator with it on the stand. It is therefore useful for the evaluator to learn whether such evidence exists so that he or she can consider its implications prior to trial and consider dealing with the relevant issues in the report.

12.4.3 The attorney thinks the evaluator weighed the factors incorrectly

Most custody cases are not black and white: some factors tend to tilt towards one parent, and some to the other. Consider a case in which joint custody is unworkable, and the evaluator finds a young child is significantly more attached to the less capable parent. The evaluator will need to weigh disrupting the child's primary attachment against the future effects of being raised with poorer parenting. There is no general solution to this problem: the evaluator will have to base his or her conclusions on particular details of the case, and might reasonably expect that the reasoning will be attacked in cross-examination. In anticipation of this line of questioning, it is important that the evaluator spell out the reasoning process in the report.

12.4.4 Insufficient empirical basis for making recommendations

As discussed above, there is limited research in the area of custody decision-making, and the applicability of general research findings to the particular case before the court is often questionable. For example, even if one accepts that research supports a general finding that there are group data suggesting joint custody is better if parents show some capacity to work together, this does not imply that given the particulars of the case before the court, 50–50 joint custody is better than 70–30. Therefore, cross-examination may attempt to show that recommendations are not evidence-based, with the implication that they reflect simply the whims or biases of the evaluator.

One way of responding to this line of questioning is to acknowledge the limitations in the research, perhaps pointing out that it is unlikely that we will ever have studies that utilize random assignment to various custodial arrangements, and so the best we can do is apply general principles that do have research support, including principles of general child development, in the context of reasoned clinical judgment that takes into account the particulars of the case. The evaluator then lays out a detailed rationale for why the proposed recommendations seem better than the alternatives. In anticipation of this line of questioning, it is useful to have given this detailed rationale in the report itself.

12.5 Conclusion

Custody evaluations are difficult, and writing custody reports is time-consuming. A well-constructed report that is compelling in its reasoning has a high likelihood of promoting settlement of a highly contested situation and leading to the best available outcomes for the children involved. Custody evaluators can take satisfaction in knowing that few decisions in a child's life have as much impact on a child's development and subsequent adult life as developing a good plan regarding the child's contact with the most important people in his or her life.

Acknowledgements

In order to obtain a wider perspective on the range of custody reports being prepared by experts in the field, the author solicited sample reports from several child and adolescent psychiatrists known for their work in this area. The author would like to acknowledge and thank Elissa P. Benedek, MD, William Bernet, MD, Stephen P. Herman, MD, and Matthew M. Soulier, MD, for providing sample reports for review.

References

American Academy of Child and Adolescent Psychiatry (Herman S. P. principal author). (1997) Practice parameters for child custody evaluation. *Journal of the American Academy of Child and Adolescent Psychiatry* **36**: 57S–68S.

American Psychological Association Committee on Professional Practice and Standards (COPPS) (1994) Guidelines for child custody evaluations in divorce proceedings. *American Psychologist* **49**: 677–680.

Ash, P. & Guyer, M. (1986) The functions of psychiatric evaluations in contested child custody and visitation cases. *Journal of the American Academy of Child Psychiatry* **25**: 554–561.

Association of Family and Conciliation Courts Task Force (2007) Model standards of practice for child custody evaluation. *Family Court Review* **45**: 70–91.

Bernet, W. (2002) Child custody evaluations. *Child and Adolescent Psychiatric Clinics of North America* **11**: 781–804.

Bow, J. N. & Quinnell, F. A. (2001) Psychologists' current practices and procedures in child custody evaluations: Five years after American Psychological Association guidelines. *Professional Psychology Research and Practice* **32**: 261–268.

Bow, J. N. & Quinnell, F. A. (2002) A critical review of child custody evaluation reports. *Family Court Review* **40**: 164–176.

Galatzer-Levy, R. M. & Kraus, L. (2009) *The Scientific Basis of Child Custody Decisions*, 2nd edn. Hoboken, NJ: J. Wiley.

Ludolph, P. S. (2009) Child custody evaluation. In *Principles and Practice of Child and Adolescent Forensic Mental Health*, ed. E. P. Benedek, P. Ash, & C. L. Scott. Washington, DC: American Psychiatric Publishing, Inc., pp. 155–165.

Michigan Child Custody Act (1993) *MCL* 722.23 sec. 3.

Tippins, T. M. & Wittmann, J. P. (2005) Empirical and ethical problems with custody recommendations: a call for clinical humility and judicial vigilance. *Family Court Review* **43**: 193–222.

Uniform Marriage and Divorce Act sec. 402 (1987) Uniform Marriage and Divorce Act sec. 402, 9A ULA 561.

United States Commission on Child and Family Welfare (1996) *Parenting Our Children: In the Best Interest of the Nation: Report of the US Commission on Child and Family Welfare.* Washington, DC: The Commission.

Chapter 13

Employment: disability and fitness

Robert P. Granacher, Jr.

13.1 Introduction

Within the United States, employment litigation is extremely common and comprises a high percentage of the reports completed by psychiatrists for forensic purposes. As American employment has become more complex, the issues within employment claims are also more complex. The areas of dispute in employment litigation are often extremely complicated and can be quite extensive. This chapter will cover the provision of reports of (1) disability evaluations, (2) workers' compensation evaluations, (3) evaluation of readiness to return to work (fitness for duty), and (4) special considerations as they pertain to the police and fire services.

Table 13.1 outlines the legal entities from which an employment cause of action may arise and thus lead to a request for a psychiatric evaluation. The Americans with Disabilities Act of 1990 (ADA) was established to protect workers from discrimination due to a disability. Disability is broadly defined within this Act to include either a physical or mental impairment that substantially limits major life activities. Mental impairment is defined to include any mental or psychological disorder, such as mental retardation, organic brain syndrome, emotional or mental illness, and specific learning disabilities. Thus, a claim against an employer could arise from an assertion that an employee was being discriminated against because of affliction with bipolar affective illness, for instance.

In contrast to the ADA, anti-discrimination laws are embodied in the Civil Rights Act of 1964 and in parallel state statutes. Claims made under the ADA and Title VII of the Civil Rights Act are somewhat dissimilar. Title VII of the Civil Rights Act of 1964 prohibits discrimination based on gender, race, national origin, and other issues of personal and civil status. These claims are most likely to be brought to an Equal Employment Opportunity Commission and thus the psychiatrist would be performing an employment examination based not on whether the claimant has a mental illness leading to workplace discrimination or lack of accommodation, but whether or not the claimant has a mental disorder, injury, or harm as a result of discrimination due to his or her personal or civil status.

Citizens can be insured for inability to work due to illness or injury through the Social Security Administration, commercial insurance, or both. The psychiatrist may receive a request for examination from an individual who is seeking Social Security Disability or who is seeking benefits under a commercial insurance policy bought by the worker to insure against inability to work. State Workers' Compensation statutes vary widely, but in general all are based upon a no-fault principle that covers injuries in the workplace. The employee

The Psychiatric Report, ed. Alec Buchanan and Michael A. Norko. Published by Cambridge University Press. © Cambridge University Press 2011.

Table 13.1 Potential employment claims

Americans With Disabilities Act of 1990 (ADA, 42-USC §§ 12101–12213)

Civil Rights Act of 1964-Title VII (42 USC Chapter 21)

Equal Employment Opportunity Commission (EEOC)

Public or private disability insurance (e.g., Social Security or commercial insurance)

State Workers' Compensation statutes

Tort claims (e.g., wrongful termination, negligence, etc.)

must waive the various defenses available in a civil claim in most instances (Melton et al. 1997). The psychiatrist may be requested to examine an injured worker with a claim of mental injury by either the employer or the worker's lawyer. On occasion, the examination may be requested by the Administrative Law Judge overseeing the claims process in State Worker's Compensation.

Lastly, tort claims in employment are brought through a civil court. These can include mental damages due to product liability, wrongful termination, injury through employer negligence outside of Workers' Compensation statutes, etc.

13.2 Special considerations in the conduct of the evaluation

13.2.1 Disability evaluations

The conduct of the evaluation, and the elements contained therein, is driven by the goal of the examination. For a disability evaluation, the questions to be answered will depend on the agency requesting examination. Public disability insurance, such as that provided by the Social Security Administration, will fall into two general categories: Social Security Disability or Supplemental Security Income. The criteria for disability are the same regardless of whether the examination is for Social Security Disability or Supplement Security Income. Mental disorders come under Social Security listing number 12.00 (42 USC, § 423). The listings for mental disorders are arranged in eight diagnostic categories as noted in Table 13.2.

Each of the categories under listing 12.00 has specific criteria for a finding of the mental disorder under the Social Security Act. Paragraph A for each of the listings of mental disorders requires the examiner to medically substantiate the presence of a mental disorder. This would require documenting the persistence of at least one of the following: (1) disorientation to time and place; (2) either short-term or long-term memory impairment; (3) disturbances of perception or thinking; (4) changes in personality; (5) disturbances in mood; (6) emotional debility; and (7) loss of measured intellectual ability of at least 15 IQ points from premorbid levels.

Paragraph B under each mental listing requires medical evidence to be present, defining at least two of the following: (1) marked restriction of activities of daily living; (2) marked difficulties maintaining social functioning; (3) deficiencies of concentration, persistence, or pace causing failures to complete tasks in a timely manner; and (4) repeated episodes of deterioration or inability to compensate in work or work-like settings (42 USC, § 423). The existence of a medically determinable impairment of the required duration must be established by medical evidence consisting of clinical signs, symptoms, and/or laboratory or

Table 13.2 Social Security listing 12.00 mental disorders

12.02: Organic Mental Disorders

12.03: Schizophrenic, Paranoid, and Other Psychotic Disorders

12.04: Affective Disorders

12.05: Mental Retardation and Autism

12.06: Anxiety Related Disorders

12.07: Somatoform Disorders

12.08: Personality Disorders

12.09: Substance Addiction Disorders

psychological test findings. Paragraph C for mental disorders under Social Security Disability examinations requires the psychiatrist to assess the level of severity, which is determined in terms of the functional limitations imposed by the impairment.

The financial criteria to qualify for Social Security Disability require that the individual has paid into the Social Security Administration at least 40 quarters of payments from employment income. Those who do not meet these criteria may qualify for Supplemental Security Income, which is reserved for the aged, blind, and disabled. Some individuals may meet the criteria for both Social Security Disability and Supplemental Security Income (SSI). An example could be a blind person or mentally retarded person, who is employed, and who has worked at least 40 quarters. Monies for this program (SSI), while administered under the Social Security Administration, are derived from general tax revenues of the United States rather than payroll deductions for Social Security Disability benefits.

Adjudication of a claimant's application for benefits under either Social Security Disability or Supplemental Security Income is performed by a federal administrative law judge. To qualify for disability under either federal program, the individual must be unable to work at all and likely to be unable to engage in work for substantial gain for at least 12 months. The examiner is not asked or expected to determine whether the claimant is disabled. The examiner is asked and expected only to report on the mental disorder as impairment. In contrast, disability under private or commercial insurance is defined on an individual basis within the policy contract purchased by the employee.

13.2.2 Workers' compensation evaluations

With regard to workers' compensation examinations, the criteria for disability are defined by state statute and administered individually by each of the 50 states. Adjudication of work-related disability is performed by an administrative law judge at the state level. In some states, disability determination requires the examiner to apply a percentage rating of impairment, regardless of whether the impairment is physical or mental. As a practical matter, the *Guides to the Evaluation of Permanent Impairment*, 6th edition (Rondinelli 2008) are used for the evaluation of medical impairment within most areas of workers' compensation or employment litigation, with the exception of disability under the Social Security Administration. The development of the most recent *Guides* derives from an editorial process using an evidence-based foundation when possible and a modified Delphi panel approach to consensus building of those who contributed to the volume. This new methodology applies terminology and adopts an analytical framework based on the World Health Organization's International

Classification of Functioning, Disability, and Health (ICF) (WHO 2001) as discussed below (Rondinelli & Duncan 2000). The *Guides* currently carry the weight of authority of the American Medical Association, and at present no other systems of impairment classification are routinely used in American medical practice for disability determination. Many State Workers' Compensation systems statutorily require the use of the *Guides*. The 6th edition of the *Guides* has taken physicians in an entirely new direction within the history of American impairment rating, with substantial changes from the prior five editions.

At the present time, there is no accepted reasonable alternative to using the *Guides* for measurement of impairment. The 6th edition of the *Guides* strengthens the ability to provide accurate impairment assessments with a number of new features. For instance, a standardized approach across organ systems and chapters has been adopted. The most contemporary, evidence-based concepts and terminology of disablement have been taken from the ICF. As the *Guides* were developed, the editors and authors used the latest scientific research and evolving medical opinions provided by American and internationally recognized experts. A unified methodology has been adopted to help physicians calculate impairment ratings through a grid construct and this promotes consistent scoring of impairment ratings. A more comprehensive and expanded diagnostic approach to organ systems is used. Precise documentation of functional outcomes, physical findings, and clinical test results are used as modifiers of impairment severity. For psychiatric examinations, this could include the use of psychological testing and neuropsychological testing as outlined in Chapter 14 of the *Guides*.

There is an increased transparency in precision of the impairment ratings relative to prior editions of the *Guides*. Physician interrater reliability has improved. These features allow for the standardized assessment of activities of daily living (ADL), which are used in the assessment of functional capacity in mental impairments. Functional assessment tools are used to validate impairment rating scales and, in particular for the psychiatrist, the *Guides* use the Brief Psychiatric Rating Scale, the Impairment Score of Global Assessment of Functioning Scale from the DSM-IV-TR (APA 2000), and a slightly modified Psychiatric Impairment Rating Scale. Considerable attention in the *Guides* is paid to the use of these three scales for psychiatric assessment and a percentage of psychiatric impairment is then calculated by the examiner (Rondinelli 2008). In workers' compensation cases, it will be necessary for the psychiatrist to determine whether the *Guides* are statutorily required as this requirement varies from state to state. For those psychiatrists performing disability evaluations where the AMA *Guides* are required, there are five new axioms of the 6th edition that must be kept in mind (Rondinelli 2008). Those are outlined in Table 13.3.

The ICF is a comprehensive model of disablement, within which classification consists of three key components: (1) loss or deviation of body functions and body structures, which are referred to as impairments; (2) activity limitations or difficulties the individual may experience carrying out task execution; and (3) participation restrictions which are barriers to the person experiencing involvement in life situations. These components comprise functioning and disability in this model (WHO 2001). The AMA *Guides* have adopted this disablement model.

For psychiatric disability evaluations, the examiner will use Chapters 13 and 14 of the AMA *Guides*. Chapter 13 covers the central and peripheral nervous system and will be used for examinations of persons with brain-based conditions which produce mental impairment in the following functional brain areas: (1) arousal and sleep disorders (section 13.3c); (2) mental status, cognition, and highest integrative function (section 13.3d);

Table 13.3 Five new axioms of the AMA *Guides*, 6th edition (Rondinelli 2008)

The *Guides* adopt the terminology and conceptual framework of disablement as put forward by the International Classification of Functioning, Disability, and Health (ICF).

The *Guides* become more diagnosis based with these diagnoses being evidence based when possible.

Simplicity, ease-of-application, and following precedent, where applicable, are given higher priority, with the goal of optimizing interrater and intrarater reliability.

Rating percentages derived according to the *Guides* are functionally based, to the fullest practical extent possible.

The *Guides* stress conceptual and methodological congruity within and between organ system ratings.

(3) communication impairments: dysphasia and aphasia (section 13.3e); and (4) emotional or behavioral impairments (section 13.3f). For example, a psychiatric examination for impairment due to traumatic brain injury or carbon monoxide poisoning resulting in a cognitive disorder and depression may require the use of Chapter 13 rather than the use of Chapter 14 of the *Guides*.

Chapter 14 of the AMA *Guides* covers mental and behavioral disorders. It deviates substantially from the examination techniques of the previous five editions of the AMA *Guides*. In particular, the use of selected psychological assessment tools in adults is stressed in this chapter. These assessment tools include psychological tests such as the Minnesota Multiphasic Personality Inventory (Graham 1993) and the Personality Assessment Inventory (Morey 1996). Intellectual assessment is advised using the Wechsler Intelligence Scales (Wechsler 1997). Academic assessment suggests use of instruments such as the Wide Range Achievement Test-3 (Wilkinson 1993) or the Wechsler Individual Achievement Test-II (Wechsler 2001), and others. In particular, where a neuropsychological evaluation is required, the AMA *Guides* state: "The exam should include assessment of the following: (1) intelligence, (2) academic achievement, (3) learning and memory, (4) attention and concentration, (5) language, (6) visuospatial functioning, (7) sensorimotor ability, (8) planning, reasoning, and problem solving, and (9) personality and mood" (Rondinelli 2008).

The *Guides* offer no recommendations to the psychiatrist in order to determine when to refer for psychological testing. However, to a psychiatrist, psychological testing is another standardized laboratory metric such as a white blood cell count, serum lithium level, or electrocardiograph. Thus, it may be wise to consult with a psychologist where measurement of mental function can add precision to the psychiatric examination. This could include queries such as the level of intelligence needed for certain occupations, cognitive examinations in questions of brain injury, the presence of malingering or symptom magnification in the case, or the presence of a personality disorder. Chapter 14 of the *Guides* stresses that if the physician examiner utilizes the services of a psychologist to perform psychological testing, the physician should review all test results to insure that the testing was done by a trained examiner and not merely co-signed by a supervising psychologist. Test findings must be internally consistent. The tester should document which materials were reviewed, and testing results should be consistent with information in the record. The review should determine that patient baseline/premorbid level of function was adequately explored and documented. Appropriate normative data should be listed for each test. The testing performed should contain two or more symptom validity tests (to determine effort, symptom magnification, or malingering). These admonitions charge the psychiatrist, or other physician, with oversight of psychological quality control. Therefore, it is wise for the psychiatrist to develop a professional consulting relationship with a trusted psychologist.

Moreover, Chapter 14 gives examples of use by the psychiatric examiner of the Brief Psychiatric Rating Scale (BPRS), the Global Assessment of Functioning Scale (GAF), and the Psychiatric Impairment Rating Scale (PIRS). It is incumbent upon psychiatric examiners performing disability examinations requiring or utilizing the AMA *Guides*, Chapter 14, to become thoroughly familiar with the scoring methods for determining impairment of mental status as the BPRS, GAF, and PIRS impairment scores are used to determine a percentage of mental impairment (Overall, & Gorham 1962; American Psychiatric Association 2000; Rondinelli 2008).

Overall, the AMA *Guides* provide operational definitions of impairment, disability, and impairment rating. Impairment is defined as a significant deviation, loss, or loss of use of any body structure or body function in an individual with a health condition, disorder, or disease. Disability is defined as activity limitations and/or participation restrictions in an individual with a health condition, disorder, or disease. Impairment rating is defined as a consensus-derived percentage estimate of loss of activity reflecting severity for a given health condition, and the degree of associated limitations in terms of ADLs (Rondinelli 2008).

13.2.3 Fitness-for-duty evaluations

Fitness-for-duty or fitness-to-work examinations are objective assessments of the mental health of an employee in relation to his or her specific job function. The purpose of the examination generally is to determine whether the individual can perform the job and to determine if the individual will be a hazard to self or others. It is critical that fitness-for-duty examinations should always be conducted by referring to the specific job description the worker holds or is intending to hold if returned to work. As we shall see below, with specificity to police and firefighters, fitness-for-duty examinations may occur at the time of application or consideration for entry into employment and assignment to a specific job (pre-placement). With the exception of this type of pre-employment examination, fitness-for-duty examinations generally are performed before an employee is returned to work after illness, injury, or after administrative removal from the work environment (e.g., dangerousness). For pre-employment fitness for duty, an employer may not offer a job contingent upon the individual passing a medical examination that indicates the employee would be able to perform the job and will not be a hazard to self or others while working in that job. The employee may be refused the job only if the health of the employee is not compatible with the working conditions, and the job requirements cannot reasonably be altered. Among an infinite number of possible outcomes following a fitness-for-duty examination, the US Government suggests six possible clinical judgments that can be made following a fitness-for-duty examination. These recommendations stem from the National Guidelines Clearinghouse, a public resource for evidence-based clinical practice guidelines. These guidelines are an initiative of the US Department of Health and Human Services. Table 13.4 lists these potential judgments and their definitions (www.guideline.gov, 2009).

The key elements of a fitness-for-duty examination, if performed under the Americans With Disabilities Act, are: (1) determine the presence or absence of a permanent mental impairment that substantially limits one or more major life activities; (2) evaluate the patient's

Table 13.4 Categories of fitness for duty

Fit: This judgment means that the employee is able to perform the job without danger to self or others, and without reservation or restrictions.

Temporarily fit: This category can be used for all types of medical assessments except pre-placement.

Fit subject to work modifications: A judgment in this category indicates that the employee could be a hazard to self or others or an impediment to other employees in the workplace if placed in the job as described, but would be considered fit to do the job if certain working conditions were modified or certain restrictions were put in place. The modifications recommended by the examiner must be described. If the employer can accommodate these recommendations, the employee is considered fit for the modified job. If the modifications cannot be reasonably accommodated, the employee is deemed temporarily or permanently unfit.

Temporarily fit subject to work modifications: "Temporarily" means that if the person's condition improves with time, the requirements for work modifications may be lifted.

Temporarily unfit: "Temporarily" means that the medical condition may improve with time, thus allowing return to work or transfer to some other job.

Unfit: This category describes the employee as unable to perform the job without being a hazard to self or others or markedly interfering with the orderly function of the business (see "Fit subject to work modifications" noted above). "Permanently" unfit usually means that the employee will never be fit for the job and that no modification of the working condition is reasonably possible or medically relevant. If "permanently" means that the employee is unable to do any available job, with or without work modifications, a statement to this effect should be made in the comments section of the report.

work capacity (mental) and delineate workplace restrictions; (3) assess workplace demands (mental) and essential functions of the job; and (4) ascertain the patient's ability to perform the essential functions of the job with, or without, accommodations (www.guideline.gov, 2009).

There is a special category of psychiatric fitness for duty when evaluating physicians. The American Psychiatric Association Council on Psychiatry and the Law and Corresponding Committee on Physician Health, Illness, and Impairment issued guidelines which were adopted by the Joint Reference Committee of the American Psychiatric Association in June 2004 (Guidelines for Psychiatric "Fitness for Duty"; APA 2004). The reader of this chapter is invited to review those guidelines where psychiatric evaluations of physicians are made to determine fitness for duty.

Fitness-for-duty evaluations are often seriously resisted by employees and their attorneys. However, the courts have universally agreed that, even where a person has an ADA-defined disability, the employer can compel an employee to undergo psychiatric evaluation if there is probable cause to believe that an employee's mental state is dangerous to the employees at large, or dangerous to the employee (*Porter* v. *United States Alumoweld*, 1996; *Yin* v. *State of California*, 1996; *Ahern* v. *O'Donnell*, 1997; *Houck Jr.* v. *City of Prairie Village*, 1997). In particular, for police officers, courts have ruled that they can be required to undergo fitness-for-duty examinations, even if claiming a disability under the ADA, as "a fitness-for-duty examination is job-related and consistent with business necessity" (*Watson* v. *City of Miami Beach*, 1999).

Disability examinations under Chapter 14 of the AMA *Guides* contain a substantial addition to the 6th edition of the AMA *Guides*, in section 14.3c. This section covers motivation and malingering. The examiner is advised to "always be aware of this possibility when examining impairments. The possibility of avoiding responsibility and/or obtaining monetary awards increases the likelihood of exaggeration and/or malingering." Section 14.3c points out that malingering occurs along a spectrum, from embellishment to exaggeration, to outright fabrication (Rondinelli 2008). Gutheil and Simon have advised that not to consider malingering within a forensic psychiatric examination is substandard practice (Gutheil & Simon 2002).

Police officers and firefighters

Psychiatrists may participate in the examination of police officers and firefighters at two important points in employment. The first place is the pre-employment examination as often required by many police and fire departments and the second likely encounter is a fitness-for-duty examination of either a police officer or a firefighter. With regard to the evaluation of public safety applicants (e.g., police or firefighters), as a practical matter, most pre-employment evaluations of public safety applicants are performed by psychologists. Generally, if a significant mental disorder is detected, then the psychiatrist is asked to perform a supplemental examination. The International Association of Chiefs of Police (AICP) is a vigorous organization that constantly develops policies for police departments. It has developed guidelines for pre-employment psychological evaluation. If psychiatrists are involved in these types of evaluations, it is probably useful to go to the IACP website and obtain further information (www.theiacp.org, 2009). Specific guidelines for the psychological evaluation of public safety applicants have been prepared and ratified by the IACP (Curan & Saxe-Clifford 2004). Psychiatrists performing fitness-for-duty evaluations of police and firefighters need a focus somewhat slightly different than that toward fitness-for-duty evaluations of civilian employees. For instance, some police and fire departments have special provisions for those individuals exposed to a critical incident. Some departments require that subsequent to a critical incident the police officer or firefighter be evaluated by a mental health professional. A critical incident is usually defined in these circumstances as any event that has a stressful impact that proves sufficient to overwhelm the usually effective coping skills of the individual. Critical incidents may include line-of-duty shootings, death, suicide, serious injury of co-workers, homicides, hostage situations, terrorist events, etc. (McNally & Solomon 1999).

With regard to fitness-for-duty examinations in police and firefighters, these usually will be triggered by a critical incident such as described above. The examiner should conduct the fitness-for-duty evaluation along suggested guidelines as noted above. Certain critical issues should be explored. Police appear to be at greater risk of posttraumatic stress reactions and job burnout than the general population. Both of these increase the risk of psychosocial difficulty, work adjustment, and in particular suicide (Stuart 2008). There is recent empiric data on police suicide from all 50 states in the United States if the reader wishes to pursue this (O'Hara & Violanti 2009). Rarely, the examiner may be confronted with a police officer for examination who has attempted to commit "suicide by cop." While this is a rare phenomenon, there is a recent study that has examined these issues and, interestingly, the demographic and situational stress factors for police are very similar to civilians who attempt suicide by cop (Arias et al. 2008).

While conducting a fitness-for-duty examination of a police officer who is demonstrating stress responses or suicidal ideation, it is worthwhile to look carefully for traits of anger which may have predated the critical incident. Traits of anger are correlated with the production of posttraumatic stress disorder symptoms in police officers (Meffert et al. 2008).

The examiner should also take a careful history of pre-critical incident life events and other traumas in the police officer's life as these are highly correlated with the development of depression in police officers (Hartley et al. 2007). Within the recommendations section of the report itself as noted below, the examiner might recommend peer-based assistance programs, in addition to the examiner's recommendations for psychiatric and psychological treatment. Peer-based assistance programs were very effective for New York City police officers following the 9/11 incidents in the United States (Dowling et al. 2006).

Like police officers, the literature on stress responses among firefighters is international as well. Multiple studies have shown a relationship between psychiatric impairment and natural disasters, fires, and other critical incidents to which firefighters are exposed. In contrast to what may be a common sense conclusion, psychiatric impairment in firefighters following critical incidents seems to be related more to their level of distress after the fires than to the severity of their exposure and losses (McFarlane 1988). Firefighters may bring significant vulnerabilities to their profession and the prevalence of posttraumatic stress disorder among professional firefighters is higher than one might suspect (Wagner et al. 1998). In this German study, the current prevalence rate of PTSD symptoms among 402 professional firefighters from Rheinland-Pfalz was 18.2%. Of the recruited subjects, 27% had a mental disorder according to the general health questionnaire. Predictors for the extent of traumatic stress were longer job experience and the number of distressing missions during the previous month. In the United States, the Oklahoma City bombing provides us with further information regarding PTSD behavior in firefighters. After the Oklahoma City bombing, a volunteer sample of 181 firefighters who served as rescue and recovery workers was assessed with a structured diagnostic interview. This study indicates that firefighters are not very likely to turn to social supports, seek mental health treatment, or take medication as a coping response following a disaster (North et al. 2002). As with police officers, it is worthwhile to look carefully for traits of anger in firefighters that may have predated the critical incident.

13.3　The report

The elements of the psychiatric report that were described in Chapter 7 and that warrant distinctive treatment in reports on disability and fitness are shown in Box 13.1.

The report of findings in disability, fitness for duty, and other pertinent employment issues should be written in a comprehensive, detailed, precise, clearly written, and well-substantiated style (Wettstein 2004). The purpose of the employment report is to convey to the trier of fact the examiner's conclusions and supporting data after the individual claimant or examinee is evaluated. It is critical that the report stand on its own merits. In other words, the report should be sufficiently detailed, sufficiently documented, and sufficiently referenced that it can be used in support of the litigation, and not necessarily require a deposition.

It is critical that the report be well organized, contain appropriate subject headings, report accurately data sources used in the analysis, delineate all available records that were reviewed by the examiner, and report relevant history. The report should also include any collateral data or collateral interviews that were performed, the mental status examination, test results if any, diagnoses, expert conclusions/opinions, and the bases for those conclusions/opinions.

13.3.1　Purpose of report

This should be clearly stated at the outset of the report after the salutatory section. For a disability evaluation, the report should state the nature of the examination and the questions to

---

Box 13.1 Topics warranting distinctive treatment in disability and fitness reports

Table 7.1 Structure of the psychiatric report

1. **Preliminary and identifying information**

2. **Introduction**

Section 13.3.1 —————— Why the report is being written, the circumstances of the request and the questions that are being addressed

Dates and duration of interviews with the subject

Section 13.3.3 —————— Sources of information used in the report

Section 13.3.2 —————— Information given to the subject at time of interview, including information regarding confidentiality

List of appended material

3. **Body of report**

Section 13.3.4 —————— Background information

Section 13.3.5 —————— Current events (the crime in a sentencing report; the events leading to the claim in a civil action), the circumstances surrounding those events, and relevant sequelae

Section 13.3.6 —————— Findings on examination

Psychological and other test results

Section 13.3.7 —————— 4. **Opinion**

5. **Concluding material**

Signature of author

Name, qualifications, and current post

Date of signing

---

be answered. A fitness-for-duty evaluation should likewise describe the nature of the examination as requested by the agency, human resources officer, or appropriate person asking that fitness for duty or fitness for work be determined. If the individual or agency hiring the examiner has stated specific questions, these questions should be included within the report. If there are a large number of questions, as is often asked in workers' compensation cases, it might be best to save these toward the end of the report and specifically state each question in a tabular fashion with the appropriate answer under the question.

13.3.2 Description of warning regarding confidentiality

The forensic examiner is ethically obligated to clearly indicate in the body of the report that a warning of non-confidentiality was given to the examinee. In clear language, the report should state that the person being evaluated was warned of the nature of the examination, the purpose of the examination, and that it is a non-confidential evaluation. Since no doctor–patient relationship exists in these types of evaluations, the person being examined should never be described as a "patient." More appropriate terms for the examinee are the litigant, plaintiff, defendant, claimant, examinee, or other non-patient-oriented descriptor. On the other hand, Resnick and Soliman (see Chapter 6) suggests it is better to humanize examinees by using their names and appropriate titles (e.g., Dr., Captain, Mr., Ms., etc.).

13.3.3 Sources of information

It is recommended that the examiner list all sources of information in a tabular fashion. For instance, specific medical records should be listed. All depositions read should be listed with the date of the deposition and the deponent. If auditory recordings or video recordings are reviewed, those should be clearly stated with appropriate identifying dates. The reader of the report should be able to tell by reviewing the list of information whether the data are from a medical source, legal source, lay source, internet website, etc. The writer of the report should convey transparency in all sources of information.

13.3.4 Background

For a medical examination, this generally follows the schema of the standard medical practice of reporting information such as past medical history, family history (genetic), social history, legal history, employment history, military history, and review of systems. The information regarding sexual abuse, psychotherapy, counseling sessions, etc. should probably not be detailed in a fitness-for-duty report going to the individual's employer. This information may be relevant for disability determination where causation must be opined.

13.3.5 Current events/circumstances

These factors will be particularly important in police officer and firefighter examinations. If a critical incident has occurred, the psychiatric examiner should delineate as carefully as possible the nature of the incident, what the investigation has revealed about the facts of the incident, and the behavior and activity of the police officer or firefighter during and after the incident.

In any examination, where posttraumatic stress disorder is an issue, the circumstances of the trauma event should be clearly described and conclusions regarding the causation of posttraumatic stress disorder should convincingly be linked to the nature of the trauma stress and the likelihood that the trauma stress would produce a posttraumatic stress disorder in any reasonable person.

For disability evaluations, it is important to delineate the functional capacities of the individual (mental) and their relationship to the examinee's performance of activities of daily living or ability to work. There should be a clear intellectual link between the opinion of impairment level and the documented inability to perform certain functions due to mental difficulty.

13.3.6 Examination findings

Since these employment reports are psychiatric in nature, obviously the mental status examination should form a core component of the examination findings. This section of the report should be written in clear language without jargon or "psycho-babble." The elements of the mental status examination should be clearly stated and the specific findings of the examiner, with appropriate examples, may be useful. It is probably wise to follow a standard text for the expression of a mental status examination (Trzepacz and Baker 1993). The mental status examination should clearly correlate with the psychiatrist's expressed opinions in the report.

If laboratory tests are ordered as part of the psychiatric examination (e.g., thyroid studies, automated chemistries, urine drug screen, etc.), these should be reported with appropriate language, measuring units, and normal values for comparison. When neuroimaging is obtained, the statements of the nuclear medicine physician or radiologist should be included in the report. The same is true for reporting electroencephalographs, electrocardiographs, etc. Psychological testing is required by some commercial disability insurance carriers and for certain Social Security disability determinations. If psychological testing is ordered by the psychiatrist, a summary of the psychologist's findings should be included within test reporting (see responsibilities of psychiatrist when using psychological testing above).

13.3.7 Conclusions and recommendations

The conclusion section of the report should state three major findings: (1) mental diagnoses in current DSM Axis format; (2) each conclusion, in a numbered tabular form, expressed by the psychiatric examiner; and (3) the bases for each conclusion. With regard to specific conclusions, in a disability evaluation for Social Security purposes, the examiner might state: "John Claimant lacks the mental capacity to engage in any and all work due to major depression and his incapacity is likely to persist for greater than twelve months."

In the bases for conclusion section of the report, it would be expected that the psychiatric examiner would clearly delineate each reason for mental incapacity that prevents John Claimant from engaging in work. It also is generally necessary to state why the psychiatric examiner believes Mr. Claimant will not regain suitable mental capacity to return to work within a year.

In a fitness-for-duty evaluation, the conclusion might appear in the following manner: "In my opinion, within reasonable medical probability, Officer Claimant lacks the mental capacity, by virtue of the illness schizophrenia, to meet the performance duties of his job description and it is not safe for him to carry a sidearm." The bases for this conclusion should be clearly stated with each and every element of mental impairment that precludes the police officer's ability to meet the duties of his job description and the specific mental reasons why it is not appropriate for Officer Claimant to carry a weapon.

Of course, these are only suggested examples and whatever particular style the examiner chooses should be used. However, if there are multiple conclusions necessary, each should be explicitly stated, within reasonable medical probability (and/or medical certainty, depending on appropriate local statutes), and there should be a clear link between the bases for conclusions and the explicit stated conclusions.

With regard to recommendations, these are generally not expected in disability examinations for the Social Security Administration or in workers' compensation cases unless explicitly requested. On the other hand, fitness-for-duty evaluations often require that recommendations for treatment, patient monitoring, and return-to-duty standards be stated within the report. These usually will be presented to the examiner by the person or agency requesting the fitness-for-duty examination. With regard to public safety officers such as police and firefighters, the request for the evaluation will generally state what recommendations the police department or fire department is requesting before returning the officer or firefighter to duty. Recommendations should be clearly stated and appropriate to the locale and job description. Oftentimes, it is requested that the psychiatrist give a timeline for treatment and likelihood of the police officer or firefighter being returned to full duty.

13.4 Frequently asked questions in cross-examination

Social Security evaluations rarely require psychiatric testimony. Workers' compensation evaluations often do require testimony. Cross-examination questions in workers' compensation claims will generally focus on a few main issues. The first and most important issue is whether or not there is a causal relationship between the claimant's psychiatric illness and a work accident. Thus, the psychiatrist will be expected to clearly answer the causal nexus between, for instance, a major depressive disorder and a crush injury of the right hand in an offset press. The second major area of cross-examination in a Workers' Compensation claim will center on the level of impairment. As noted above, many states require that the impairment rating be expressed in percentage terms. It is therefore incumbent upon the psychiatrist to clearly understand how impairment ratings are derived (Rondinelli 2008). If the claimant has applied for total disability, the psychiatrist can expect cross-examination on the mental disease and why it presents a level of impairment so high that the worker is precluded from returning to employment. Lastly, the psychiatrist may receive cross-examination on the current psychiatric treatment being offered to the worker and the likelihood of a positive response. In order to answer this line of questioning, it is necessary for the psychiatrist to understand response rates to commonly used psychiatric medications and treatments.

Fitness-for-duty examinations sometimes lead to legal testimony. The claimant may have hired a lawyer to represent his or her desire to return to work and the employer may also have hired a lawyer to determine whether or not it is appropriate for the employee to return to work with an active mental disorder. In particular, if dangerousness or suicidality is an issue, the psychiatrist should be prepared for questions regarding dangerousness risk, suicide risk, appropriateness for the employee to return to the previous level of employment, and to provide recommendations to the trier of fact for managing the mental disorder of the employee or accommodating the individual at work.

13.5 Conclusions

Employment reports cover multi-variant areas of potential examination as noted in Table 13.1. Examinations conducted within the arena of employment law should be based squarely on the questions asked specific to the individual's employment duties. Psychiatrists who determine impairment in examinations for disability should provide sufficient evidence-based psychiatric data so that triers of fact can adjudicate whether or not disability is present. Fitness-for-duty evaluations are designed to determine whether the employee can be returned safely to work and whether or not the individual's accommodations or treatment to improve his or her ability to be employed. Examinations of police officers and firefighters have special needs due to the significant nature of stress imposed upon these public safety employees and also due to the significant likelihood of critical incidents which may be life threatening.

References

Ahern v. *O'Donnell* (1997) 109 F.3d 809.

American Psychiatric Association (APA) (2000) *Diagnostic and Statistical Manual of Mental Disorders-IV, Text Revision*. Washington, DC: American Psychiatric Association.

American Psychiatric Association (2004) *Guidelines for Psychiatric "Fitness for Duty": Evaluation of Physicians, Resource Document*. Arlington, VA: American Psychiatric Association.

Americans with Disabilities Act of 1990, 42 USC §§ 12101–12213.

Arias, E. A., Schlesinger, L. B., Pinizzotto, A. J., et al. (2008) Police officer commits suicide by cop: a clinical study with analysis. *Journal of Forensic Sciences* 53: 1455–1457.

Civil Rights Act of 1964-Title VII 42 USC Chapter 21.

Curan, S. F. & Saxe-Clifford, S. (2004) *Psychological Evaluation of Public Safety Applicants: The 2004 Revised Guidelines of the Police Psychological Services Section*. Los Angeles, CA: IACP Police Psychological Services Section.

Dowling, F. G., Moynihan, G., & Genet, B., et al. (2006) A peer-based assistance program for officers with the New York City Police Department: Report of the effects of Sept 11, 2001. *American Journal of Psychiatry* **163**: 151–153.

Graham, J. R. (1993) *Assessing Personality and Psychopathology*, 2nd edn. New York: Oxford University Press.

Gutheil, T. G. & Simon, R. I. (2002) *Mastering Forensic Psychiatric Practice: Advanced Strategies for the Expert Witness*. Washington, DC: American Psychiatric Press.

Hartley, T. A., Violanti, J. M., Fekedulegan, D., et al. (2007) Associations between major life events, traumatic incidents, and depression among Buffalo police officers. *International Journal of Emergency Mental Health* 9: 25–35.

Houck Jr. v. *City of Prairie Village* (1997) 978F Supp. 1397.

McFarlane, A. C. (1988) Relationship between psychiatric impairment and national disaster: the role of distress. *Psychological Medicine* 18: 129–139.

McNally, V. J. & Solomon, R. M. (1999) The FBI's critical incident stress management program. *The FBI Law Enforcement Bulletin* 68: 20–26.

Meffert, S. M., Metzler, T. J., Henn-Haase, C., et al. (2008) A prospective study of trait anger and PTSD symptoms in police. *Journal of Traumatic Stress* 21: 410–416.

Melton, G. P., Petrila, J., Poythress, N. G., et al. (1997) *Psychological evaluations for the courts. A Handbook for Mental Health Professionals and Lawyers*, 2nd edn. New York: Oxford University Press.

Morey, L. C. (1996) *An Interpretative Guide to the Personality Assessment Inventory (PAI)*. Odessa, FL: Psychological Assessment Resources.

North, C. S., Tivis, L., McMillen, J. C., et al. (2002) Coping, functioning, and adjustment of rescue workers after the Oklahoma City bombing. *Journal of Traumatic Stress* 15: 171–175.

O'Hara, A. F. & Violanti, J. M. (2009) Police suicide – a web surveillance of national data. *International Journal of Emergency Mental Health* 11: 17–23.

Overall, J. E. & Gorham, D. R. (1962) Brief psychiatric rating scale. *Psychological Reports* 10: 799–812.

Porter v. *United States Alumoweld* (1996) 125 F.3d 243.

Rondinelli, R. D. (Ed.) (2008) *Guides to the Evaluation of Permanent Impairment*, 6th edn. Chicago, IL: American Medical Association.

Rondinelli, R. D. & Duncan, P. W. (2000) The concepts of impairment and disability. In *Impairment Rating and Disability Evaluation*, ed. R. D. Rondinelli & R. T. Katz), Philadelphia, PA: WB Saunders Company.

Social Security Act 42 USC, § 423.

Stuart, H. (2008) Suicidality among police. *Current Opinion in Psychiatry* 21: 505–509.

Trzepacz, P. T. & Baker, R. W. (1993) *The Psychiatric Mental State Examination*. New York: Oxford University Press.

Wagner, D., Heinrichs, M., & Ehlert, U. (1998) Prevalence of symptoms of posttraumatic stress disorder in German professional firefighters. *American Journal of Psychiatry* 155: 1727–1732.

Watson v. *City of Miami Beach* (1999) 177 F.3d 932.

Wechsler, D. (1997) *Wechsler Adult Intelligence Scale*, 3rd edn. San Antonio, TX: Psychological Corporation.

Wechsler, D. (2001) *Wechsler Individual Achievement Test-II*. San Antonio, TX: Psychological Corporation.

Wettstein, R. M. (2004) The forensic examination and report. In *American Psychiatric Publishing Textbook of Forensic Psychiatry*, ed. R. I. Simon & L. H. Gold. Washington, DC: American Psychiatric Publishing, Inc.

WHO (2001) International Classification of Functioning, Disability, and Health: ICF. Geneva: World Health Organization.

Wilkinson, G. S. (1993) *Wide Range Achievement Test-3: Administration Manual*. Wilmington, DE: Wide Range.

www.archives.gov, Civil Rights Act of 1964, Title VII, site accessed November 17, 2009.

www.guideline.gov, fitness for duty, site accessed August 19, 2009.

www.theiacp.org, site accessed August 21, 2009.

Yin v. *State of California*, 95F. 3d 864 (9th Cir. 1996).

Chapter 1

Writing for the US federal courts

Sally Johnson, Eric Elbogen, and Alyson Kuroski-Mazzei

14.1 Introduction

This chapter outlines standards and statutes governing psychiatric reports for the federal courts. Federal courts adjudicate disputes arising under the United States constitution, federal statutes and regulations, and the federal common law at three different levels: (1) federal district courts for each state or federal territory, grouped under twelve sets of appellate courts called circuits; (2) circuit courts providing appellate review of district court decisions; and (3) the US Supreme Court providing appellate review of circuit court decisions. The US Supreme Court also has limited "original jurisdiction," for example, in cases brought by one state against another. There is a right to appeal any final decision rendered by the district court to the circuit court. Appellate cases heard by the Supreme Court are discretionary. If four justices agree to hear the case the Court issues a "writ of certiorari," beginning a process of written and oral argument.

Federal law is contained in federal statutes and rules (Federal Rules of Criminal Procedure; Federal Tort Claims Act; The American with Disabilities Act; The Civil Rights Act; The Federal Rules of Civil Procedure; The Social Security Act; United States Criminal Code) and evolves through judicial decisions. An ongoing process exists in which federal district court judges interpret the law and those interpretations are then reviewed by the respective circuit court. If a circuit court rules on the issue, all district courts in that circuit must abide by that ruling; however, no district court ruling is binding on the other district courts in that circuit or any other. There is no guarantee that different district courts will interpret the same issue in the same manner, and there is also no guarantee that different circuits will rule similarly in similar cases. It is possible at any one time to have differences in application and interpretation across districts and between circuits pending further and final review at the Supreme Court, whose decisions are binding in all courts. When conducting forensic evaluations for federal courts, the evaluator must seek clarification not only on the applicable statutes and standards, but also on the case precedents applicable to the issue at hand in the specific jurisdiction.

Most commonly evaluations will be requested by the attorneys involved in the federal case. All federal cases, both civil and criminal, are prosecuted by the Department of Justice through United States Attorneys. Federal criminal cases are defended by federal public defenders or private attorneys who may be privately retained or publicly appointed in indigent cases. The district judge may also elect to request an evaluation directly.

Psychiatrists may be tasked with reviewing individuals or systems and these reviews and the subsequent reports that are generated can involve criminal or civil issues. Criminal issues can arise at the pre-trial, pre-sentencing, or post-conviction phase. Civil issues can arise within the criminal area, such as commitment of criminal defendants, but they more commonly arise in response to alleged violations of an individual's constitutional rights. This chapter will briefly review the types of forensic evaluations and forensic expert testimony in the federal system, and the critical components of federal forensic reports, emphasizing how mental health professionals can assist the federal courts in dealing with psychiatric forensic issues.

14.2 Testimony

The evaluator must be accepted as an expert by the federal court prior to delivering expert testimony. The determination as to whether an evaluator will be qualified as an expert and allowed to testify is ultimately a determination by the judge. If there is a challenge to the credentials of the expert, a *voir dire* hearing on this issue takes place outside of the presence of the jury. Review of a recognized expert's credentials and experience is generally placed before the jury on direct examination of the expert and is subject to cross-examination by opposing counsel.

Admissibility of expert testimony in federal cases is governed by the Federal Rules of Evidence 702–706. Rule 701 addresses opinion testimony by lay witnesses (Fed. R. Evid. 701). It is possible that a psychiatrist may be asked to testify as a lay witness. In that situation testimony is limited to opinions or inferences which are based on the witness's perceptions (rather than being based on specialized knowledge) and are helpful in the determination of a fact at issue. Rule 702 addresses testimony by expert witnesses (Fed. R. Evid. 702). A witness, qualified as an expert based on knowledge, skill, experience, training, or education may offer an opinion if "scientific, technical, or other specialized knowledge will assist the trier of fact to understand the evidence" and if "the opinion is based on sufficient facts" and is the "product of reliable principles or methods applied to the facts."

Rule 703 clarifies that the facts upon which the expert bases their opinion may become known to the expert before or during the hearing, and need not be admissible in evidence in order for the expert's opinion to be admitted (Fed. R. Evid. 703). Rule 704 permits the expert to offer an opinion on an ultimate issue except in regard to rendering an opinion on insanity at the time of the offense (Fed. R. Evid. 704). Rule 705 states that the expert can give an opinion without first testifying to the underlying facts, but can be required to disclose the underlying facts on cross-examination (Fed. R. Evid. 705). Rule 706 discusses the ability of the court to appoint experts, either with the agreement of the parties involved or simply through its own selection provided the expert agrees to serve as an expert (Fed. R. Evid. 706). Experts' findings are usually submitted in writing but may be required to be stated at deposition or through court testimony subject to cross-examination.

The application of these rules is guided by a series of Supreme Court decisions beginning with *Daubert* v. *Merrill Dow Pharmaceuticals* (1993). *Daubert* provides guidelines for judges to consider in determining whether to admit expert testimony. These include whether a theory has been tested, subjected to peer review, or published in a scientific journal; the rate of error of the technique; and general acceptance of the scientific community. Later, *General Electric* v. *Joiner* (1997) established that an abuse of discretion standard of review was appropriate for appellate review of a trial judge's decision on admissibility. This means that only in rare cases would the district court judge's opinion be overturned. *Kumho Tire* v. *Carmichael* (1999) clarified that *Daubert* governs all expert testimony (scientists and non-scientists)

A number of authors have explored the potential implications of these decisions on expert testimony (Grove & Barden 1999; Gutheil & Stein 2000; Youngstrom & Busch 2000). Scholars generally conclude that one cannot apply the *Daubert* standard to mental health assessment as a broad category; rather, different diagnoses (e.g., schizophrenia versus dissociative disorder) and different assessment techniques (e.g., objective versus projective personality tests) may have varying degrees of scientific consensus and empirical foundation. In practice, however, admissibility of evidence on psychiatric issues is infrequently challenged, unless the material presented is novel or peripheral to mainstream understanding of diagnosis, prognosis, or treatment intervention (Roberts 1996; Gutheil & Sutherland 1999; Slobogin 1999; Slobogin et al. 2001). Interesting examples of admissibility debates have centered on testimony about syndromes that do not neatly fit into accepted diagnostic categories (Biggers 2005; Dahir et al. 2005; Amato & Packer 2006). More commonly, debate on an issue is addressed through cross-examination, the introduction of additional experts, and judicial instruction.

Not every evaluation results in the completion of a written report. The preparation of a report is at the discretion of the retaining attorney. All court-ordered evaluations, however, do require that a written report be prepared, and distributed pursuant to the court's instructions. Testimony is not required in every case in which a report is completed. The judge may find the content of the report sufficient to assist in determination of the issue at hand. If testimony is required, the expert is usually contacted by the person who has retained them to complete the evaluation. In court-ordered evaluations, the expert is usually contacted by the side supported by the expert opinion. Occasionally, at a later stage of the process, an expert may be contacted by the other side, if information from the initial report is viewed as potentially useful regarding an issue that is being addressed. The expert can request that a subpoena be issued by the court requiring their testimony if this is not automatically issued. This may facilitate payment and also avoids the appearance of the expert being overly invested in the outcome of the case.

Although Rule 706 states that experts are entitled to reasonable compensation for their time (Fed. R. Evid. 706), the definition of reasonable can vary. At the outset, the expert should clarify the source of payment and determine whether usual fees can be paid by the court. In court-ordered evaluations of indigent defendants, there may be a set maximum compensation unless payment in excess is certified by the court because the services are of an unusual character or duration, and the amount of the excess payment is approved by the chief judge (United States Code). Other special fee situations can exist, such as the Ninth Circuit's policy in capital cases that limits the hourly fee that can be paid to an expert (Judicial Council of the Ninth Circuit Amended CJA Capital Habeas Costs Policy 2008). More commonly an expert is asked to estimate the cost of the evaluation and a set amount of funding is pre-approved. The expert is asked to complete an agreement for services and advised that any costs above those approved must be requested before expended. Travel funds for hotel and meals are covered at the federal per diem rates available at www.gsa.gov.

14.3 Evaluations in federal criminal cases

A variety of criminal evaluations can be conducted under federal law and are outlined in detail in 18 USC §§ 4241–4248. Crucial to writing reports on criminal issues is an understanding of 18 USC § 4247, which defines terms and discusses psychiatric or psychological examinations and reports. 18 USC § 4247 defines broad categories of what should be included in any report. Each report must include:

1. the person's history and present symptoms;
2. a description of the psychiatric, psychological, and medical tests that were employed and their results;
3. the examiner's findings; and
4. the examiner's opinions as to diagnosis, prognosis, and the specific issue addressed by the section of the statute under which the evaluation was ordered.

The law dictates that the examiner, who may be a psychiatrist or psychologist, must be licensed or certified and designated by the court, and identifies the time frames permitted for the initial evaluation. License or certification may be by any state or recognized jurisdiction. In cases that involve re-evaluation or evaluation by multiple interviewers, the court may identify different time frames for submission of reports. The reports prepared are filed with the court with copies provided to the counsel for the person examined and to the Assistant United States Attorney handling the case.

14.3.1 Competence to stand trial

Initial competency to stand trial evaluations are ordered under 18 USC § 4241. As defined in the statute, the issue to be addressed is whether the person is suffering from "a mental disease or defect rendering him mentally incompetent to the extent that he is unable to understand the nature and consequences of the proceedings against him or to assist properly in his defense." Interpretation continues to be guided by *Dusky* v. *US* (1960), which established the core issues to be whether the defendant has "sufficient present ability to consult with his attorney with a reasonable degree of rational understanding and whether he has a rational as well as factual understanding of the proceedings against him." Recent decisions continued to define and refine the level of competence needed to enter a plea or represent oneself. For example, *Indiana* v. *Edwards* (2008) moved beyond *Godinez* v. *Moran* (1993) in differentiating between the level of competence to stand trial and that required to represent oneself.

By statute, 30 days are allowed for the initial competency evaluation with a 15-day extension permitted (and routinely requested) pursuant to approval of a request made to the court. Evaluations by additional evaluators often occur consecutively, delaying the time period before a competency hearing is scheduled and the expert is potentially called to testify. If the court finds by a preponderance of the evidence that the defendant is not competent to stand trial, the defendant is committed to the custody of the Attorney General (the Federal Bureau of Prisons) pursuant to 18 USC § 4241(d) for a period of up to 4 months, "to determine whether there is a substantial probability that in the foreseeable future he will attain the capacity to permit the proceedings to go forward." From a practical standpoint this means that the defendant is committed to a federal prison psychiatric facility.

Reports must then be submitted every 6 months, or sooner if the competence appears to have been restored. These address whether competence has been restored and, if not, whether it can be restored in the future. If competence has not been restored, commitment may be extended for as long as the court finds a "substantial probability that within such additional period of time the defendant will attain the capacity to permit the proceedings to go forward" (18 USC). If the examiner determines that the defendant's competence cannot be restored, the examiner must evaluate whether the defendant's release would create a "substantial risk of bodily injury to another or serious damage to the property of another" (18 USC).

An opinion that the defendant's release would pose a danger then requires a report pursuant to 18 USC § 4246. The report is submitted to the clerk of the court for the district in which the defendant is confined, along with a certificate prepared by the director of the facility in which the defendant is housed, with a copy of the packet sent to the court of original jurisdiction. A hearing to determine commitment is then held and the examiner may be subpoenaed to testify. The examiner and the facility in which the defendant is held are required to determine whether a suitable state placement is available for the defendant (as an alternative to commitment to the Bureau of Prisons), and this information, including details of any efforts to establish such a placement, should be included in the report.

Defendants may remain committed under 18 USC § 4241(d) for extended periods of time, especially if they are charged with serious crimes, or if treatment is contested. States are unlikely to assume custody of an inmate who is still facing federal charges.

Experts are frequently asked to address the issue of medicating a defendant for the purpose of competence restoration. *Sell* v. *US* (2003) outlines four issues to be addressed prior to authorization for involuntary treatment: (1) the court must find that important government interests are at stake (this is directed at review of the seriousness of the crime); (2) the court must conclude that involuntary medication will significantly further those state interests; (3) the court must conclude that involuntary medication is necessary to further those interests and any alternative, less intrusive treatments are unlikely to achieve substantially the same results; and (4) the court must conclude that administration of the drugs is medically appropriate. Any report addressing the need for competence restoration should focus on the last three issues (Heilbrun & Kramer 2005; Mitrevski & Chamberlain 2006; Paul & Noffsinger 2008). Rendering an opinion on whether the government interests are sufficient to outweigh the individual's protected interests in refusing medication is beyond the expertise of a psychiatrist.

The question of competence to proceed in the legal process is not restricted to the pretrial stage. It can be raised by any party at any point in the process, including during the trial, at the pre-sentencing stage, or even post sentencing. Death penalty cases can present the psychiatric expert with the question of competence to be executed. The American Medical Association's Council on Ethical and Judicial Affairs (CEJA) has issued an opinion (CEJA Opinion 2.06) regarding capital punishment which provides guidance to clinicians in this area (AMA 1993). The opinion states that testifying (1) in competence to stand trial hearings, (2) to medical aspects of aggravating or mitigating circumstances during the penalty phase of a capital case, and (3) to medical diagnoses as they relate to the legal assessment of competence for execution do not constitute physician participation in execution.

The Supreme Court in *Ford* v. *Wainwright* (1986) found that the Eighth Amendment prohibited executing the insane, and clarified that defendants in death penalty cases must be able to understand the sentence that is being imposed and the reason it is being imposed. This was further reviewed in *Panetti* v. *Quarterman* (2007) where the Court held that a defendant with a long history of mental illness, who understood the nature of his crime and knew that the state's stated reason for his execution was because of the murders he had committed, could not be executed because his delusional belief that the state actually intended to execute him in order to carry out a satanic conspiracy against him precluded him having a rational understanding of the reason for his execution. This raised the importance of at least considering a broader interpretation of the meaning of understanding. The above referenced CEJA Opinion cautions that physicians should not determine legal competence to be executed, stating that a " physician's medical opinion should be merely one aspect of the information taken into account by a legal decision maker such as a judge or hearing officer."

Psychiatrists can also be asked to address an individual's competency to give up their appeals in the post-sentencing phase of a death penalty case. Here the question involves the individual's competency to waive their rights, and should focus on whether the waiver of rights is knowing, competent, and voluntary (Carvalho 2006; Shapiro 2008).

14.3.2 Insanity

Federal insanity evaluations are ordered pursuant to 18 USC § 4242, which asks whether the person was insane at the time of the offense charged (Federal Rules of Criminal Procedure). The standard is defined in 18 USC § 17 as "an affirmative defense to prosecution under any Federal Statute that, at the time of the commission of the offense, the defendant, as a result of severe mental disease or defect, was unable to appreciate the nature and quality or the wrongfulness of his acts." Mental disease or defect does not otherwise constitute a defense. The defendant has a right to competent, independent psychiatric assistance in insanity cases (*Ake* v. *Oklahoma*, 1985). The court routinely commits the person to the custody of the Attorney General for a period of up to 45 days for the evaluation. A 30-day extension can be requested. Of note, the current concept of insanity has been shaped by federal legislation. The Insanity Defense Reform Act of 1984, passed by Congress and signed into law in the wake of the Hinckley attempt to assassinate President Ronald Reagan, narrowed the defense. Specifically, this law shifted the burden of proof on the defendant to establish the insanity defense by clear and convincing evidence, limited the scope of expert psychiatric testimony on ultimate legal issues, and modified the insanity standard to require that the defendant suffer from a severe mental disease or defect.

In the report, the examiner can opine as to the ultimate issue, but as noted in Rule 704 (Fed. R. Evid. 704), cannot testify to this opinion in a jury trial. This can present a challenge for the expert as there is no consistency in how testimony is elicited and how near to outlining the ultimate opinion the examiner can go (Buchanan, 2006). The expert should ask the court for direction if they feel that their response may cross the boundary as outlined in Rule 704 (Fed. R. Evid. 704).

If the defendant is found to be not guilty only by reason of insanity, they are committed to a suitable facility (one that is able to provide care or treatment given the nature of the offense and the characteristics of the defendant; i.e., a federal prison medical center) as defined by 18 USC § 4247, for a period of 45 days (with a possible 30-day extension) to undergo yet another evaluation. The issue to be addressed is whether the person is suffering from a mental disease or defect as a result of which their release would create a substantial risk of bodily injury to another person or serious damage to the property of another.

Because the statute requires the examiner and the facility where the individual is housed to try to place them in a suitable state facility or in a conditional release program, evaluators should assess the individual for reasonable release conditions. These evaluations are, in essence, comprehensive risk assessments, the details of which should be outlined in the evaluation report. If, after a hearing, the court determines that the person's release would cause a danger, then they are committed to the custody of the Attorney General and detained in a Federal Bureau of Prisons psychiatric hospital facility until such time as they are no longer mentally ill or dangerous. The issue of suitability for release with or without conditions must be revisited at least annually in the form of a written report.

14.3.3 Pre-sentencing evaluations

Pre-sentencing evaluations focused on psychiatric issues can be conducted pursuant to 18 USC § 4244. Within 10 days of a finding of guilt but before sentencing, the court may order an evaluation to determine whether the person is suffering from a mental disease or defect as a result of which care or treatment at a suitable facility is required. The examination can also be ordered under 18 USC § 3552, as part of a pre-sentence investigation, with the evaluator being asked to make recommendations as to how the mental condition of the defendant should affect the sentence (focusing on issues outlined in 18 USC § 3553). The time allowed for a 4244 evaluation is 30 days with a 15-day extension. The time allowed for a 3552 evaluation is 60 days with a possible 60-day extension. Under 4244 if the examiner concludes that the defendant is in need of care or treatment at a suitable facility, the court may hospitalize the defendant under the care of the Attorney General in lieu of sentencing at that time. When the examiner determines that the defendant has recovered from mental illness and is thus no longer in need of custody for care or treatment, a report is filed, along with a certificate from the director of the facility, and the defendant can then move to final sentencing.

Diminished responsibility defenses at sentencing, under federal law, are only allowed for non-violent crimes (Parry & Drogin 2007). The concept of diminished responsibility is considered after an individual is convicted but before he is sentenced. Under Federal Sentencing Guidelines, which are no longer considered mandatory (*United States* v. *Booker*, 2005), punishment may be reduced due to mental disability. There have been some differences among circuits as to which crimes should be considered non-violent and thus eligible for a downward departure of sentencing. Appellate courts have also overturned cases in which mental impairments have been used to reduce sentences and affirmed them when they have enhanced punishment (ABA 2009).

14.4 Involuntary commitment of incarcerated individuals

18 USC § 4245 allows for hospitalization of an imprisoned person suffering from mental disease or defect, thus serving as the involuntary commitment statute for federally incarcerated individuals. In contrast to typical state commitment laws that focus on danger to self or others, federal commitment specifically addresses only a need for treatment or the risk of serious harm to others or to the property of others (18 USC). The question to be addressed, as in 18 USC § 4244, is whether the person is suffering from a mental disease or defect as a result of which he is in need of care or treatment at a suitable facility. The time frame for this evaluation is 30 days with a possible 15-day extension.

18 USC § 4246 provides for hospitalization of a person due for release but suffering from mental disease or defect. The question here, as in 18 USC § 4243, is whether the person is suffering from a mental disease or defect as a result of which their release would create a substantial risk of bodily injury to another person or serious damage to the property of another. The time frame for this evaluation is 45 days with a 30-day extension.

18 USC §4248, which came into existence with the passage of the Adam Walsh Act in 2006, provides for civil commitment of a sexually dangerous person. A psychiatric or psychological report on this issue addresses whether the person is a sexually dangerous person

(18 USC). Supreme Court cases (*Kansas v. Hendricks*, 1997; *Seling v. Young*, 2001; *Kansas v. Crane*, 2002) have described this as including uncontrollable behavior and the presence of a mental abnormality. The time frame for this evaluation is 45 days with the possibility of a 30-day extension. If the court finds by clear and convincing evidence that the person is a sexually dangerous person, the individual can be committed to the custody of the Attorney General until such time as they are no longer dangerous or a state assumes responsibility for care, custody, and treatment. (*US v. Comstock*, 2010; *US v. Tom*, 2009).

18 USC §§ 4243, 4246, and 4248 allow for conditional releases to be established that allow individuals who have been hospitalized through commitment into the federal system and for whom plans have been established to manage their risk, to leave the prison system but remain under federal supervision. The evaluator may be asked to determine whether a conditional release would be appropriate, and if so what the conditions should be. Subsequently, if conditions are violated, the examiner may again be asked to opine, in a report, on current dangerousness and need for revocation of or modifications to the release plan (Caffrey 2005; Morris 1997).

Commitment pursuant to any of these sections does not, in itself, authorize involuntary treatment with psychotropic medication. This may require an internal administrative review (*Washington v. Harper*) for convicted individuals or formal court review in pretrial cases. Neither of these precludes treatment in emergency situations. As noted, the law is evolving in regard to involuntary treatment for the purposes of restoration of competency to stand trial (*Sell v. US*, 2003) and courts are grappling with how to apply the Sell guidelines to individual cases.

For convicted inmates, the courts have recognized the internal administrative procedure developed within the Federal Bureau of Prisons as outlined in 28 CFR 549.43 Involuntary psychiatric treatment and medication. This involves review of the issue by a hearing officer (a psychiatrist not involved in the treatment); assignment of a staff representative to assist the inmate in contesting the proposed treatment; notice of the hearing; testimony by the treating clinician as to the rationale for treatment, proposed treatment plan, and anticipated response; and review of any additional testimony or witnesses identified or offered by the inmate. The hearing officer renders an opinion as to whether treatment is necessary. The inmate can appeal the decision to the institution mental health division administrator. The hearing officer then assures that periodic ongoing reviews of any involuntary treatment being rendered occur.

There is a provision to allow for the videotaping of any federal evaluation process (18 USC). This has been handled in various ways in various jurisdictions. Videotaping each individual interview is not the usual practice; more commonly, a single comprehensive interview focusing on the questions of the evaluation is videotaped during the latter part of the evaluation period and that videotape is provided at the time that the report is submitted. If videotaping is requested, the evaluator should determine what is reasonable without unduly interfering with the evaluation process, seek any needed clarification with the court if this is not viewed as acceptable to the parties involved, and ascertain any special requirements as to format. The courts recognize that videotaping can potentially intrude on the process of a forensic evaluation, yet under certain circumstances (e.g., when hypnosis is used) videotaping may be strongly recommended or even required (AAPL Task Force 1999).

The court may choose to conduct certain hearings via video conferencing. This occurs most often in regard to commitment proceedings pursuant to 18 USC §§ 4245 and 4246, but can be utilized in other types of hearings if authorized by the court. This too can present unique challenges to the expert, such as the video conferencing setup placing the clinician at a different site than the attorney who is eliciting their testimony on the issue, and technical limitations that prevent attending to all the parties equally. These hearings can also, however, save considerable time for the expert and expense to the court, and avoid the security concerns of transporting and housing seriously mentally ill inmates for the time period necessary for more traditional courtroom proceedings.

Initial federal evaluations pursuant to 18 USC §§ 4241–4248 are usually conducted within the Federal Bureau of Prisons (BOP; 2004). The BOP develops regulations which are eventually codified in the Code of Federal Regulations. These outline procedures for implementing 18 USC §§ 4241–4247. Review of applicable regulations provides additional detail for the evaluator conducting evaluations under these statutes. The BOP operates several federal medical centers with psychiatric units that conduct evaluations, and has identified mental health evaluators at other facilities who are available to complete certain types of evaluations. If a psychiatric evaluation is ordered by the court, the option exists to send the individual for an inpatient evaluation at one of the federal medical centers.

Women facing federal charges undergo evaluations at the Federal Medical Center in Carswell, Texas. Male offenders may be sent to any of the other Federal Medical Centers (Butner, NC; Springfield, MO; Rochester, MN; or Devens, MA) for evaluations. If the nature of the evaluator (psychiatrist or psychologist) is not specified, the case may be referred to a non-medical center institution for evaluation. The decisions as to where inmates will be sent for the various types of evaluations are handled through the Central Office of the BOP. Which institutions are conducting which types of evaluations can change over time, but can be determined by contacting the Designations Office or reviewing the BOP website at www. bop.gov.

Additional evaluations, by experts outside of the BOP, can be requested under any of the statutes described above, and are routinely authorized. These may take place in federal prisons or in a jail or detention facility. It is useful for the external evaluator, when evaluating someone in federal custody, to be aware of the types of records that are routinely established within the BOP, and to request them by name or type. A general request for medical records will not routinely provide all available or useful data. The evaluator should specifically request the medical record, Medication Administration Records, the Central File, the psychology file (PDS), any personal notes by evaluators or therapists, seclusion observation records, and logbook entries from any area in which the person has been housed. Movement, housing and commissary purchase records, as well as records of visitors and recordings of non-attorney phone conversations are also available, and can be extremely helpful in the evaluation process.

The US Marshall Service, Federal Bureau of Information, the US Secret Service, and Federal Probation Services all are potential sources of collateral information in federal cases. Written documents are routinely established during investigation and monitoring, and should be requested. Direct interview of agents or officers can provide clarification of information and can be a crucial source of behavioral observation to assist the evaluator in completing a comprehensive report.

14.5 Forensic evaluations in federal civil cases

The doctrine of sovereign immunity limits the ability to file suit against both federal and state government. There are exceptions, the most common of which are waivers of this immunity (e.g., through laws passed by federal or state governments allowing tort or contract suits against the government) (Federal Tort Claims Act) and abrogation of state immunity by exercise of federal powers under Article 5 of the Fourteenth Amendment. The Fourteenth Amendment created new constitutional rights including citizenship, voting rights, equal protection, and due process. Article 5 gives Congress the power to enforce the provisions of this amendment; thus Congress can authorize citizens to sue states in federal courts for deprivation of the rights created by the Fourteenth Amendment. In general, immunity is circumvented by bringing suit against individuals in their official government capacity (*Bivens* v. *Six Unknown Named Agents*, 1971). Even though the government itself is immune, government officials acting illegally or unlawfully, outside of their scope of employment, and in violation of the Constitution, are stripped of their position's power of protection, and are eligible to be sued as individuals.

Civil suits can be filed by institutionalized persons, including prisoners, regarding their conditions of confinement, care or treatment, if there is reason to believe that such conditions, care or treatment have fallen below a level defined by statute or the Constitution. Although there are many avenues under which these complaints can be addressed (Emergency Medical Treatment Act), one of the more common ways is to pursue action under the Civil Rights Act. 42 USC § 1983 provides that any person who, under color of any statute, deprives another of any rights secured by the Constitution and federal statutes, shall be liable to the person injured. The Supreme Court, in *Estelle* v. *Gamble* (1976) and again with *Farmer* v. *Brennan* (1994), viewed deliberate indifference to serious medical needs as cruel and unusual punishment, setting the standard to establish liability for medical maltreatment or negligence of convicted persons. *Bell* v. *Wolfish* (1979) did the same for pretrial inmates but utilized a due process argument. Individuals are expected to utilize reasonable professional judgment in the care and treatment of institutionalized persons. It is difficult to establish liability under this standard unless there is gross neglect or substantial departure from accepted standards or practice as was held by the court in *Youngberg v. Romeo* (1982).

Invitation to clinicians to be involved in a review may be initiated by the Department of Justice Civil Rights Division, after they have identified an institution or system that is suspect for falling below constitutional standards. These reviews involve intensive and extensive review of records, site visits to institutions, and direct interviewing of inmates and staff (Metzner 2002a, 2002b). The reports that are generated do not initially go directly to the court. They are used as resource and supporting documents in the process of federal review of state services. They are aimed not only at identifying weaknesses and deficiencies, but at describing the functional aspects of the operation. Suggestions for change, restructuring, and service enhancement or modification are included. The goal in these cases is correction of problems and improvement of conditions and care. The evaluator may be asked to commit to periodic reviews and submission of updated reports over a period of several years. Specifically the evaluator may be asked to identify when sufficient improvement/change has occurred to reasonably conclude that the problem does not need continued federal oversight.

The Prison Litigation Reform Act (1995) was implemented to restrict the number of frivolous lawsuits filed by inmates. It requires exhaustion of administrative remedies before a lawsuit can be filed, implements a number of provisions to penalize inmates who make inappropriate use of the system, and gives the court more discretion to dismiss suits (Belbot 2004). It also prohibits inmates from filing mental health claims unless physical injury has occurred and been documented by a medical provider. The psychiatrist's role, however, is limited to addressing the mental health claim.

The inmate can also petition the federal court for a writ of habeas corpus, in accordance with 28 USC § 2241, the granting of which is discretionary. Psychiatric experts are often retained to evaluate whether there are mental health issues that were not adequately explored at the time of the original trial. Reports here are provided directly to retained defense counsel and the report itself or its content may then be assimilated into a habeas petition. The Antiterrorism and Death Penalty Act of 1996 has impacted the ability of inmates to have habeas corpus review in the federal courts. The major impacts are outlined in Title 1 of the Act and include: a bar on federal habeas reconsideration of legal and factual issues ruled upon by state courts in most instances; creation of a general 1-year statute of limitations within which habeas petitions must be filed after the completion of direct appeal; creation of a 6-month statute of limitation in death penalty cases; encouragement for states to appoint counsel for indigent state death row inmates during state habeas or unitary appellate proceedings; and a requirement of appellate court approval for repetitious habeas petitions (PL 104–132, 110 Stat.1214).

The Federal Rules of Civil Procedure generally require that all experts must prepare written reports that form the basis for their opinions. Reports must set forth the expert's qualifications, including publications, opinions, the facts and data relied on, and the reasons for conclusions. If the expert is qualified as such by the judge, the report is admitted into evidence and the expert is subject to direct and cross-examination. The civil party retaining the expert must produce, in discovery, all reports prepared by its experts. The trial judge has considerable discretion to apply these rules.

Rule 26 (Federal Rules of Civil Procedure) also requires that the identity of any experts that may be used at trial be disclosed along with the written report, prepared and signed by the expert. This disclosure must occur at the time directed by the court. The report for a trial expert must also contain a complete statement of all opinions the witness will express and the basis and reasons for them; the data or other information considered by the witness in forming them; any exhibits that will be used to summarize or support them; the witness's qualifications, including a list of all publications authored in the previous 10 years; a statement of compensation to be paid for the study and testimony in the case; and a list of all other cases in which the witness testified as an expert at trial or by deposition during the previous 4 years.

14.6 Producing the report and clarifying your opinion

Federal guidelines do not dictate the format of the psychiatric report. The evaluator can request that the court order that the parties involved promptly provide requested collateral information. Although many types of federal evaluations have a time frame for completion outlined in statute, there is some flexibility in interpreting when the evaluation period actually begins. With notification to the court, most judges will approve that the evaluation process start at the time the defendant is made available to the evaluator. The goal of the report is clarity and completeness for the audience. Although federal rules allow for them, depositions in criminal cases are not the norm. Federal Rules of Civil Procedure 74 and 76 provide general guidance. The court does maintain the authority to order that a deposition be taken without the consent of all parties. The court may also order that the deposition transcript serve as the expert witness report.

14.7 Conclusion

Although writing reports for the federal courts involves familiarity with many of the details, rules, and regulations outlined above, the process, regardless of whether the issue is criminal or civil, involves attention to the core issues outlined throughout this text. Conducting evaluations in federal cases, however, can also lead experts into areas where specialized knowledge is needed outside the realm of that usually encountered in other evaluation settings or even in the general practice of psychiatry. There are certain types of crimes, individuals, and settings that come under federal jurisdiction that bring with them unique cultural, international, or agency-related issues, and the onus is on experts to familiarize themselves sufficiently with such issues to be able to apply their psychiatric expertise accurately and appropriately.

Federal evaluations may focus on terrorists, spies, hijackers, presidential threateners, kidnappers, drug traffickers, sex offenders, tax evaders, or counterfeiters, or on crimes of the airways, seas, borders, internet, or reservations. Evaluations of individuals involved in any of these unique criminal areas present opportunities for psychiatrists to explore issues of national and international concern. Likewise, addressing issues such as what are the minimal constitutional standards or rights to evaluation or care in institutions, or how competent is competent enough to proceed through the criminal justice system, can ultimately assist in enhancing psychiatric services and shaping the law and public policies affecting the mentally ill.

References

AAPL Task Force (1999) Videotaping of forensic psychiatric evaluations. *Journal of the American Academy of Psychiatry and the Law* 27: 345–358.

ABA (2009) American Bar Association Commission on Mental & Physical Disability Law Digest: Criminal Diminished Responsibility.

Adam Walsh Act, Title III §302.

Ake v. *Oklahoma* 470 US 68 (1985).

AMA (1993) Physician Participation in Capital Punishment: Opinion 2.06. *Journal of the American Medical Association* 270: 365–368.

Amato, J. M. & Packer, I. K. (2006) Battered-child syndrome. *Journal of the American Academy of Psychiatry and the Law* 34(3): 414–416.

Americans with Disabilities Act 42 USC Section 12101 et. seq.

Belbot, B. (2004) Report on the Prison Litigation Reform Act: what have the courts decided so far? *The Prison Journal* 84(3): 290–316.

Bell v. *Wolfish*, 441 US 520 (1979).

Biggers, J. R. (2005) The utility of diagnostic language as expert witness testimony: should syndrome terminology be used in battering cases? *Journal of Forensic Psychology Practice* 5(1): 43–61.

Bivens v. *Six Unknown Named Agents*, 403 US 388 (1971).

Buchanan, A. (2006) Psychiatric evidence on the ultimate issue. *Journal of the American Academy of Psychiatry and the Law* 34(1): 14–21.

Caffrey, M. (2005) A new approach to insanity acquittee recidivism: redefining the class of truly responsible recidivists. *University of Pennsylvania Law Review* 154: 399.

Carvalho, V. (2006) Competence for waiver of appeals in the death penalty: timing, standard and standing. *Journal of the American Academy of Psychiatry and the Law* **34**(1): 120–122.

Civil Rights Act, USC Section 1983.

Dahir, V. B., Richardson, J. T., Ginsburg, G. P., et al. (2005) Judicial application of Daubert to psychological syndrome and profile evidence: a research note. *Psychology, Public Policy, and Law* **11**(1): 62–82.

Daubert v. *Merrell Dow Pharmaceuticals Inc.*, 61 USLW 4805, 113 S.Ct. 2786 (1993).

Dusky v. *US*, 362 US 402, 80 S.Ct. 788 (1960).

Emergency Medical Treatment Act 42 USC § 1395dd.

Estelle v. *Gamble*, 429 US 97 (1976).

Farmer v. *Brennan*, 511 US 825 (1994).

Federal Rules of Evidence 701, 702, 703, 704, 705, 706.

Federal Bureau of Prisons (2004) Guidelines for Forensic Evaluations: Clinical Practice Guidelines.

Federal Rules of Civil Procedure.

Federal Rules of Criminal Procedure, Rule 12.2.

Federal Sentencing Guidelines, USSG section 5K2.13.

Federal Tort Claims Act, 28 USC Ch. 171, ss. 1346, 2671.

Ford v. *Wainwright*, 477 US 399, 106 S.Ct. 2595 (1986)

General Electric Co. v. *Joiner*, 118 S.Ct. 512 (1997)

Godinez v. *Moran*, 113 S.Ct. 2680 (1993).

Grove, W. M. & Barden, R. C. (1999) Protecting the integrity of the legal system: the admissibility of testimony from mental health experts under Daubert/Kumho analyses. *Psychology, Public Policy, and Law* **5**(1): 224–242.

Gutheil, T. G. & Stein, M. D. (2000) Daubert-based gatekeeping and psychiatric/psychological testimony in court: review and proposal. *Journal of Psychiatry and the Law* **28**(2): 235–251.

Gutheil, T. G. & Sutherland, P. K. (1999) Forensic assessment, witness credibility and the search for truth through expert testimony in the courtroom. *Journal of Psychiatry and the Law* **27**(2): 289–312.

Heilbrun, K & Kramer, G. M. (2005) Involuntary medication, trial competence, and clinical dilemmas: Implications of Sell v. United States for psychological practice. *Professional Psychology: Research and Practice* **36**(5): 459–466.

Indiana v. *Edwards*, 554 US 208 (2008).

Judicial Council of the Ninth Circuit Amended CJA Capital Habeas Costs Policy October 2008. Available at www.azd.uscourts.gov.

Kansas v. *Crane* 534 US 407 (2002).

Kansas v. *Hendricks* 521 US 346 (1997).

Kumho Tire Co., Ltd. v. *Carmichael*, 119 S.Ct. 1167 (1999).

Metzner, J. (2002a) Class action litigation in correctional psychiatry. *Journal of the American Academy of Psychiatry and the Law* **30**: 19–29.

Metzner, J. (2002b) Prison litigation in the USA. *Journal of Forensic Psychiatry* **13**(2): 240–244.

Mitrevski, J. P. & Chamberlain, J. R. (2006) Competence to stand trial and application of sell standards: involuntary medication allowed in a nondangerous defendant, to restore competence to stand trial. *Journal of the American Academy of Psychiatry and the Law* **34**(2): 250–252.

Morris, G. H. (1997) Placed in purgatory: conditional release of insanity acquittees. *Arizona Law Review* **39**: 1061.

Panetti v. *Quarterman*, 127 S.Ct. 2842 (2007).

Parry, J. & Drogin, E. (2007) *Mental Disability Law, Evidence, and Testimony: A Comprehensive Reference*. Chicago, IL: American Bar Association.

Paul, R. & Noffsinger, S. (2008) Involuntary medication to restore competence to stand trial: Sell revisited. *Journal of the American Academy of Psychiatry and the Law* **36**(4): 583–585.

PL 104–132, 110 Stat.1214.

Prison Litigation Reform Act of 1995, Pub. L. No. 104–134.

Roberts, P. (1996) Will you stand up in court? On the admissibility of psychiatric and psychological evidence. *Journal of Forensic Psychiatry* **7**(1): 63–78.

Seling v. *Young* 531 US 250, 254–55 (2001).

Sell v. *US*, 539 US 166, 123 S.Ct. 2174 (2003).

Shapiro, P. (2008) Are we executing mentally incompetent inmates because they volunteer to die?: A look at various states' implementation of standards of competency to waive post-conviction review. *Catholic University Law Review* **57**: 567.

Slobogin, C. (1999) The admissibility of behavioral science information in criminal trials: From primitivism to Daubert to voice. *Psychology, Public Policy, and Law* **5**(1): 100–119.

Slobogin, C., Frost, L. E., & Bonnie, R. J. (2001) *Psychiatric Evidence in Criminal Trials: A 25-year Retrospective. The Evolution of Mental Health Law*. Washington, DC: American Psychological Association, pp. 245–276.

Social Security Act 42 USC Ch. 7.

United States Code, Title 18, Chapter 201, § 3006A.

United States Criminal Code 18 USC Ch. 1 et. seq.

United States v. *Booker*, 543 US 220 (2005).

US v. *Comstock*, 130 S. Ct. 1949 (2010).

US v. *Tom*, 558 F. Supp. 931, 941 (2009).

Washington v. *Harper*, 28 CFR 549.40.

Youngberg v. *Romeo* 457 US 307, 323 (1982).

Youngstrom, E. A. & Busch, C. P. (2000) Expert testimony in psychology: ramifications of Supreme Court decision in Kumho Tire Co., Ltd. v. Carmichael. *Ethics and Behavior* **10**(2): 185–193.

Chapter 15

Incorporating psychological testing

Madelon V. Baranoski

Although psychological testing is not required in psychiatric evaluations, it is often included as an adjunct to clinical assessments or forensic psychiatric assessments. As part of psychiatric and forensic assessments, psychological testing explains dysfunction and disruptive behaviors. It analyzes thinking and behavior beyond the diagnosis of disorders and can include objective measures of cognitive functioning, standard indicators of effort and of feigning, a comparison of individual characteristics to population norms, and simulation of real situations to test ranges of concentration and emotional control in ways beyond usual clinical assessments. In forensic assessments, the addition of psychological testing can bolster the foundation of the psychiatric assessment and contribute to the expert's demonstration of a comprehensive approach to the work (Baranoski 2010).

Psychological testing is a subspecialty in psychology and includes a wide array of measures that have established psychometric properties (i.e., established reliability and validity, as well as limits to the generalizability and application of each test) and standardized methods of administration, scoring, and interpretation. Tests vary in form, from standardized measures of cognitive, perceptual, and motor capacities to projective tests that offer impressions of critical issues and coping style. Psychological evaluations include a battery of tests that collectively describe cognitive and memory capacity, personality profiles and characteristics, and problem-solving approaches. Subspecialties of psychological evaluations include neuropsychological batteries and assessments of autism.

Psychological tests are selected for administration based on the question to be answered, the history, and the purpose of the evaluation. For example, IQ and achievement tests would be used as part of career counseling for a person with no history of head trauma. With a history of a brain injury, however, the testing would need to include a neuropsychological battery to identify the specific deficits that may interfere with usual learning and to suggest ways to accommodate for the impairment. In forensic assessments and in diagnostic clinical assessments, psychological testing usually consists of a standard battery that includes cognitive and personality assessments as well as measures of effort and of feigning.

A review of all types of psychological testing is beyond the scope of this chapter but is available elsewhere (Melton et al. 2007). The purpose of this chapter is to describe the integration of psychological assessments into the psychiatric report and to identify ways to address inconsistent testing results from collateral sources. This chapter will begin with a brief discussion of the advantages and limitations of psychological testing and what should

The Psychiatric Report, ed. Alec Buchanan and Michael A. Norko. Published by Cambridge University Press. © Cambridge University Press 2011.

be expected from a psychological evaluation and report and then consider the advantages of different methods of including psychological assessments in psychiatric reports.

15.1 Advantages of psychological testing

All psychological tests include standardized material, administration, and interpretation. That is, any given test includes the same items presented to every person tested in the same way and scored in the same way, regardless of the context or history of the person. This standardization provides a set of norms by which to compare the person tested with the population of persons similar in age, primary language, education, and sometimes gender. Many of the tests identify strengths, deficits, and abnormalities in terms of deviations from the established norms. For example, intelligence testing compares the individual's cognitive ability to a normed distribution of scores from the samples upon which the tests were developed. The normed tests are similar to physiological measures such as blood tests, in which values obtained for an individual are compared to distributions of values determined through population studies. A so-called abnormal finding is one that falls out of the range of values for healthy controls. One difference with the normed scores on psychological tests that measure various capacities (in contrast to blood tests) is that rather than outcomes described as normal and abnormal the results are presented in terms of standard deviations from the average score in the population and as such describe strengths when the score is significantly higher than average and deficits when the score is significantly lower than the mean. The bi-dimensional characteristic of testing results in a profile of strengths and weaknesses that adds to a diagnostic profile and can inform treatment decisions. For example, a person with a psychotic disorder who demonstrates higher-than-average short- and intermediate-term memory would likely benefit more from cognitive interventions to enhance coping skills than would a patient with the same diagnosis who has below-average memory ability.

In addition to identifying different levels of capacity, psychological testing results also indicate dysfunction, such as formal thought disorder, deficits in attention and concentration, performance anxiety, and psychomotor, language, and perceptual deficits. When combined, the results of different tests can offer treatment strategies that address the disorders by building on the strengths of the individual, tailoring the interventions to maximize function. For example, psychological testing for patients in an intensive outpatient program for patients with schizophrenia helped to identify activities best suited for each client. Those with strengths in pattern recognition and visual motor integration and deficits in abstract reasoning participated in groups that used visual arts and craft work to express emotional states; those whose strength was in verbal skills but not in visual and manual skills were in groups that used writing and "talk" to explore issues in daily living. The success of the approach culminated in a play produced for staff and family in which all had a part in the production, from stage and scenery art to acting. The psychological testing allowed staff to see beyond the diagnosis to the individual's problem-solving style and personality.

Psychological testing can mimic challenges of everyday life and thereby elicit responses not apparent in a clinical interview. The standardization of the tests provides a yardstick for comparing the individual to the theoretical peer group to enhance the assessment of strengths and weaknesses. For example, in a forensic competency to stand trial evaluation, a defendant was irritable and marginally cooperative, responding with sarcastic answers that mocked the evaluation, the psychiatrist, and the court. When asked the role of the defense attorney, the defendant answered, "He don't know nothin, he don't do nothin." Throughout the interview, his responses varied little in tone, his usual response being "I don't know and I don't care." His behavior and the lack of collateral data made it difficult to draw a conclusion. The psychiatrist requested psychological testing to help determine whether the lack of cooperation reflected willful obstruction or some deficit. The testing revealed a cognitive deficit (an IQ of 74) and a guarded style in which the young man answered only when he knew the answer or thought he did. What was revealed on the testing is that he was eager to show off his ability but was shamed by his limitation. The psychological testing added a quantification of the man's intellectual capacity, revealing his uncooperative façade to be an effort to preserve his dignity. For example, when asked, *How many eggs in a dozen?* he answered with a smile, "I know this! Six eggs in a small dozen and in a big dozen, eight. I go shopping and I do my own money. My worker lets me hold the change." When the questions got harder and the man was aware that he did not know the answers, behavior similar to that which he displayed in the competency interview emerged. When asked on what continent Belgium is located, he answered, "That is a stupid question. I don't know and I don't care." The testing results were useful in identifying the cognitive deficit but also in providing a strategy for eliciting his understanding of the court proceedings and for teaching him what he needed to know.

15.1.1 Diagnostic clarification

Psychological testing aids in diagnostic formulation and can help to reconcile disparate symptoms relevant to different diagnoses. For example, testing can help to identify whether distractibility is the result of an attention deficit disorder or of psychotic intrusions into thinking. Cognitive testing can also estimate the level of premorbid functioning and thereby give some estimate of the severity of the current impairment as well as an indication of what range of function to expect with treatment and recovery interventions. The standardized measures also provide a yardstick for tracking changes in function as well as in the effectiveness of treatment. For example, interval assessments of memory and language for patients with dementia help to define the trajectory of decline.

15.1.2 Assessment of feigning and malingering

Assessment of malingering (Box 15.1) is another area that is aided by psychological tests. The diagnosis requires intentional feigning of symptoms motivated by external incentives. Psychological tests have been designed to assess effort, feigning, and exaggerated style of responding, such as over-reporting of symptoms or the denial of problems. These assessments are used for two purposes: to assess the validity of the rest of the testing and to measure directly the feigning of specific symptoms. In all testing situations, the examiner wants to be certain that the results reflect honest effort so that the scores are valid indicators of ability. Many measures – the Minnesota Multiphasic Personality Inventory is one example – include validity indicators that determine the extent to which the scores are meaningful. Results that are invalid cannot be interpreted. On cognitive tests, full effort is required to assess intellectual capacity.

Specific tests assess effort and feigning. Two common tests used in psychological assessments are the Validity Indicator Profile (VIP) (Frederick 1997), a measure of effort and of feigning cognitive impairment, and the Test of Memory Malingering (TOMM) (Tombaugh 2009), which evaluates intentional faking of memory deficits. The Structured Interview

Box 15.1 Malingering

Malingering is a subclass of feigning. Feigning is the willful reporting of fake symptoms. The diagnosis of malingering requires that feigning be motivated by external incentives.

of Reported Symptoms (SIRS) assesses the validity of reported psychotic symptoms and identifies patterns associated with feigning and with actual psychosis (Rogers 1992, 2002). Incorporating the results of these tests can inform an assessment of feigning beyond the information provided in a clinical interview. The structured and relatively lengthy tests in particular can reduce the risk of false-positive assessments of exaggeration or feigning. By structure and length they are able to reduce the effect of over-emphasis that frequently occurs when patients and defendants are concerned that their distress is not being acknowledged.

In forensic assessments, tests of feigning and malingering are essential components of psychological assessments because of the obvious external incentive related to the outcome of the legal matter. The inclusion of the psychological assessment enhances the psychiatric formulation because of the formality of the malingering assessment.

15.1.3 Supporting and identifying forensic issues

In forensic evaluations, psychological testing offers additional advantages. A psychological assessment buttresses even the most certain and supported psychiatric opinion and gives further evidence of comprehensiveness in the use of all means available to answer the legal question. In both forensic and clinical cases, results of psychological testing usually suggest psychological issues worthy of further exploration; thus, the psychiatrist may find it beneficial to meet again with the person after learning the results of the psychological evaluation.

In addition, psychological testing identifies vulnerable areas in a formulation that might require more collateral information or more discussion. For example, consider the case of a man who stabbed to death another man, during a fight in which the victim threatened the defendant with a shovel, after the defendant hit the victim's car while parking. The defendant claimed self-defense, citing fear that the victim was about to hit him with the shovel. His story seemed implausible since he would have had to approach quite close to a shovel-wielding person to strike him with a screwdriver. Psychological testing revealed marked deficits in pattern and spatial recognition in contrast to average ability on the other tests. The results were suggestive of parietal lobe and pre-frontal trauma, although the man had reported none. The psychiatrist investigated further and found hospital records that confirmed the defendant had sustained head trauma and was unconscious after a fight while incarcerated in another state. Although the defendant had no recollection of the event, a brain scan showed evidence of scar tissue in the pre-frontal cortex. The history of head trauma and its location made the defendant's account more plausible.

15.2 Questions psychological testing cannot answer

Three issues that are common in forensic psychiatry in particular and in psychiatry in general cannot be answered by psychological testing: the etiology of the deficit, the veracity of the client's account, and the cause of a specific behavior in the past (Box 15.2).

Testing can define the parameters of the deficit, not the etiology. For example, in a civil suit involving compensation for damages after an auto accident, psychological testing can estimate the extent of impairment but cannot determine the connection between the

---

Box 15.2 Questions psychological testing cannot answer

Psychological testing *cannot* determine:
- What caused a deficit.
- Whether a person is lying or telling the truth.
- State of mind at a given time in the past.

---

accident and the decreased function. Collateral data such as pre-accident educational and employment records are more relevant. The testing, however, can be useful in formulating an opinion about whether the past level of performance is consistent with the degree of injury and current level of impairment.

Psychological testing cannot determine whether someone is lying about a specific topic. Even if testing establishes that a person has feigned symptoms on the testing, and even whether the personality profile is one associated with lying in general, the testing cannot determine if lying occurred in the particular case. Even habitual liars sometimes tell the truth, and the most honest of humans has probably lied. Indeed, one of the validity questions on a personality test requests an honest answer to a question about whether the individual ever told a lie. Although the testing results may address the likelihood of an opinion that someone was honest or not, no psychological testing report should include an opinion (based on testing) about the veracity of a discrete event or statement.

In a similar way, psychological testing cannot determine the cause of any past behavior, since behavior can have many different and interactive causes. Even during a psychotic episode, not every behavior is the result of psychosis. What psychological testing can do is to bolster or refute the likelihood of a behavioral cause that involves a psychiatric illness. In the same way that knowledge of climate makes a weather reporter's forecast for a particular day more or less likely, psychological testing can describe the parameters of cognition and personality that include likely behaviors. Just as there are record-setting weather events that occur understandably within a climate context, a person's unusual behavior may be understood better within a psychological context informed by testing.

15.3 The referral for psychological testing

The most useful psychological assessment begins with an appropriate referral that specifies the questions to be answered and the context of the case. Psychological assessments cannot be completed without history, situational context, and a clinical assessment by the psychologist. The psychologist requires a clear question and background information to choose the correct tests, an understanding of the context in order to describe the conditions of confidentiality of the evaluation, and a detailed assessment to garner confirmation that the testing results are a valid reflection of the individual. The confirmation occurs in an assessment of symptoms, daily activities, and collateral information from knowledgeable contacts, educational, psychiatric, and medical records. The psychologist arrives at conclusions by integrating testing results and the individual's presentation, daily life, and past history.

Because psychological assessments are less effective when conducted without adequate information, communication between the psychiatrist and psychologist is critical and should be ongoing throughout the testing before the final report is prepared. In this way conflicting findings can be explored with further sessions or collateral information by both the psychiatrist and psychologist. The least effective referral is one in which the psychological testing is requested as a pro forma addition to the psychiatric evaluation, without being integrated into the evaluation or the final report.

The referral for psychological testing initiates collaboration on the assessment between the psychiatrist and psychologist. Through that collaboration, the referral question is refined, the limits of testing are examined, and a discussion of preliminary findings and impressions guide the next phases of the evaluation. The effort is not to shape the two evaluations to force agreement, but rather to use the findings in each assessment to inform and direct the work of both professionals (Campbell & Baranoski 2008).

15.4 Incorporating the psychological assessment

On request by a psychiatrist, psychological testing is done by a psychologist who generates an independent signed report. The psychologist can act without referral as the sole clinician or forensic expert, but this chapter will address report writing when the psychologist is responding to a referral by the psychiatrist. The incorporation of the psychological findings into the psychiatric report can be accomplished in a number of ways, each with advantages and disadvantages.

15.4.1 Including the entire psychological report

One of the less common approaches involves the incorporation of the entire psychological report into the psychiatric report. Under a separate heading (e.g., Report of Psychological Testing), the psychiatrist introduces the psychologist's report and sets it off so that the print is visually distinguishable from the rest of the psychiatric report (e.g., in italics or another font).

The advantage of this method for the psychiatrist is that the psychological report becomes a subsection of the psychiatric report and not an independent assessment. The psychiatrist in this way takes ownership of the assessment and indicates the primacy of the psychiatric formulation and conclusion. Similar to incorporating the results of a brain scan or blood work, the incorporation directs attention to the psychiatric conclusion.

The disadvantages of this method are the flipside of the advantages. Taking ownership of the psychological report means that the psychiatrist will be asked to defend and explain another professional's thinking and methods. In forensic cases and in testimony, the psychiatric expert may be asked about minutiae of testing or about the limitations of the tests and be unable to answer. In one forensic case, the psychiatrist included the entire psychological report in which the psychologist had quoted the computer-generated report for the MMPI-2. The psychiatrist was asked on cross-examination why only one quotation was included and what had been left out. She was challenged about picking the favorable quotations and hiding that which went against her opinion. Her inability to guess what the psychologist had been thinking undermined her credibility on the stand. Had the psychologist been asked the same question, the ready answer was that the computer-generated reports included irrelevant material, and it was part of the testing, scoring, and interpretive process to review the computer assessment against collateral data.

An uncommon variation of this method that takes care of this disadvantage is for both the psychologist and psychiatrist to sign the report and enter it as a team document in which both endorse the whole opinion but take responsibility for explaining different parts of the document.

> **Box 15.3 Conditions of testing**
> - Date(s) of session(s)
> - Total contact time
> - Medication, substance, and alcohol use at and around time of testing
> - Special accommodations (interpreter, hearing aid, etc.)

Whenever the psychological report is incorporated into the psychiatric report, there must also be a separate report signed by the psychologist. Since a signature on a document declares ownership, endorsement, and responsibility, a psychological report without the preparer's signature would have no standing in court.

15.4.2 Including a summary prepared by the psychologist

A more common method of incorporating the psychological assessment is to ask the psychologist to prepare a jargon-free summary of the testing conditions (see Box 15.3), records reviewed and collateral sources, conclusions drawn from the testing, and implications for day-to-day behavior.

In addition to the conditions of testing, the summary should include a brief statement of the purpose of the evaluation (the question or questions that the psychological testing is designed to answer), a description of the presentation and attitude toward the testing of the person tested, and a summary of mental status during the session. In forensic reports, a section on malingering should be included in the summary.

Testing conclusions should be expressed as brief statements about the areas of testing, formatted so as to highlight the separate findings. For example, consider a hypothetical forensic case in which a man was arrested for carrying a gun into the bank where he had been a financial manager and threatening the official who had laid him off. A psychiatrist was assessing Mr. Doe for state of mind and had opined that he was suffering from a psychotic depression at the time of the event and was suicidal. Psychological testing was completed and the following summary of conclusions was provided by the psychologist:

> Mr. Doe was cooperative with the testing and showed no evidence on the testing of malingering or exaggerating symptoms or impairments. He put forth honest effort to answer correctly as evidenced on the validity scales and malingering tests. Mr. Doe demonstrated average intellectual capacity and showed no evidence of a thought disorder. However, he processed information at a slow rate, a finding that is consistent with depression. On personality testing, he produced a profile associated with obsessive-compulsive characteristics and a level of suspiciousness that at times can reach paranoid proportions. These characteristics did not reach the level of a personality disorder on the testing. He showed evidence of anxiety and major depression but without suicidal intention or preoccupation. He has a strong attachment to his family and links his identity and value to his ability to provide for them. At this time, he is filled with shame and views himself as a failure.

The last part of the summary should address strengths and vulnerabilities, make inferences about daily functioning based on the testing, and state whether the testing is or is not congruent with collateral information. For example, based on the previous hypothetical conclusions, the summary might have noted further the following:

> Considering Mr. Doe's past success as a banking manager for over 25 years and the information provided by his wife about the change in his behavior since he was laid off during a bank

merger in the economic downturn, I conclude that the suspiciousness and the paranoid and obsessive-compulsive personality characteristics evident from the testing are more a product of his depression than of any enduring personality characteristics. The testing suggests that Mr. Doe reacts to stress, depression, and anxiety with heightened attention to detail, the loss of the "big picture," and distrust of others. When his acute distress subsides, he is likely to show significantly less obsessive thinking or paranoia. The finding of no thought disorder on cognitive testing and the absence of a personality disorder even in the presence of depression indicate that he does not have a primary psychotic disorder. However, at the time of the testing he was on an antipsychotic medication and one for depression. Therefore, without treatment and in the presence of major depression, his paranoia and rigid thinking will likely be more pronounced and may reach psychotic proportions, interfering with his perception of reality. Mrs. Doe's description of her husband's change in behavior indicates that he was less able to make decisions even about simple things, was concerned that others viewed him as a failure, worried that his resume would be lost by the postal service, and believed he was singled out by the bank president because he was older than others and had disagreed with the policy of the bank in a meeting 10 years before. These behaviors demonstrate the heightened obsessive-compulsive characteristics, suspiciousness, and paranoia that were described in the personality profile of the testing.

In the example, the conclusion does not address the specific event at the bank, but rather links the testing results to everyday behavior that indicates the applicability of the testing. Moreover, the conclusion is presented in a way that can explain why a man who had never had a psychiatric diagnosis in the past could have a psychotic episode under the right conditions.

The advantage of the psychologist-produced summary is that the information provided is relevant to the assessment and can be utilized in a way that highlights the main results. At the same time, the summary does not include aspects of the methodology that the psychiatrist cannot explain. So although the tests are listed, the psychiatrist is not expected to defend or explain them, since the report summary does not include particulars about the tests themselves. Of course, the psychiatrist and psychologist should discuss the findings and conclusions before the summary is prepared. The psychiatrist has the final say about whether the summary is included in the psychiatric report.

A disadvantage is that the psychiatrist can still be held accountable for wording or ideas prepared by someone else. It is also the case that slightly different wording in the psychiatric formulation and the psychological summary may be distracting, especially in a forensic case, where judges, attorneys, and juries may be confused by clinically meaningless differences. The inclusion of the summary attests to the independence of the two evaluations. To emphasize the distinction between the two reports, the psychiatrist can append the complete psychological report signed by the psychologist.

15.4.3 Summarizing the psychological report

Another common approach is for the psychiatrist to create a summary from the original psychological report. The advantage here is that the psychiatrist chooses what is relevant and restates the findings in his or her own words. There will be continuity within the language of the report, and the psychiatrist will have full ownership over what is included and therefore be able to account for what is summarized.

The disadvantage is that the restatement might be challenged along with the psychiatrist's choice of what to exclude and what to highlight. When this method is used, the report of the psychologist should always be appended if it does not go directly to the requester of the psychiatric evaluation.

15.4.4 Excluding the psychological content

The least supportable and least common method of dealing with a psychological evaluation in a forensic case is to note that one was completed but include no data or discussion of the psychological testing results. The one exception when this method is the only alternative is the occasion when the psychiatrist and psychologist have been hired separately and complete their assessments and write-ups separately and concurrently without conferring with each other. Otherwise, the usual progression is for the psychological assessment to be available for the psychiatrist as he or she is writing the final formulation.

Psychiatrists who have included no information from the psychological testing in their report have the advantage of offering the court two completely independent assessments that concur. However, a disadvantage is that the two reports address different questions, and to the extent that the psychiatrist had requested psychological testing, ignoring the findings suggests that the testing was not relevant.

15.5 When results conflict

When the psychological findings support the psychiatric formulation, the incorporation of the testing requires attention to wording and the elimination of jargon. A very different challenge exists when the psychological testing does not support the conclusion. This can happen when the findings identify a disorder that was not evident in the psychiatric assessment or when they identify feigning but the psychiatric assessment indicates that real illness exists. Under these circumstances, reconciling the disparate findings falls to both the psychiatrist and psychologist. In clinical cases, conflicting reports may lead to competing treatment recommendations. Such cases call for a general discussion of the different findings and how the clinician might collect evidence to verify one or the other formulation or some combination of them. For example, in a case where the testing results indicate a greater degree of psychosis than is evident in the psychiatric assessment that found a bipolar disorder, a helpful resolution to the difference would be to describe the impact of emotional instability on rational thinking. Less useful are two reports that offer different diagnoses.

In forensic cases, however, conflicting reports from the same team undermine the effectiveness of the experts. Such conflict needs to be resolved before the final report is prepared. An effective resolution is rarely a simple choice of one formulation over the other. Far more effective is a discussion of how the conflict arose and an explanation of why it reasonably exists. To the extent that the psychological testing was administered properly, scored accurately, and interpreted appropriately, then the conflicting findings may be the result of different conditions under which the evaluations were done. For example, if the psychiatric examination was done before medication was begun and the psychological testing after, the effect of the medication needs to be considered. In that case, the psychiatrist may need a re-visit, or the psychologist may need to emphasize the potential effects of medication on various symptoms and on the results of the testing.

Another common explanation of differences is the nature of what is measured in psychological testing compared with a psychiatric interview. Consider a case in which a man with schizophrenia is incarcerated after killing his father. Although medicated, the man continues to have hallucinations and delusions but is much calmer than he was reported to be in the days surrounding the event. The psychiatrist interviews the man for many hours and notes that he is slow to answer and echoes the questions posed. The psychiatrist formulates the case based on evidence of psychosis and the man's delusional belief that his father had made him impotent by inserting electrical charges into his body while he slept. The psychiatrist also notes that the man is intellectually slow. The psychological testing finds that the man has higher-than-average intellectual endowment but is psychotic. The psychiatric evaluation identified the functional effect of the psychosis on cognition. The psychological evaluation can also assess the intellectual capacities, such as vocabulary and past learning, that are spared despite the disorder. In this example the resolution is relatively easy – the psychiatric formulation that explains the criminal behavior does not turn on intellectual ability but on psychosis. Indeed, changing the formulation to include the psychological finding of strong intellectual endowment can actually bolster the psychiatrist's opinion that the psychotic illness has reduced functional capacity as well as contributed to the violent behavior.

Some conflicts cannot be resolved, because although there is agreement about the data, their meaning is contested. In these cases, if discussion fails to resolve the differences, both experts need to acknowledge in the written report that opinions can vary, and both ought to be explicit about their reasoning. In forensic cases, the psychiatrist is responding to questions posed by an attorney or the court. The psychologist, on the other hand, is responding to questions raised by the psychiatrist.

When a psychiatrist requests psychological testing to aid in a diagnosis or forensic formulation, the psychologist has the responsibility to avoid any conflict in the formulation of the case. The psychologist must report the testing results as they are and interpret them accurately, but should stop short of discussing the implications with regard to the legal question (e.g., competency, state of mind) if his or her opinion differs from the referring psychiatrist's, since the application of the testing results to the legal question and formulation of the case goes beyond the scope of testing and a psychological assessment. In discussions, the psychologist and psychiatrist ought to advocate for their own opinions, but in the final writing the ultimate formulation rests with the psychiatrist who requested the testing.

15.6 Psychiatrist-administered psychological tests

Psychiatrists, like licensed psychologists, have a credential that gives access (with appropriate training) to standard psychological tests such as the MMPI-2, the Millon Clinical Multiaxial Inventory and their standard scoring and computerized interpretations. The application of these tests can enhance the psychiatric assessment and report. There are, however, several caveats. First, tests should be scored using the standard programs (e.g., Q Local through Pearson Assessments); home-made or pirated scoring should be avoided, especially in forensic cases where all methodology can be questioned.

A second concern is that no one psychological test is adequate to explain behavior, a caveat applicable to all testing. Since psychiatrists generally will not be administering a battery of tests, the addition of one test, like the MMPI, may result in more conflicting findings than in useful data. A battery of tests is used to assess congruity across testing. Variation in one test cannot establish a diagnosis. One striking example occurred in a case of a woman who was incarcerated on charges that she neglected her 3-year-old, who was found nearly naked in the street in winter. She was incarcerated in a prison where all inmates were administered the short-form of the MMPI in a group administration upon entry to confinement. The tests were computer scored and entered into the medical record. This woman produced an invalid MMPI. When she was referred to the clinic by a correctional officer who had observed her appearing dazed, the invalid MMPI in her chart alerted the staff that she was likely malingering. Finally, during a court appearance, her attorney learned that she was illiterate and had received services for her intellectual impairment. She had lived with her mother who had died weeks before. Left to her own devices, she was unable to care for herself or her child. The inappropriate administration and interpretation of the MMPI had contributed to an inadequate assessment.

A third caveat applies to forensic cases. The psychiatrist needs to know the limits and properties of the tests that are administered. For the standardized personality inventories, such as the MMPI, the interpretation of the test also should be followed closely. The results do not declare a direct measure of the person tested (as with an IQ test or a blood test); they describe a pattern that has been defined in the development of the test. These patterns identify discrete profiles that correlate with styles and disorders. For the person being tested, the profile must be clinically or individually correlated before it can be accepted as valid. For example, if a person produces a profile that suggests a pattern of somatization, then before that finding is considered valid, evidence in the background or in the interview is sought to confirm the testing result. Therefore, reports of the testing should not describe the person as having any particular symptom based on the test; rather, the following qualifier should be included in the report: *On the MMPI, Ms. Doe answered in a way that produced a profile associated with somatic complaints, and a denial of social anxiety and inhibition of aggression. The profile is consistent with Ms. Doe describing that she greatly enjoys being the "center of attention," although her frequent migraine headaches and stomach problems often interfere with her enjoying herself. She noted that although she has had frequent physical examinations for her difficulties, all medical tests turn up negative.* In this case, the report identifies characteristics that are supported by descriptions of Ms. Doe in real life.

15.7 The Daubert Standard: special considerations in forensic cases

Federal and state courts have standards for the admissibility of expert evidence in forensic cases. The Daubert Standard, from the decision by the US Supreme Court in *Daubert* v. *Merrell Dow Pharmaceuticals, Inc.*, 509 US 579 (1993), and subsequent related cases defined guidelines for what can be considered valid science to support an opinion. Under the *Daubert* decision, the judge can decide whether evidence or testing results meet the threshold of acceptable science to present to a jury. The principles that the judge uses include evidence of reliability and validity, peer-review through publication, and presentation and knowledge of the limitations of the test or error rates. Established psychological tests meet these criteria. New ones may not. And although there are many interesting surveys and instruments around, they may not have the psychometric properties that can justify their use in a forensic case. In some cases, the instruments have been used in research and not in a clinical population. Including such a measure in a report can undermine the rest of the testing and credibility of the formulation. For example, an instrument was developed to test the hypothesis that psychopathy involved immunity to anxiety. An instrument was developed and tested on college students that demonstrated that those who had a low regard for rules and had a previous infraction at the school were more likely to take higher risks on a test that involved picking up coins in the face of exposure to electric shock. Although the test made theoretical sense in research, it was disallowed by a court because of its novelty and because it had not been administered to a clinical population and, therefore, was viewed as irrelevant as evidence in the case.

Although novel tests in clinical assessments may generate diagnostic hypotheses and lead to new formulations, variation from the established testing runs the risk of undermining a solid opinion in a forensic case. Testing, therefore, should include assessment tools that have already met the standard in court. Even established batteries are subject to scrutiny if a *Daubert* hearing is requested and granted. The challenge, however, will more likely be met for tests that have a track record.

15.8 Conclusion

Psychological testing can augment a psychiatric assessment, enrich diagnostic and forensic formulations, and buttress an expert psychiatric opinion (Box 15.4). Integration of the psychological assessment into the psychiatric report will maximize the benefits of the testing. The goal is to create in the final formulation a logical argument that incorporates the results of testing into the overall diagnostic and formulation narrative. The testing, as an independent source of data, supports the clinical or forensic assessment and adds credibility to the opinion.

Ideally, in the psychiatric report, the psychological assessment is first presented as the separate evaluation it is, but in the final formulation the results are woven into a coherent and logically connected account that links the objective, empirical results with the individual's characteristics and the events particular to the case. Like diagnoses, psychological testing results create the psychiatric framework through which behaviors can be organized and explained.

References

Baranoski, M. V. (2010) Psychological testing in forensic psychiatry. In *Textbook of Forensic Psychiatry*, 2nd edn., ed. R. I. Simon & L. H. Gold. Washington, DC and London: American Psychiatric Publishing, pp. 617–658.

Campbell, W. H. & Baranoski, M. V. B. (2008) Psychological testing for forensic psychiatrists.

Presented at the 39th annual meeting of the American Academy of Law and Psychiatry, Seattle, WA, October 2008.

Frederick, R. I. (1997) *Validity Indicator Profile Manual*. Minneapolis, MN: National Computer Services.

Melton, G. B., Petrila, J., Poythress, N. G., et al. (2007) *Psychological Evaluations for the Courts: A Handbook for Mental Health Professionals and Lawyers*, 3rd edn. New York, London: Guilford Press.

Rogers, R. (1992) *Structured Interview of Reported Symptoms*. Odessa, FL: Psychological Assessment Resources.

Rogers, R. (2002) *Clinical Assessments of Malingering and Deception*. New York: Guilford Press.

Tombaugh, T. N. (2009) *Test of Memory Malingering*. Princeton, NJ: Pearson Education.

Reasonable medical certainty

Gregory B. Leong, J. Arturo Silva, and Robert Weinstock

The concept of "reasonable medical certainty" has been recognized by the US Supreme Court in *Addington* v. *Texas*, 441 US 418, 430 (1979), and has been in widespread use elsewhere in the US legal system. Reasonable medical certainty has been in use for the duration of the professional lives of all currently practicing physicians and attorneys in the United States.

The concept of reasonable medical certainty has assumed critical importance for psychiatric expert witnesses. The psychiatric-legal opinions provided by the psychiatric expert witness in the courtroom are expected to meet the threshold for reasonable medical certainty. By extension the forensic psychiatrist's psychiatric-legal opinions offered in the written psychiatric report would also need to meet this threshold, especially since only a small fraction of cases involving forensic psychiatric assessment proceed to trial. Further, there is the distinct possibility that the forensic psychiatric report will serve as a significant, if not primary, basis for the decision by the trier of fact.

In this chapter, the origin and evolution of the concept of reasonable medical certainty is described. After exploration of this concept, suggestions for achieving reasonable medical certainty are explored.

16.1 Definition of reasonable medical certainty

The literal meanings of the three words, "reasonable medical certainty," essentially constitute an oxymoron (Lewin 1998). The word "reasonable" indicates that there is a range of acceptable solutions to an inquiry, i.e., the focus of the forensic psychiatric assessment. In contradistinction, the word "certainty" connotes an absoluteness (Lewin 1998). So "reasonable certainty" would defy a precise meaning, since the adjective "reasonable" negates the absoluteness of "certainty" and imputes a range of acceptable solutions. The middle word "medical" does not add or subtract from the definition per se, since any other field of scientific study could be added here, such as reasonable "dental" certainty.

16.2 The origins of reasonable medical certainty

The appearance of the use of the concept of reasonable medical certainty in the courtroom dates back less than a century ago. Lewin traced the origins of the concept of reasonable medical certainty in the courtroom to sometime between 1915 and 1930 in the Chicago, Illinois area, as a result of efforts generated by the local bar to deal with two inconsistent rules of evidence that had been adopted by the Illinois Supreme Court nearly concurrently

The Psychiatric Report, ed. Alec Buchanan and Michael A. Norko. Published by Cambridge University Press. © Cambridge University Press 2011.

during the early twentieth century (Lewin 1998). The "reasonable-certainty" rule prohibited expert witnesses from expressing speculative opinions about damages; and the "ultimate-issue rule" prohibited expert witnesses from "invading the province of the jury" by expressing definitive opinions on the issue. By 1931, the phrase "reasonable medical certainty" was in use statewide in Illinois, though there is no substantiation of its use outside of Illinois courtrooms prior to 1940. The historical cases reviewed by Lewin involved claims of civil damage. However, once used outside of Illinois, reasonable medical certainty gradually appeared in more states, with use in at least 22 states by 1960. By 1970 the phrase "reasonable medical certainty" appeared in all but two states in published opinions (Lewin 1998). Since this zenith in the use of reasonable medical certainty, the adoption of the Federal Rules of Evidence and the subsequent US Supreme Court decision in *Daubert* v. *Merrell Dow* have more recently affected the role of reasonable medical certainty in regard to expert witness input.

16.3 The interpretations of reasonable medical certainty by contemporary forensic psychiatrists

The exploration of reasonable medical certainty by forensic psychiatrists appears to be of relatively recent origin, spanning approximately the past quarter of a century. While undoubtedly psychiatrists and other physicians involved in the legal arena had at least thought about the significance of reasonable medical certainty prior to this time period, there appears to have been no significant discussion in the psychiatric literature prior to the views presented by three contemporary forensic psychiatrists: Seymour Pollack, Jonas Rappeport, and Bernard Diamond.

16.3.1 Seymour Pollack

Pollack utilized three principles in the formulation of the forensic opinion: legal dominance, reasonable medical certainty, and reasonable probability (Pollack 1982). Pollack's principle of legal dominance describes the primacy of the legal context in which the forensic psychiatrist works, including forgoing the therapeutic bias that might influence the forensic psychiatrist's opinion. Pollack recognized the difficulty in achieving neutrality and objectivity in arriving at the forensic opinion and advocated acknowledgement of therapeutic and other biases to address in part this potential conundrum.

Pollack conceptualized the principle of reasonable medical certainty as a basis for defining a threshold for the level of confidence required for psychiatric opinions in the legal context. In other words, the principle of reasonable medical certainty depends on the principle of legal dominance for its operationalization. Pollack offered that reasonable medical certainty relies on a "level of probability that is intimately associated with the contemporary state of medical art and with the degree of sophistication of current acceptable strategies of medical practice" (Pollack 1982, p. 34). However, he did not elaborate on what he meant in this prior description of reasonable medical certainty, nor did he offer a specific definition of reasonable medical certainty elsewhere. Instead, he described the parameters of reasonable medical certainty as used in the clinical context and a general guideline as to how to apply it in the legal context.

Pollack recognized that reasonable medical certainty as used in the clinical context differed from that subsumed by a more rigorous scientific methodology and was based largely on shared professional experiences, i.e., from a combination of empirical medical data and clinical experience. To achieve the threshold of reasonable medical certainty in the legal context, Pollack advocated collecting a substantial database to support the psychiatric opinion. Pollack's practice of forensic psychiatry and formulation of the principle of reasonable medical certainty took place prior to the diagnostic methodology introduced by the *Diagnostic and Statistical Manual of Mental Disorders*, Third Edition (DSM-III; APA 1980), so a significant portion of his focus on the principle of reasonable medical certainty dealt with making the appropriate psychiatric diagnosis. Pollack cautioned that the forensic psychiatrist should take care in recognizing what comprises the database and what comprises clinical inferences drawn from the database.

Pollack's third principle of reasonable probability for forensic evaluation serves to clarify the lack of a specific definition of reasonable medical certainty. This principle functions as a guideline for an acceptable level of confidence in making clinical forensic opinions. This principle of reasonable probability required the level of conviction for the forensic psychiatric opinion to be greater than a possibility, with the "lowest possible risk of error," and "given with a substantial degree of confidence." Pollack cautioned that reasonable probability did not translate to the "legal concept of burden of proof" to be considered by the trier of fact's decision-making. To achieve the reasonable probability, Pollack stressed the importance of demonstrating the psychiatric expert's reasoning in arriving at the forensic opinion, including explaining the lower probabilities for alternative hypotheses and recognition of the limitations of the forensic opinion.

From a contemporary and retrospective view, Pollack's principle of reasonable probability could be combined with the principle of reasonable medical certainty into a single principle of reasonable medical probability. However, when combining the two principles, a conceptualization of reasonable medical probability cannot be abstracted beyond how to approach the forensic evaluation process with a sufficient and substantial database followed by unbiased, neutral, and objective reasoning. It remains unclear as to whether Pollack called his second principle "reasonable medical certainty" out of deference to the use of reasonable medical certainty in the courts and as such he only described this general approach to forensic psychiatric evaluation. Pollack further did not define probability as more likely than not (as it is generally used in either everyday or legal settings). He only noted in his principle of reasonable probability that a forensic opinion be the most likely of all the possibilities. Pollack did not address the potential for experts to arrive at varying opinions, especially when these opinions are approximately equally likely. Pollack's principles of reasonable medical certainty and reasonable probability would therefore allow two forensic psychiatric experts using an identical database to arrive at different opinions offered with reasonable probability and not be in violation of his principles for arriving at forensic opinions.

16.3.2 Jonas Rappeport

Rappeport acknowledged his uncertainty about what the legal concept of reasonable medical certainty meant to physicians. Rappeport first explored how medical decisions in clinical practice take place. Medical decisions often occur in the face of reasonable doubt as the presence of other factors such as risk and harm come into play in medical decision-making. Rappeport then extended this clinical paradigm to the concept of reasonable medical certainty. He considered the threshold of reasonable medical certainty to be "more likely than not" along with this modification: "that level of certainty which a physician would use in making a similar clinical judgment" (Rappeport 1985, p. 9). Rappeport's modification allows for the "more likely than not" threshold to change and be subject to interpretation by different forensic psychiatric expert witnesses based on what similar clinical situation is selected. For example, when assessing a criminal defendant for the insanity defense under the American Law Institute (ALI) rule, there does not appear to be a similar situation encountered in clinical psychiatric practice that is analogous to the determination of whether an individual lacks substantial capacity to conform his or her behavior to the requirements of law. Rappeport's conceptualization of reasonable medical certainty would allow for differing and even conflicting forensic psychiatric opinions to be offered with reasonable medical certainty.

Rappeport concluded his manuscript with the caveat that forensic opinions be given "within the limits of your honesty and integrity" (Rappeport 1985, p. 14). As honesty and integrity have been identified as two important ethical precepts in the practice of forensic psychiatry (Candilis et al. 2007; Candilis 2009), Rappeport has placed ethical forensic psychiatric practice as a component in defining reasonable medical certainty. Rappeport's addition of ethical contours for forensic psychiatric practice – while important for forensic psychiatrists to follow – would not add clarity to identifying the threshold for reasonable medical certainty.

16.3.3 Bernard Diamond

Diamond held that forensic opinions offered with reasonable medical certainty should be expressed with the "psychiatrist's highest level of confidence in the validity and reliability of his opinion," with the level of confidence deriving from "the validity of the underlying scientific knowledge about the issue in question and the validity and reliability of the application of that scientific knowledge to the particular case" (Diamond 1985, p. 123). Diamond posited that reasonable medical certainty cannot be translated into a legal standard of proof and it is the trier of fact's responsibility to make the translation in arriving at the ultimate decision. Diamond cautioned that in some cases the psychiatric expert would not be able "to reach that level of confidence implied by reasonable medical certainty," but added, "I do not think the law requires a higher level of proof from the psychiatric expert than he would normally use in clinical practice" (Diamond 1985, p. 125). Diamond concluded that "the phrase reasonable medical certainty is a valid and valuable expression of the level of confidence maintained by the psychiatric expert witness for his opinions. It is a clinical concept with the roots in both the relevant fund of scientific knowledge and the specific clinical observations of the psychiatrist" (Diamond 1985, p. 127).

Although Diamond's conceptualization of reasonable medical certainty incorporates the reliability and validity of scientific knowledge, Diamond defaults to a clinical standard Rappeport embraced and at one point appears to inadvertently consider reasonable medical certainty a "clinical concept." As with Pollack and Rappeport, Diamond's conceptualization of reasonable medical certainty allows for differing and conflicting forensic psychiatric opinions to be offered with reasonable medical certainty. Diamond refined Pollack's conceptualization of reasonable medical certainty in his closing remark as he proposed that the phrase "reasonable medical certainty" be replaced with "reasonable medical probability" to more accurately reflect scientific reality.

Although "probability" would be more consistent with clinical reality than "certainty" and more closely reflect the generally dimensional perspective of psychiatry versus the generally categorical perspective of the law, in actuality there probably exists little distinction between the two. However, like Pollack and Rappeport, Diamond does not describe or define the threshold for what constitutes "reasonable."

16.4 Other interpretations of reasonable medical certainty

Reasonable medical certainty can be interpreted only in a limited number of ways. The common interpretations by courts and commentators have ranged from more likely than not (equivalent to a preponderance of the evidence standard of proof) to near the vicinity of absolute certainty (roughly equivalent to a beyond a reasonable doubt standard of proof) (Miller 2006). The prevailing view held by the courts and commentators alike is that reasonable medical certainty would minimally be at a threshold level of more likely than not, i.e., a probability and not merely a possibility. Some courts have made a distinction between expert opinions expressed with "reasonable (medical) certainty" and "reasonable (medical) probability" while others have considered them equivalent (Hullverson 1986–1987).

The lack of a clear-cut methodology and threshold for determining reasonable medical certainty (or probability) by the medical expert witness has led to the incantation of "reasonable medical certainty" as ritualistic and rising to a talismanic status (Lewin 1998), or as one commentator writes, an "indispensable abracadabra of expert proof" (Hullverson 1986–1987, p. 577).

16.5 Rethinking reasonable medical certainty at the millennium

A science-based threshold for reasonable medical certainty would be difficult to ever satisfy, as scientific advances depend on testing of the null hypothesis or findings that exclude the possibility of chance. But to offer opinions with this kind of scientific precision would seem especially difficult to attain in the forensic context for any scientific field of study, including psychiatry.

Equating the standard of proof for a legal decision with that of the degree of accuracy of an expert opinion might appear to be a solution, but lacks any known mathematical relationship or logic behind this. For example, consider the US Supreme Court case of *Addington* v. *Texas* (1979) in which the standard of proof required for (long-term) involuntary civil commitment is clear and convincing evidence. Would this mean that in order for an individual to be civilly committed the examining psychiatrist would have to offer an expert opinion at a clear and convincing level of proof? There are no guidelines on how a psychiatrist can offer an opinion on the relevant considerations with a clear and convincing level of proof. Similarly, there are no guidelines on what "clear and convincing" would correspond to in terms of a mathematical probability, assuming a method for accurately quantifying such a probability could even be developed.

Recent developments from both the legal and clinical vantage points appear to have relevance to the conceptualization of reasonable medical certainty. Two important developments include the US Supreme Court case of *Daubert* v. *Merrell Dow* (1993) and the concept of evidence-based medicine.

Although *Daubert* v. *Merrell Dow* can be considered to simply endorse the Federal Rules of Evidence as the basis for admissibility of expert testimony into the courtroom, it has often been viewed as defining a methodology to exclude "junk science" from expert witness testimony and, by extension, in the expert's written report. *Daubert* v. *Merrell Dow* outlined those factors that the court should consider in determining admissibility based on the consideration as to whether the expert scientific testimony is based on valid scientific methodology and whether other scientists in the field have accepted the science behind the expert opinion. The Supreme Court specifically mentioned knowing the error rate as important information to know in considering admissibility.

Daubert v. *Merrell Dow* does not, however, address reasonable medical certainty and has the potential to become the focal point for influencing forensic psychiatric assessment rather than for the undefined concept of reasonable medical certainty. Moreover, the weak link in the analysis by the Supreme Court involves whether the trial court has the ability to actually determine admissibility, or more specifically what constitutes acceptable science for the case at hand, especially in the presence of competing or conflicting expert opinions.

Nonetheless, *Daubert* v. *Merrell Dow* might be a viable way to refine previous conceptualizations of reasonable medical certainty. Of course, the rejection of the admissibility of expert opinions is probably an infrequent event, with judges generally permitting the jury to consider all expert opinions. As such, the *Daubert* v. *Merrell Dow* admissibility test per se would not eliminate the need to consider reasonable medical certainty. Nonetheless, the constructs highlighted in *Daubert* v. *Merrell Dow* of exposure of the scientific methodology (reasoning) and description of the potential error rate could assist in refining the conceptualization of reasonable medical certainty.

Poythress, a psychologist, discussed the effect of *Daubert* v. *Merrell Dow* on meeting "reasonable medical certainty" in regard to evaluations involving the insanity defense where a fair body of clinical knowledge and research has been achieved (Poythress 2004). Poythress thought that if sufficient funds could be available to fund research to answer the question of the validity (accuracy) of a retrospective forensic evaluation of insanity, the admissibility of the forensic opinion under *Daubert* could be satisfied (Poythress 2004). Poythress, however, did not explain how, even if the validity question can be answered, this would specifically enlighten the conceptualization of reasonable medical certainty.

The clinical world of medicine has in recent years embraced the phrase "evidence-based medicine" to convey thoughtful scientific proof to medical treatment, including mental health care (Drake et al. 2003). Systematic reviews or meta-analyses represent the gold standard for medical treatment (McHugo & Drake 2003). They are used to locate the optimal clinical approaches or define "best practices" in clinical treatment, as opposed to utilizing a lower level of scientific evidence such as single case reports. For those with a science background, this type of inquiry should have always been the practice, so it is unclear as to the reason evidence-based medicine has generated so much attention, though it certainly has been embraced by third party payers as a way to contain health care costs.

Evidence-based medicine finds its principal utility as identifying the most effective clinical intervention(s) for a medical condition. Evidence-based medicine is not a specific methodology, but functions as a guide to evaluating the scientific evidence for specific treatment interventions (Drake et al. 2003; McHugo & Drake 2003). Although relying on the scientific evidence from systematic reviews would arguably be the optimal choice when selecting a treatment intervention, relying on clinical knowledge from single case studies is not prohibited. In fact, treatment guidelines generally operate in a similar fashion, allowing the medical practitioner to select from a range of options based on varying sources of scientific evidence. Nonetheless, evidence-based medicine does not provide any specific guidance for forensic psychiatric evaluations, unless the evaluation involves a treatment issue.

In sum, *Daubert* v. *Merrell Dow* and the concept of evidence-based medicine offer valuable suggestions on how to provide psychiatric expert opinions with the highest possible levels of accuracy. Nonetheless, the phrase "evidence-based medicine" has been bandied around to impute clinical significance similar to how "reasonable medical certainty" has been utilized in forensic reports and testimony, i.e., the proclamation carries a similar talismanic meaning, since evidence-based medicine varies from scientifically rigorous systematic reviews to a single case report.

16.6 Real world issues with reasonable medical certainty

The types of clinical questions that arise in forensic psychiatric evaluation, whether in the criminal or civil arena, span the gamut of psychiatric knowledge. An encyclopedic work would be needed to attempt coverage of each forensic topic. A sampling of issues relevant to reasonable medical certainty follows in this section to illustrate some of the challenges encountered in forensic psychiatric practice.

16.6.1 Competency to stand trial

Forensic psychiatric evaluation for competency to stand trial has been explored in considerable depth. Practice guidelines for competency to stand trial evaluations have been developed (Mossman et al. 2007). Moreover, assuming the examining forensic psychiatrist has the requisite clinical skills to perform an adequate assessment, the competency to stand trial evaluation should be among the most accurate assessments performed by forensic psychiatrists since it depends on an individual's present mental status and is not subject to the increasing inaccuracy due to assessing past (retrospective) mental states. Following the American Academy of Psychiatry and the Law competency to stand trial practice guidelines (Mossman et al. 2007) and paying attention to potential areas of inaccuracy (particularly the manufacture, exaggeration, and/or denial of actual mental symptoms) should improve the forensic psychiatrist's accuracy and increase the likelihood of reaching a competence opinion with reasonable medical certainty, however that is defined.

Despite the extensive knowledge base regarding competency to stand trial (including many psychometric-like tools to assist in the evaluation) measurement of the accuracy of the outcome of the forensic psychiatric evaluation can be elusive. Take, for example, the case of *United States* v. *Gigante* (1997) in which 11 forensic experts (nine psychiatrists and two psychologists) participated. All of the experts were well known, with four of the psychiatrists having been a past President of the American Academy of Psychiatry and the Law, and several of the expert witnesses having contributed extensively to the professional psychiatric or psychological literature. There were psychiatrists and a psychologist supporting the position that Gigante was competent as well as the position that Gigante was not competent. Of interest was the judge's commentary on the expert witnesses (*United States* v. *Gigante*, p. 199):

> All of the experts assisting the court in dealing with the difficult questions surrounding diagnosis of defendant's mental condition were able, ethical, and candid. They all met the standards of *Daubert* v. *Merrell Dow Pharmaceuticals*. That the court did not credit the conclusions of those experts tendered by the defendant constitutes no suggestion of lack of confidence in their professional skills and veracity.

The judge specifically mentioned that all the forensic experts met the admissibility standards of *Daubert* v. *Merrell Dow* and complimented the experts in their evaluations. However, the judge had to ultimately make a choice between competent or incompetent. The judge's decision would imply that the judge accepted the opinion of one side as having been at least more likely or perhaps more "reasonable" than the opinion of the other side. This would not disallow the possibility that both the opinion supporting competence and the opinion supporting incompetence could have been offered with reasonable medical certainty. Nonetheless, in the end, would this mean that the judge considered that only the competence opinion expressed by one side reached the threshold of reasonable certainty while the other did not?

16.6.2 Mild traumatic brain injury

Traumatic brain injury (TBI) has received increasing scrutiny outside of the medical field, particularly with the media attention paid to US veterans sustaining such injuries in recent international conflicts. The degree of injury from TBI plays a significant role in determining how the TBI ultimately interacts with the forensic opinion, with cases involving mild TBI (mTBI) creating the most ambiguity. The current state of the research finds sparse literature on functional neuroimaging and its application to mTBI as well as the lack of clinical correlation between functional neuroimaging and mTBI and behavioral, neuropsychological, or structural neuroimaging findings (Granacher 2008). As such, forensic opinions in cases of mTBI would largely lack an objective scientific basis and rely more upon subjective data (Granacher 2008). Moreover, with a high base rate of malingering or symptom exaggeration among those with mTBI (Mittenberg et al. 2002), defining the threshold for reasonable medical certainty in mTBI cases would be a challenging endeavor.

In his analysis of neuroimaging in evaluating mTBI cases, Granacher posits that neuroimaging technologies, presently PET and SPECT, would fail to meet the *Daubert* v. *Merrell Dow* criteria in reference to the error rates and general acceptance among the relevant scientific community (Granacher 2008). Lack of admissibility of neuroimaging data in mTBI cases may automatically signify that the use of neuroimaging data to support the forensic opinion at issue does not meet the threshold for reasonable medical certainty. The lack of admissibility suggests that such data could be considered not to have reached the reasonable medical certainty threshold based on objectively derived error rates. Additionally, should the error rates decrease and neuroimaging data became routinely admissible into the courtroom proceedings, then forensic opinions based on these data could be considered to be given with increasing medical certainty.

16.6.3 Malpractice cases

In assessing malpractice, the forensic expert has to consider, among other things, the standard of care. Simon has noted that the standard of care not only varies across jurisdictions, but also is dependent on an array of factors, including, but not limited to the forensic expert's opinion, practice guidelines, the extant psychiatric literature, hospital policies and procedures, and state and federal regulations (Simon 2005). In reference to practice guidelines, Simon noted the rapid changes these guidelines undergo along with findings in some courts that negligence cannot be excused just because other physicians practice similarly (Simon 2005). Simon posed the question as to what then constitutes reasonable or adequate medical care, particularly since the standard of care does not require utilization of "best practices" or even "good" practice (Simon 2005). Given these ambiguities in defining the standard of care, determining what constitutes reasonable medical certainty when providing expert opinions in malpractice cases remains elusive.

16.7 Describing reasonable medical certainty at the beginning of the twenty-first century

Reasonable medical certainty has gradually spread to courtrooms across the United States from its Illinois-based origin nearly a century ago and has become the standard by which forensic medical experts offer their opinions. Individual courts have defined reasonable medical certainty as a threshold starting from just over 50% probability to an upper limit approaching 100% probability, mirroring the legal standards of proof of preponderance of the evidence and beyond a reasonable doubt (Miller 2006).

As noted above, the semantic use of reasonable certainty borders on the oxymoronic. Moreover, there has been no prevailing legal definition for reasonable medical certainty. So is an operationalization of reasonable medical certainty attainable?

The contributions by forensic psychiatrists to the forensic psychiatric literature are basically those from contemporary forensic psychiatrists Pollack, Rappeport, and Diamond from about a quarter century ago, and more recently a review by Miller. None of these forensic psychiatrists could clarify or pinpoint either a clinical or legal definition for reasonable medical certainty. The important concepts offered by Pollack, Rappeport, and Diamond can be synthesized to the forensic evaluation process in general, namely, collection of an adequate database to answer the forensic psychiatric question at issue, considering the validity and reliability of the various data points (including vigilance for data distortion due to malingering, dissimulation, and/or exaggeration of history or symptoms), and arrival at the forensic psychiatric opinion through a reasoning process that includes consideration of alternative hypotheses and the reasons behind the ranking of the opinions considered.

Rappeport highlighted the psychiatrist's medical perspective as a clinician in arriving at the forensic opinion, while Diamond favored the use of probability instead of certainty. Nonetheless, what these three forensic psychiatrists discussed was the general process and procedure for performing adequate forensic psychiatric evaluations and arriving at the resultant opinions (whether written in the report or provided orally via courtroom testimony), and that following such a paradigm for forensic psychiatric evaluation more readily achieves reasonable medical certainty. Still, a precise definition eluded these three forensic psychiatrists and so far others. Of course, none of the descriptions of reasonable medical certainty by Pollack, Rappeport, Diamond, or any one else would necessarily prohibit the possibility that the forensic opinions authored by psychiatric expert witnesses on opposing sides of a legal case could not both be offered with reasonable medical certainty.

The case of *Daubert* v. *Merrell Dow* and the development of evidence-based medicine do not directly involve the reasonable medical certainty concept, but do illuminate the notion of having an acceptable level of science behind the forensic opinions. The specific message from *Daubert* v. *Merrell Dow* and evidence-based medicine appears to be the need for continuing scientific advances in psychiatry, so the error rate or uncertainty further diminishes.

The definition of reasonable medical certainty might be best considered a moving target, but the approach to reasonable medical certainty as collated from the models of Pollack, Rappeport, and Diamond along with the principles derived from *Daubert* v. *Merrell Dow* and evidence-based medicine could serve as a general guideline to offer professionally competent and ethical opinions in the forensic report or testimony.

References

Addington v. *Texas*, 441 US 418 (1979).

American Psychiatric Association (APA) (1980) *Diagnostic and Statistical Manual of Mental Disorders, Third Edition*. Washington, DC: American Psychiatric Association.

Candilis, P. J. (2009) The revolution in forensic ethics: narrative, compassion, and a robust professionalism. *Psychiatric Clinics of North America* 3: 423–435.

Candilis, P. J., Weinstock, R., & Martinez, R. (2007) *Forensic Ethics and the Expert Witness*. New York: Springer.

Daubert v. *Merrell Dow Pharmaceuticals, Inc.*, 509 US 579 (1993).

Diamond, B. L. (1985) Reasonable medical certainty, diagnostic thresholds, and definitions of mental illness in the legal context. *Bulletin of the American Academy of Psychiatry and the Law* 13: 121–128.

Drake, R. E., Rosenberg, S. D., Teague, G. B., Bartels, S. J., & Torrey, W. C. (2003) Fundamental principles of evidence-based medicine applied to mental health care. *Psychiatric Clinics of North America* 26: 811–820.

Granacher, R. P. Jr. (2008) Commentary: Applications of functional neuroimaging to civil litigation of mild traumatic brain injury. *Journal of the American Academy of Psychiatry the Law* 36: 323–328.

Hullverson, J. E. Jr. (1986–1987) Reasonable degree of medical certainty: A tort et a travers. *St. Louis University Law Review* 31: 577–598.

Lewin, J. L. (1998) The genesis and evolution of legal uncertainty about "reasonable medical certainty." *Maryland Law Review* 57: 380–504.

McHugo, G. J. & Drake, R. E. (2003) Finding and evaluating the evidence: a critical step in evidence-based medicine. *Psychiatric Clinics of North America* 26: 821–831.

Miller, R. D. (2006) Reasonable medical certainty: a rose by any other name. *Journal of Psychiatry and Law* 34: 273–290.

Mittenberg, W., Patton, C., Canyock, E. M., & Condit, D. C. (2002) Base rates of malingering and symptom exaggeration. *Journal of Clinical and Experimental Neuropsychology* 24: 1094–1102.

Mossman, D., Noffsinger, S. G., Ash, P., et al. (2007) AAPL practice guideline for the forensic psychiatric evaluation of competence to stand trial. *Journal of the American Academy of Psychiatry the Law* 35 (4, suppl): S3–S72.

Pollack, S. (1982) Principles of forensic psychiatry for reaching psychiatric-legal opinions: Application. In *The Mental Health Professional and the Legal System*, ed. B. H. Gross and L. E. Weinberger. San Francisco, CA: Jossey-Bass Inc, pp. 25–44.

Poythress, N. G. (2004) "Reasonable medical certainty": Can we meet *Daubert* Standards in insanity cases? *Journal of the American Academy of Psychiatry and the Law* 32: 228–230.

Rappeport, J. R. (1985) Reasonable medical certainty. *Bulletin of the American Academy of Psychiatry and the Law* 13: 5–15.

Simon, R. J. (2005) Standard-of-care testimony: best practices or reasonable care? *Journal of the American Academy of Psychiatry the Law* 33: 8–11.

United States v. *Gigante*, 996 F. Supp. 194 (1997).

Violence risk assessment

Alec Buchanan and Michael A. Norko

17.1 Introduction

Courts, social services, jails and prisons, probation services, and attorneys all request psychiatric reports addressing the risk someone poses to other people. They do so in a range of circumstances (see Shah 1978). Table 17.1 lists the most frequent. Psychiatric reports written for other purposes, for instance to assess fitness for work, sometimes address the risk of harm to others as part of their larger inquiry (see Chapter 13). The degree to which the principles outlined in this chapter then govern the structure and content of the report will depend on the contribution of the assessment of risk to the psychiatric evaluation as a whole.

Older approaches to risk assessment frequently began with the premise that people who acted violently fell into types, such as the "culturally violent" and the "institutionally violent" (Spencer 1966; see also Greenland 1985). For the most part, these groupings have not been validated. They have been replaced by an emphasis on the "transactional" aspects of violence. Dangerousness is now seen as an attribute of situations, not just individuals (see Skeem & Mulvey 2002). As a result, risk assessments and the reports they generate now focus, not just on people, but on the circumstances in which those people find themselves (Royal College of Psychiatrists 2008a).

Risk assessment is an area where the provision of a psychiatric opinion can damage what the person being assessed sees as their best interests. Courts sometimes increase the length of a prison sentence, for instance, in response to evidence on risk. The conflict with *primum non nocere* may be deeper than is sometimes implied because the Latinized injunction probably prescribes helping, not merely avoiding harm (Veatch 1981; Tuohey 1989; Burt 2009). Two justifications have been offered for the continued provision by doctors of risk assessments to courts. The first sees psychiatrists and psychologists in forensic settings not as clinicians but as evaluators, guided by an alternative, "forensic", ethic based on respecting others and truthfulness (see Appelbaum 1990, 1997; Mullen & Ogloff 2009).

The second justification notes that a doctor has duties not only to the patient but also to the medical profession and to society as a whole (Royal College of Psychiatrists 2008b). These duties have to be balanced according to the circumstances of the case. Depending on the outcome of this balancing, it may still be ethical to report the results of a medical evaluation even if the subject of the evaluation regards this as contrary to his or her interests. These dilemmas, particularly acute where the opinion concerns risk of harm to others, are related to broader questions concerning the provision in a forensic setting of a psychiatric

The Psychiatric Report, ed. Alec Buchanan and Michael A. Norko. Published by Cambridge University Press. © Cambridge University Press 2011.

Table 17.1 Contexts in which psychiatric risk assessment reports are commonly requested

Setting	Circumstance
Criminal	Bail applications
	Plea bargaining
	Pre-sentence reports on convicted defendants
	Pre-release reports at the request of prisons and parole boards
Civil	Child custody disputes
	Malpractice cases
Mental health	Sex-offender commitment
	Civil commitment
	Commitment to hospital of insanity acquittees
	Management of insanity acquittees committed to hospital, including conditional release

opinion that the subject regards as unhelpful. These broader questions are discussed in detail in Chapters 4 and 19.

The attempt in this chapter to identify the principles at work in the best risk assessments is not intended to imply that there is a single best way to present the results. The principles at work in psychiatric risk assessment derive from clinical psychiatry, where the results are entered in medical records, communicated verbally or, perhaps most often, used to inform clinical management without ever being articulated (see Heilbrun et al. 1999). As with clinical assessments, when writing for the courts, the context affects the way in which an opinion is communicated.

17.2 Conducting the evaluation

17.2.1 Approaches to risk assessment

Otto (2000) has reviewed the range of risk assessment approaches that are available. These approaches include clinical, anamnestic, structured clinical, actuarial, and adjusted actuarial. From what is sometimes a contentious literature, none emerges as consistently superior. With one exception, the important differences between the methods lie on one of two dimensions. The first dimension is whether the approach reaches its conclusions by attending to statistical correlations or by means of a more cause-based analysis. The second is the degree to which the approach provides a structure for the assessor to follow.

The exception is anamnestic assessment, which seems capable of contributing to both correlation- and cause-based approaches. Anamnestic assessment uses patterns in a person's life history to predict the circumstances under which violence may recur (see Dvoskin 2002; Melton et al. 2007). As a consequence, its application to cases where the person being evaluated has no history of violence seems problematic (although most approaches can be expected to struggle in these circumstances). The predictive validity of anamnestic assessment has not yet been established. If its emphasis on patterns proves helpful, however, those patterns will probably not emphasize crime type. Mentally disordered offenders when they seriously reoffend usually do not commit the same type of crime (Buchanan et al. 2003). Structured versions of anamnestic assessment have been offered as alternatives to traditional, unstructured, ones (see Borum et al. 1996).

17.2.2 Correlation and cause in risk assessment

Correlation-based approaches assess risk by looking for variables associated with violence. They therefore benefit from the numerous epidemiological data now available describing the relationship between mental disorder and crime. When structured approaches combine those variables into risk assessment instruments they have the additional benefit of allowing the author of a report to make the results transparent: with the necessary information on how items were completed and combined the reader can see how the conclusions were arrived at. Because they are empirically based, correlation-based approaches typically exclude symptoms and signs, including the Capgras phenomena (Christodoulou 1978; Tomison & Donovan 1988; Silva et al. 1989) and "over-identification with the child" (Resnick 1969), that have been reported to be linked to violence but are either rare or difficult to define operationally.

Correlation-based criminological data suggest that psychiatric patients differ in some respects from the general population. The tendency for violent acts to be conducted by men is less evident, first offenses occur later, and the likelihood of acting violently does not fall off so rapidly with advancing age (Häfner & Boker 1973). The protective effect of stable relationships may be less (McNiel et al. 1988; Mullen 1997), particularly for people whose overall functioning is poor (Swanson et al. 1998). In other respects, however, the correlates of offending in the general population seem to apply also to the mentally disordered (see Bonta et al. 1998).

Thus crimes of violence are more likely to be committed by younger males and recidivism for violent crimes is much less than for property crime. Substance abuse is associated with both violent and non-violent crime in both mentally disordered and non-mentally disordered populations. The more serious the crime, generally speaking, the lower the risk of repetition. Recidivism rates for homicide are particularly low, even allowing for the effects of incapacitation. First offenders, on average, do better than people with extensive criminal records. Unemployment, living in a high-crime neighborhood, and having antisocial peers all add substantially to risk.

Causation-based approaches work differently. They assume that violence happens for reasons and that clinicians can use their understanding of those reasons to prevent it:

> The skillful clinician assessing dangerous behavior formulates and tests a series of clinical hypotheses to define patterns of violence in the individual's history. Once defined, these patterns can be applied to the explanation and prediction of violence in that individual (Pollock et al. 1989, p. 105; see also Marra et al. 1987).

Causation-based approaches have to rely heavily on inference. Future conditions will never exactly mimic the conditions in which past behavior occurred, and some means has to be found to assess the relevance of past patterns to future behavior.

In addition to testing a series of hypotheses, clinicians trying to work out what might cause future violence presumably use the same prototypes, cognitive schemas and scripts that they learn in training and develop in their clinical practice (see Garb 1998; Skeem et al. 2000). Claims that these ways of thinking are better than correlation-based ones at predicting rare events (Sreenivasan et al. 2000) have not been confirmed. Instead, their persistence when clinicians think about risk may relate to the fact that many of the other judgments

Table 17.2 Structured risk assessment instruments

Type, name, and reference	Target population
Actuarial	
VRAG (Quinsey et al. 2006)	General psychiatry, forensic
SORAG (Quinsey et al. 2006)	Sexual offenders
Static 99 (Hanson & Thornton 1999)	Sexual offenders
COVR (Monahan et al. 2006)	General psychiatry
PCL-R (Hare 1991)	General psychiatry, forensic
PCL-SV (Hart et al. 1995)	General psychiatry, forensic
Structured professional judgment	
HCR 20 (Webster et al. 1997)	General and forensic
SARA (Kropp et al. 1999)	Spousal assault
SVR-20 (Boer et al. 1997)	Sexual offenders
RSVP (Hart et al. 2004)	Sexual offenders

required in medicine are also causation-based: establishing why someone has symptoms, for instance, or deciding which investigations are needed. Because clinical practice requires each of these judgments to be integrated into a single plan, it may be that clinicians find it helpful to use the same causal heuristic in assessing risk that they use in other aspects of their practice.

17.2.3 Structure in risk assessment

Structured approaches to risk assessment are sometimes treated as a category but they differ from unstructured methods in degree, not kind. Clinicians use structure, largely derived from their professional training, to take a history and to examine the patient. Structure offers the same advantages in risk assessment as it offers in other aspects of clinical practice. It assists training (see McNeil et al. 2008). It is a useful aide-memoire, particularly when the question is unusual (some risk factors apply particularly to sex offenses, for instance; Hanson and Bussière 1998). Finally, structure can order information in a familiar way and make it easier to integrate that information (Skeem et al. 1998). Structured approaches to risk assessment usually take the form of rating scales or instruments. Singh and Fazel (2010) counted 126. The most widely used are listed in Table 17.2. Some of these scales and instruments are more structured than others (see Monahan 2008). The HCR-20 contains a list of items but leaves to the assessor the task of estimating risk. The VRAG, by contrast, includes an arithmetic algorithm that allocates a case to one of nine risk categories.

Follow-up studies suggest that structured approaches have greater predictive validity than unstructured ones when risk assessments cover periods of months or years (Grove & Meehl 1996; Grove et al. 2000). It is not yet clear whether the same is true for short-term assessments. On the one hand, at least over periods longer than a few weeks, the accuracy of structured approaches does not seem to decline as the follow-up period shortens (Mossman 1994), and some actuarial approaches demonstrate good short-term accuracy (McNiel et al.

2003). On the other hand, the short-term predictions of emergency room clinicians have been shown to be as accurate as the long-term ones of structured instruments (see Lidz et al. 1993; Mossman, 1994).

The proven predictive validity of structured approaches has not led to their unqualified clinical acceptance (Litwack 2001). The reasons are probably complex. One clinician's structure is another's straitjacket. Doctors and, less often, psychologists complain that they have to respond both to risky circumstances, such as their patient obtaining a weapon, and to mitigating factors, such as the incapacitation of someone with a high actuarial score, neither of which may be included in an instrument (see Rogers 2000; Glancy 2006). One alternative would be to outline permissible exceptions, when the results of using a scale could be ignored, but this course has been opposed by the authors of some of the most accurate instruments (Quinsey et al. 2006). A related clinicians' complaint is that it is difficult to use the score on a rating scale to guide treatment when research has yet to show whether treatment changes the score, or whether the risk will then be less.

On the other hand, unstructured (sometimes called "clinical") approaches to risk assessment may not integrate straightforwardly with other aspects of treatment, either. Unstructured approaches are more vulnerable to the cognitive biases, such as attending disproportionately to recent events, that afflict many of the judgments that people make (Kahneman et al. 1982; see Shah 1978). And not all reports offer treatment recommendations. Finally, if the central task of risk assessment lies in establishing and quantifying statistical correlations, the arithmetic techniques contained in some structured approaches may be best suited to the task (Sarbin 1943).

Braitman and Davidoff (1996) list seven criteria to establish whether a validated rating scale will be useful in an individual case. Three are statistical: whether the confidence limits are acceptable, whether the scale works for all subgroups of subjects ("goodness of fit"), and whether its predictions are accurate. While the predictive accuracy of many instruments is uncontroversial, confidence intervals remain contentious (see Hart et al. 2007; Mossman & Sellke 2007). Braitman and Davidoff's non-statistical criteria include the degree to which the patient resembles patients in the validation study, the similarity between the outcome in the study and the outcome of interest to the clinician, and the availability to the clinician of data similar to those available in the study. In the absence of a resolution of the statistical debate, these non-statistical criteria are likely to be of most help to report writers.

17.2.4 Integration

Correlation-based approaches can indicate whether a subject shares some characteristics with a high-risk group, but not whether that subject can properly be seen as representative of the group and what intervention is most appropriate. Causation-based approaches can incorporate more kinds of information but offer no obvious mechanism whereby the psychiatrist can use data to compare the risk to that posed by other people. Because they offer different things, a risk assessment report that makes use of both approaches is, at least in principle, in a better position to help the reader than one that chooses between them (see Skeem & Mulvey 2002).

There is little agreement as to how such integration might be achieved. One possibility is that the psychiatrist should proceed hierarchically, reviewing the established correlates of violence that are present and using this review as a starting point for a cause-based analysis derived from an understanding of the subject and their circumstances. Correlation-based approaches, after all, generate information that courts, in particular, can usually obtain by other means, for instance from pre-sentence reports prepared by the probation service. In theory, causation-based approaches have the potential to provide something extra. Three factors are likely to govern the extent to which they can do this in practice.

The first is the degree to which the psychiatrist has had access to the patient's mental state. Where someone is willing to discuss his or her feelings, intentions, and beliefs, clinicians can incorporate this information. The second is the circumstances in which the question is asked. Where consideration is being given to treating in the community a patient who has recently acted violently, for instance, an evaluation that concentrates on identifying the population correlates of violence, such as past violence and age, is unlikely to be helpful. A more useful assessment will usually focus on the origins of recent violence and what has, and what has not, changed. Where the circumstances are liable to change, for instance when it is not known whether the subject of the evaluation will return to live with the partner he has abused, a cause-based approach that incorporates different plausible scenarios may allow the reporter to make conditional statements that are potentially helpful.

The third factor governing the availability of a causation-based approach is the period over which the assessment will apply. In emergency settings where an assessment is often required to cover days or weeks there are few correlates to guide clinicians (see Douglas & Skeem 2005), although anger (Skeem et al. 2006) and substance use (Mulvey et al. 2006) both seem to be important. Instead, risk assessments will be based on an understanding of the likely effect on a patient of the circumstances to which he or she is being discharged. Assessments designed to apply over longer periods, on the other hand, are less able to rely on this kind of understanding because mental states, circumstances and the sources of risk change. Unless they know what these changes will be, clinicians who wish to offer an estimate of risk designed to cover months or years have little choice but to concentrate on recognized risk factors, using either an unstructured approach or a validated structured instrument.

17.3 Conduct of the evaluation

17.3.1 General

The general principles of report writing contained in the first section of this book apply also to reporting on risk assessments. The psychiatrist should be able to demonstrate relevant expertise and experience and that they are maintaining their skills. They need to be able to resist pressure to address questions that are beyond their competence or that do not make sense and should understand the possible consequences of the evaluation. The subject should be informed of its nature and purpose. Consent should be obtained. Assessment should include a clinical examination, and if it does not the reasons and consequent limitations to the validity of the opinion should be described. Any limits to confidentiality need to be clarified prior to the evaluation and explained to the subject.

17.3.2 Clarifying the question

The person or agency requesting a risk assessment usually has some flexibility regarding the nature and wording of the questions posed. This flexibility can be used to ensure that the question is a helpful one. It is not usually helpful, for instance, to attempt to answer a question such as, "Does the patient present a risk?" Presumably, everybody presents some risk and the request for advice implies that there is already some concern. An alternative question, which is usually closer to what the person or agency wants to know, is, "How much of a risk does the patient present?" This acknowledges the quantitative aspect of risk, and is easier for a psychiatrist to address.

This second alternative, however, still makes no allowance for the qualitative aspects of risk: what kinds of behavior are of concern in this case, and in what circumstances would their occurrence be most problematic? In addition, it makes no explicit provision for the psychiatrist to describe what might be done to reduce, or otherwise manage, the risk. Finally, it offers no mechanism for the psychiatrist to clarify the clinical implications of the findings or otherwise avoid a conclusion that amounts to no more than saying "a lot," or "a little."

These implications can sometimes be clarified by reference to a threshold. A patient may present too much of a risk for discharge from a hospital but still be able to move to an open ward, for instance, or require a more detailed occupational therapy assessment before living unsupervised. The most satisfactory course will often be to have these qualitative aspects of risk, therapeutic considerations, and likely implications incorporated into the request. The report can then address a question such as, "How can the risk of this man assaulting a fellow resident be managed in his supported housing complex?" This format also allows the psychiatrist to answer unasked but important, related, questions, as when he or she concludes, "It can't."

17.3.3 Obtaining background information

The categories under which information is obtained for the purposes of a risk assessment will usually follow the structure of the model report in Chapter 7.

Information from collateral sources is often crucial. These can include the client's own writing, in the form of electronic mail, diaries, and letters, as well as school and hospital records. Police reports and witness statements often provide valuable details on acts of violence. Lists of convictions by definition omit acts where the subject was never charged or was charged but not convicted, for instance following a plea bargain. When the collateral sources are people, those people sometimes ask the purpose for which the report is being produced and whether they will be able to read it; the psychiatrist should know the answers to these questions before contacting them. Collaterals may also ask whether the person being evaluated gave permission for them to be contacted. The person or agency requesting the report may have a view about who can most appropriately provide collateral information and should have the opportunity to explain that view.

The "Background" section to the report (see Chapter 7) will include information relating to the patient's personal history, characteristics, and circumstances. A number of variables from these domains have been identified by empirical research as correlated with future violence (see Bonta et al. 1998; Skeem & Mulvey 2002; Mullen & Ogloff 2009). Table 17.3 lists those variables identified most frequently in psychiatric reviews of risk assessment and risk management.

Because past violence is the strongest statistical correlate of future violence, and because the risk of future violence increases with each subsequent offense (Walker et al. 1967), risk assessments include details of the client's history of acting violently. The dates and types of violent act are important in part because criminological variables such as age of onset of violent behavior and the number of violent convictions are themselves correlates of future violence.

A cause-based analysis, however, usually requires further information. The circumstances of each act should be described in sufficient detail to allow the identification of patterns, if these exist. These circumstances include the individual's living situation, relationship to the

Table 17.3 Correlates I. Background factors and social circumstances linked to violence (see Monahan 1981, 1985; Mullen 1997; Otto 2000; Tardiff 2008; Mullen & Ogloff 2009)

	Substantial correlate	Correlate	Protective
Socio-demographics		Youth	
		Male sex	
Past behavior	History of violence if no change in person or circumstance	History of threats not acted upon	
	Recent violence		
Psychiatric and substance abuse	Substance use, especially if rising	Conduct disorder	
Social circumstances	Availability of weapons, familiarity with their use	Domestic conflict, especially if escalating	Good social networks
	Future circumstances likely to resemble those in which violence has previously occurred		
Traits	Hare psychopathy (see Table 17.5)	Impulsiveness	Fear of own potential for violence
		"Feckless" disregard for consequences in schizophrenia	Has demonstrated internal resources to cope with conflict

victim, intentions at the time they acted, mental state (and whether he or she was in treatment), and use of drugs and alcohol. The nature the victim's injury should be described; hospital treatment is often an indicator of severity. Collateral sources that can be of assistance in gathering this information include arrest records, police reports, trial transcripts, pre-sentence reports, and treatment records.

The association between substance use and violence is one of the most widely reported empirical findings in risk assessment. Moving beyond the statistical correlation to a cause-based analysis requires the report to address the details of an individual's behavior in relation to substances. Violence may be the result of intoxication and past instances of violence when using substances should be noted. It may follow an exacerbation of mental illness precipitated by drug use, in which case the history may indicate previous instances of drug-induced relapse. Finally, violence may be a consequence of involvement in a drug market where territorial conflicts are common and where weapons are carried, although this is less an issue for alcohol. The response of the subject to treatment for substance abuse problems will usually be important, especially when risk is assessed at criminal sentencing.

The report's description of the past psychiatric history should make clear the relationship, if any, between the individual's history of violence and his or her mental disorder. The nature of any treatment, the individual's compliance with treatment and their response to treatment will usually be important. The psychiatric history may also suggest what psychiatric measures have and have not been helpful previously in reducing risk. The subject's social circumstances should be described for past episodes of violence (see above), for the present, and with reference to the period over which the risk assessment is required. Attention should be paid to the presence or absence of potentially protective factors such as stable relationships, employment, and housing. The availability of likely victims, including the victims of past violence, should be noted.

17.3.4 Examining the mental state

Mental state findings relating to risk do not exist independent of circumstances. Where someone harbors delusions regarding an individual, for instance, the likelihood of his or her coming into contact with that individual and the likely nature of that contact are important. Pathological jealousy is likely to be managed differently if the jealous man plans to live with the wife he believes is being unfaithful. The mental state findings and circumstances most commonly listed by reviewers as associated with risk of harm to others are listed in Table 17.4. The weight that can appropriately be attached to mental state abnormalities depends also on the period over which the risk assessment is intended to apply. Some features listed in Table 17.4, such as threats, carry particular short-term significance. Others, such as insight into illness will usually be more relevant when the assessment is intended to cover months or years.

The description of thought content should include reference to thoughts of violence and their quality. Obsessional thoughts concerning violence in the absence of psychotic symptoms are not unusual and empirical research has not linked them to future violence. Command hallucinations have been described in association with violence but the association is inconsistent, the empirical base is limited and conflicting, and the implications at the population level uncertain (Junginger & McGuire 2004). As with other symptoms, a detailed analysis of past violence may nevertheless reveal their importance in an individual case. Violent thoughts that are pleasurable warrant particular concern, and when the pleasure has a sexual component, particular attention to the sexual history.

In describing a subject's insight into his or her past behavior, a detailed description or verbatim account will usually be more helpful than a summary statement. "Lack of remorse," in particular, can cover a range of phenomena of which a general unwillingness to take responsibility probably carries fewer implications for future dangerousness than a sense of self-justification, the persistence of a grudge, or a reference to unfinished business (see Grounds 1995). A subject's willingness to address the causes of violence should be assessed in the light of his or her response to previous interventions. Ambivalence may not always have prevented successful treatment.

17.3.5 Psychological testing

Of the psychological tests available to assess personality and general psychological functioning, only the Hare psychopathy checklist (Table 17.5; see Hare 1991) has been shown consistently to predict violence (Borum 1996).

A range of specialized risk assessment instruments are now available, however. The best validated are shown in Table 17.2. The contribution made by the results of using these scales to the Conclusion will depend on the overall approach adopted (see Section 17.2). Instruments

Table 17.4 Correlates II. Mental state features and interactions associated with risk of harm to others (see Monahan 1981, 1985; Mullen 1997; Otto 2000; Tardiff 2008; Mullen & Ogloff 2009)

	Substantial correlate	Correlate	Protective
Mental state features (including recent behaviors)	Steps taken in preparation (obtaining weapons, surveillance, putting affairs in order)	Delusions, particularly misidentification syndromes	Compliant with treatment
	Threats creating fear and concern in people who know the person making the threats	Clouding of consciousness and confusion	Responding to treatment
	Violent thoughts or intentions		Perceives treatment as effective
	Morbid jealousy where object of jealousy available		Insight into illness and need for treatment
	Delusional systems focused on individuals seen as a threat or as obstructing an important goal		
Interactions	Depressed suicidal mothers of young children	Stalking without past violence	
	Suicidal seeking revenge		
	Stalking with past violence		
	Angry and threatening with a plan to cause harm		
	Fearful with a plan to cause harm (may be pre-emptive)		

should only be used by clinicians with the proper training and experience. Descriptions of this training and experience appear in the references included in Table 17.2.

17.3.6 Opinions

The form of the Opinion will follow its function. If that function is to describe the results of using an actuarial approach then risk factors should be identified, the data supporting the presence of those risk factors listed, and the results of combining them reported. The degree of professional acceptance of the approach and any qualifications regarding its applicability to the case under discussion should be described. If more than one scale is used, the report should discuss any inconsistencies between the findings. Where a suitable scale is available,

Table 17.5 Personality traits constituting Hare psychopathy (see Hare 1991)

Glibness or superficial charm

Grandiose sense of self-worth

Need for stimulation or proneness to boredom

Pathological lying

Conning/manipulative

Lack of remorse or guilt

Shallow affect

Callous/lack of empathy

Parasitic lifestyle

Poor behavioral controls

Promiscuous sexual behavior

Early behavioral problems

Lack of realistic, long-term goals

Impulsivity

Irresponsibility

Failure to accept responsibility for own actions

Many short-term marital relationships

Juvenile delinquency

Revocation of conditional release

Criminal versatility

where the psychiatrist has been able to apply it properly, and where the base rate of offending in studies using that scale seems applicable to the subject, some psychiatrists will be comfortable offering an estimate of risk in numeric terms, perhaps as a percentage (see Quinsey et al. 2006). If this is done, the type of violence and the time span to which the numeric conclusion applies should be specified.

In many cases either no suitable scale will be available or it will not be possible to complete one. Even if it is possible to do so, identifying a population to which the subject can properly be said to belong and comparing the base rate of violence in that population with the base rate of violence in studies validating the risk assessment instrument each pose further difficulties (see Miller & Morris 1988). In these circumstances, basing an Opinion on a numerical estimate will be difficult to defend. None of the alternatives are without their own drawbacks, however. Judges are said to prefer that report writers use categories, such as "low," "medium," and "high" risk, without further elaboration (Kwartner et al. 2006). It is not clear that this does more than allow imprecision to mask the shortcomings of numerical statements made in the absence of base rate data.

A second alternative to basing the Opinion on a number is to compare the client to a reference group (see Otto 2000) such as the general population, drug-dependent offenders, or insanity acquittees (Melton et al. 2007). This assumes that the psychiatrist is familiar with the reference group and that whoever is requesting the report has the knowledge and experience to make use of such a comparison. A third alternative is to refer to a functional standard (see Section 17.3.2). A clinician might conclude that were the subject treated as a condition of probation, the risk would not be so great that hospital admission would be indicated or that if the subject was placed in the community, this should be with 24-hour nursing. Offering this type of comparison has the merit of allowing psychiatrists to testify to thresholds with which they are familiar. Clinicians know that such thresholds are seldom applied consistently, however. Decisions regarding admission and placement are made using many criteria, not just one.

In addition to describing the level of risk, a satisfactory Opinion will follow the identification of a suitable question (see Section 17.3.2). It will be probabilistic, expressed in conditional terms and make clear the level of confidence with which the opinion is held (Pollock et al. 1989). It will take into account factors that reduce the risk, as well as those that increase it (Webster 1984). It will address, in as much detail as possible, what can be done to best manage the case (Dvoskin & Heilbrun 2001). It will be informed by empirical research describing the correlates of violence. It will also, however, use the skills that psychiatrists learn in training and develop in their clinical practice. The validity of a psychiatric report is greatest where those skills can be applied. Where they cannot, for instance because the subject does not suffer from a mental disorder or for other reasons does not resemble the patients psychiatrists see and treat, the Opinion will be qualified accordingly.

17.4 Conclusion

The most commonly noted pitfalls in psychiatric risk assessment lie in departing from common sense. There is no empirical evidence to contradict the practice of identifying risk where violence has recently occurred and the circumstances are unchanged (see Litwack & Schlesinger 1987). By the same token, predicting violence in the absence of either an intention to act, a desire to harm, or a history of prior violence will always be problematic (see Kozol et al. 1972; American Psychiatric Association 1974; Weiner & Hess 1987). Given the range of possible questions, an allegiance to a single way of answering them will usually be less successful than an adaptable approach. US courts have noted that it is the quality and comprehensive form of an assessment, rather than the psychiatrist's adoption of any particular method, which represents defensible practice (*White* v. *US*; *Currie* v. *US*).

The most helpful psychiatric risk assessments probably make use of both known statistical correlations and causal explanations:

> By supplementing a knowledge of relevant risk factors with a detailed examination of an individual's mental state, it may be possible to build up some picture of the calculus of reasons on which that individual's future actions may be based and in this way to give a more precise prediction … the more [an action] is dominated by some over-riding preoccupation or delusion, the more precise will be a prediction based on a knowledge of risk factors and the individual's calculus of reasons. (Howard 1991, p. 70)

However detailed our understanding, Howard noted, we cannot predict what a person will do. One measure of the quality of a risk assessment is the degree to which it informs the important decisions that courts and clinicians nevertheless make on the basis of what that person might.

The ability to inform important decisions is not the same as predictive accuracy, but predictive accuracy is clearly important. The development of structured approaches whose predictive accuracy has been demonstrated in a range of patient groups represents the most significant research advance to have occurred in psychiatric risk assessment since the

American Psychiatric Association published its Task Force Report on psychiatric patient violence in 1974. The extent to which this research advance changes future clinical practice will properly depend on whether structured approaches can be shown to improve the quality of those decisions.

Acknowledgements

The authors thank Dr. Simon Wilson, Dr. John Meyers, Dr. Ken Hoge, Madelon Baranoski PhD, and Kate Winarski LCSW.

References

American Psychiatric Association (1974) *Clinical Aspects of the Violent Individual. Task Force Report 8.* Washington, DC: American Psychiatric Association.

Appelbaum, P. (1990) The parable of the forensic psychiatrist: ethics and the problem of doing harm. *International Journal of Law and Psychiatry* 13: 249–259.

Appelbaum, P. (1997) A theory of ethics for forensic psychiatry. *Journal of the American Academy of Psychiatry and the Law* 25: 233–247.

Boer, D., Hart, S., Kropp, P., & Webster, C. (1997) *Manual for the Sexual Violence Risk – 20: Professional Guidelines for Assessing Risk of Sexual Violence.* Vancouver, BC, Canada: British Columbia Institute Against Family Violence.

Bonta, J., Law, M., & Hanson, K. (1998) The prediction of criminal and violent recidivism among mentally disordered offenders: a meta-analysis. *Psychological Bulletin* **123**: 123–142.

Borum, R. (1996) Improving the clinical practice of violence risk assessment. Technology guidelines and training. *American Psychologist* 51: 945–956.

Borum, R., Swartz, M., & Swanson, J. (1996) Assessing and managing violence risk in clinical practice. *Journal of Practical Psychiatry and Behavioral Health* 2: 205–215.

Braitman, L. & Davidoff, F. (1996) Predicting clinical states in individual patients. *Annals of Internal Medicine* 125: 406–412.

Buchanan, A., Reiss, D., & Taylor, P. (2003) Does "like predict like" when patients discharged from high secure hospitals re-offend? An instrument to describe serious offending. *Psychological Medicine* 33: 549–553.

Burt, R. (2009) Doctors vs lawyers: the perils of perfectionism. *Saint Louis University Law Journal* 53: 1177–1188.

Christodoulou, G. (1978) Syndrome of subjective doubles. *American Journal of Psychiatry* 135: 249–251.

Currie v. *US*, 644 F. Supp 1074 (MDNC 1986).

Douglas, K. & Skeem, J. (2005) Violence risk assessment: getting specific about being dynamic. *Psychology, Public Policy and Law* **11**: 347–383.

Dvoskin, J. (2002) Knowledge is not power – knowledge is obligation. *Journal of the American Academy of Psychiatry and the Law* 30: 533–540.

Dvoskin, J. & Heilbrun, K. (2001) Risk assessment and release decision-making: toward resolving the great debate. *Journal of the American Academy of Psychiatry and the Law* 29: 2–10.

Garb, H. (1998) *Studying the Clinician: Judgment Research and Psychological Assessment.* Washington, DC: American Psychological Association.

Glancy, G. (2006) Caveat usare: actuarial schemes in real life. *Journal of the American Academy of Psychiatry and the Law* 34: 272–275.

Greenland, C. (1985) Dangerousness, mental disorder and politics. In *Dangerousness: Probability and Prediction, Psychiatry and Public Policy*, ed. C. Webster, M. Ben-Aron, & S. Hucker. New York: Cambridge University Press, pp. 25–40.

Grounds, A. (1995) Risk assessment and management in clinical context. In *Psychiatric Patient Violence. Risk and Response*, ed. J. Crichton. London: Duckworth, pp. 43–59.

Grove, W. & Meehl, P. (1996) Comparative efficiency of informal (subjective, impressionistic) and formal (mechanical, algorithmic) prediction procedures: the clinical-statistical controversy. *Psychology, Public Policy and Law* 12: 293–323.

Grove, W., Zald, D., Lebow, B., Snitz, B., & Nelson, C. (2000) Clinical versus mechanical prediction: a meta-analysis. *Psychological Assessment* 12: 19–30.

Häfner, H. & Boker, W. (1973) *Crimes of Violence by Mentally Disordered Offenders*. Cambridge: Cambridge University Press.

Hanson, K. & Bussière, M. (1998) Predicting relapse: a meta-analysis of sexual offender recidivism studies. *Journal of Consulting and Clinical Psychology* 66: 348–362.

Hanson, R. & Thornton, D. (1999) *Static 99: Improving Actuarial Risk Assessments for Sex Offenders*. Ottawa: Department of the Solicitor General of Canada.

Hare, E. (1991) *Hare R: The Revised Psychopathy Checklist*. Toronto: Multi-Health Systems.

Hart, S., Cox, D., & Hare, R. (1995) *The Hare Psychopathy Checklist: Screening Version (PCL:SV)*. Toronto, ON, Canada: Multi-Health Systems.

Hart, S., Kropp, P. & Laws, R. (2004) *The Risk for Sexual Violence Protocol (RSVP)*. Mental Health, Law, and Policy Institute, Simon Fraser University, Burnaby, BC, Canada.

Hart, S., Michie, C., & Cooke, D. (2007) Precision of actuarial risk assessment instruments. *British Journal of Psychiatry* 190: s60–s65.

Heilbrun, K., Philipson, J., Berman, L., & Warren, J. (1999) Risk communication: clinicians' reported approaches and perceived values. *Journal of the American Academy of Psychiatry and the Law* 27: 397–406.

Howard, C. (1991) The individual's calculus of reasons: forensic psychiatry and science. *Psychiatric Bulletin* Supplement 4, **70**.

Junginger, J. & McGuire, L. (2004) Psychotic motivation and the paradox of current research on serious mental illness and rates of violence. *Schizophrenia Bulletin* 30: 21–30.

Kahneman, D., Slovic, P., & Tversky, A. (ed.) (1982) *Judgment Under Uncertainty: Heuristics and Biases*. New York: Cambridge University Press.

Kozol, H., Boucher, R., & Garofalo, R. (1972) The diagnosis and treatment of dangerousness. *Crime and Delinquency* 18: 371–392.

Kropp, P., Hart, S., Webster, C., & Eaves, D. (1999) *Manual for the Spousal Assault Risk Assessment Guide*, 3rd edn. Toronto, ON, Canada: Multi-Health Systems.

Kwartner, P., Lyons, P., & Boccaccini, M. (2006) Judges' risk communication preferences in risk for future violence cases. *International Journal of Forensic Mental Health* 5: 185–194.

Lidz, C., Mulvey, E., & Gardner, W. (1993) The accuracy of predictions of violence to others. *Journal of the American Medical Association* 269: 1007–1011.

Litwack, T. (2001) Actuarial versus clinical assessments of dangerousness. *Psychology, Public Policy and Law* 7: 409–443.

Litwack, T. & Schlesinger, L. (1987) Assessing and predicting violence: research, law and applications. In *Handbook of Forensic Psychology*, ed. I. Weiner & A. Hess. New York: Wiley, pp. 205–257.

Marra, H., Konzelman, G., & Giles, P. (1987) A clinical strategy to the assessment of dangerousness. *International Journal of Offender Therapy and Comparative Criminology* 31: 291–299.

McNiel, D., Binder, R., & Greenfield, T. (1988) Predictors of violence in civilly committed acute psychiatric patients. *American Journal of Psychiatry* 145: 965–970.

McNiel, D., Gregory, A., Lam, J., Binder, R., & Sullivan, G. (2003) Utility of decision support tools for assessing acute risk of violence. *Journal of Consulting and Clinical Psychology* 71: 945–953.

McNiel, D., Chamberlain, J., Weaver, C., et al. (2008) Impact of clinical training on violence risk assessment. *American Journal of Psychiatry* **165**: 195–200.

Melton, G., Petrila, J., Poythress, N., & Slobogin, C. (2007) *Psychological Evaluations for the Courts: A Handbook for Mental Health Professionals and Lawyers*, 3rd edn. New York: Guilford.

Miller, M. & Morris, N. (1988) Predictions of dangerousness: an argument for limited use. *Violence and Victims* **3**: 263–283.

Monahan, J. (1981) *The Clinical Prediction of Violent Behavior*. Rockville, MD: US Department of Health and Human Services.

Monahan, J. (1985) Evaluating potentially violent persons. In *Psychology, Psychiatry and the Law: a Clinical and Forensic Handbook*, ed. C Ewing. Sarasota, FL: Professional Resource Exchange, pp. 9–39.

Monahan, J. (2008) Structured risk assessment of violence. In *Violence Assessment and Management*, ed. R. Simon & K. Tardiff. Arlington, VA: American Psychiatric Publishing, pp. 17–33.

Monahan, J., Steadman, H., Appelbaum, P., et al.(2006) The classification of violence risk. *Behavioral Sciences and the Law* **24**: 721–730.

Mossman, D, (1994) Assessing predictions of violence: being accurate about accuracy. *Journal of Consulting and Clinical Psychology* **62**: 783–92.

Mossman, D. & Sellke, T. (2007) Avoiding errors about "margins of error". *British Journal of Psychiatry* http://bjp.rcpsych.org/cgi/eletters/190/49/s60.

Mullen, P. (1997) Assessing risk of interpersonal violence in the mentally ill. *Advances in Psychiatric Treatment* **3**: 166–173.

Mullen, P. & Ogloff, J. (2009) Assessing and managing the risk of violence towards others. In *New Oxford Textbook of Psychiatry*, 2nd edn., vol. 2, ed. M. Gelder, N. Andeasen, J. López-Ibor, & J. Geddes. Oxford: Oxford University Press, pp. 1991–2002.

Mulvey, E., Odgers, C., Skeem, J., et al. (2006) Substance use and community violence: a test of the relation at the daily level. *Journal of Consulting and Clinical Psychology* **74**: 743–754.

Otto, R. (2000) Assessing and managing violence risk in outpatient settings. *Journal of Clinical Psychology* **56**: 1239–1262.

Pollock, N., McBain, I., & Webster, C. (1989) Clinical decision making and the assessment of dangerousness. In *Clinical Approaches to Violence*, ed. K. Howells & C. Hollin,. Chichester, UK: John Wiley, pp. 89–115.

Quinsey, V., Harris, G., Rice, M., & Cormier, C. (2006) *Violent Offenders: Appraising and Managing Risk*, 2nd edn. Washington, DC: American Psychological Association.

Resnick, P. (1969) Child murder by parents: a psychiatric review of filicide. *American Journal of Psychiatry* **126**: 325–334.

Rogers, R. (2000) The uncritical acceptance of risk assessment in forensic practice. *Law and Human Behavior* **24**: 595–605.

Royal College of Psychiatrists (2008a) *Rethinking Risk to Others in Mental Health Services. College Report CR150*. London, UK: Royal College of Psychiatrists.

Royal College of Psychiatrists (2008b) *Court Work. College Report CR 147*. London, UK: Royal College of Psychiatrists.

Sarbin, T. (1943) A contribution to the study of actuarial and individual methods of prediction. *American Journal of Sociology* **48**: 593–602.

Shah, S. (1978) Dangerousness. A paradigm foe exploring some issues in law and psychology. *American Psychologist* **33**: 224–238.

Silva, J., Leong, G., Weinstock, R., & Boyer, C. (1989) Capgras syndrome and dangerousness. *Bulletin of the American Academy of Psychiatry and the Law* **17**: 5–14.

Singh, J. & Fazel, S, (2010) Forensic risk assessment. A metareview. *Criminal Justice and Behavior* **37**: 965–988.

Skeem, J. & Mulvey, E. (2002) Assessing the risk of harm posed by mentally disordered offenders being treated in the community. In *Care of the Mentally Disordered Offender in the Community*, ed. A. Buchanan. Oxford: Oxford University Press, pp. 111–142.

Skeem, J., Golding, S., Cohn, N., & Berge, G. (1998) Logic and reliability of evaluations of competence to stand trial. *Law and Human Behavior* **22**: 519–547.

Skeem, J., Mulvey, E., & Lidz, C. (2000) Building mental health professionals' decisional models into tests of predictive validity: the accuracy of contextualized predictions of violence. *Law and Human Behavior* **24**: 607–628.

Skeem, J., Schubert, C., Odgers, C., et al. (2006) Psychiatric symptoms and community violence among high-risk patients: a test of the relationship at the weekly level. *Journal of Consulting and Clinical Psychology* **74**: 967–979.

Spencer, C. (1966) *A Typology of Violent Offenders. Research Report Number 23.* Sacramento, CA: Department of Corrections.

Sreenivasan, S., Korkish, P., Garrick, T., Weinberger, L., & Phenix, A. (2000) Actuarial risk assessment models: a review of critical issues related to violence and sex-offender recidivism assessments. *Journal of the American Academy of Psychiatry and the Law* **28**: 438–448.

Swanson, J., Swartz, M., Estroff, S., et al. (1998) Psychiatric impairment, social contact, and violent behavior: evidence from a study of outpatient-committed persons with severe mental disorder. *Social Psychiatry and Psychiatric Epidemiology* **33**: S86–S94.

Tardiff, K. (2008) Clinical risk assessment of violence. In *Textbook of Violence Assessment and Management*, ed. R. Simon & K. Tardiff. Washington, DC: American Psychiatric Publishing, pp. 3–16.

Tomison, A. & Donovan, W. (1988) Dangerous delusions: the Hollywood phenomenon. *British Journal of Psychiatry* **153**: 404–405.

Tuohey, J. (1989) Balancing benefit and burden. *Health Progress* **70** (January–February): 77–79.

Veatch, R. (1981) *A Theory of Medical Ethics.* New York: Basic.

Walker, N., Hammond, W., & Steer, D. (1967) Repeated violence. *Criminal Law Review* 465–473.

Webster, C. (1984) How much of the clinical predictability of dangerousness issue is due to language and communications difficulties? Some sample courtroom questions and some inspired but heady answers. *International Journal of Offender Therapy and Comparative Criminology* **28**: 159–167.

Webster, C, Douglas, K., Eaves, D., & Hart, S. (1997) *HCR–20: Assessing Risk for Violence (Version 2).* Mental Health, Law, and Policy Institute, Simon Fraser University, Vancouver BC, Canada.

Weiner, I. & Hess, A. (1987) *Handbook of Forensic Psychology.* New York: John Wiley.

White v. US, 780 F 2d. 97 (DC Cir 1986).

Malingering

Charles Scott and Barbara McDermott

The *American Heritage Dictionary of the English Language* defines malingering as "to feign illness or other incapacity in order to avoid duty or work." The American Psychiatric Association (2000) provides a more specific definition: malingering is "the intentional production of false or grossly exaggerated physical or psychological symptoms motivated by external incentives" (p. 739). In the psychiatric setting, that external incentive can be much more diverse than avoidance of work. It can include the procurement of financial compensation (legal settlements or verdicts, worker's compensation, disability benefits); the obtainment of prescription medications; or access to a hospital bed. The *Diagnostic and Statistical Manual of Mental Disorders – Fourth Edition*, Text Revision (DSM-IV-TR) guidelines for when to suspect malingering include (1) medico-legal evaluations, (2) when there is a marked discrepancy between a person's claimed stress or disability and objective findings, (3) when there is a lack of cooperation with diagnostic interview, and (4) the presence of Antisocial Personality Disorder (American Psychiatric Association 2000, p. 739).

In the context of this definition, Resnick (1997b, p. 131) has described the following three subcategories of malingering:

1. *Pure malingering*: A person feigns a disorder that does not exist at all.
2. *Partial malingering*: A person exaggerates existing symptoms or fraudulently alleges that prior symptoms are still present.
3. *False imputation*: A person attributes actual symptoms to a cause that the person knows has no relationship to the reported symptoms.

In disability evaluations, the examiner is often asked to comment on whether *secondary gain* is involved in the presentation of the claimant's symptoms and alleged disability. Definitions of secondary gain vary with at least three suggested definitions. Under psychodynamic theory, secondary gain represents an unconscious defense mechanism to avoid further psychic trauma. In behavioral medicine, secondary gain is used to describe situations when a provider unintentionally reinforces the patient's illness behavior. In the context of disability evaluations, "secondary gain" is sometimes used to imply that the person is intentionally fabricating symptoms for financial benefit, which in reality is an alternate way of labeling the claimant as a malingerer (Rogers & Payne 2006). In addition to secondary gain, individuals with genuine illness may also face *secondary losses* to include: a loss of power; loss of respect; loss of authority; and/or a loss of function (Wiley 1998). Because many people are not familiar with the concept of secondary loss, malingerers may fail to understand and report these important secondary loss factors. When writing forensic reports, the examiner should clarify which definition of secondary gain is being used and also address whether the claimant volunteers any secondary losses related to their reported illness (Hall & Hall 2006).

Clearly the evaluation of malingering in any medico-legal context is important. In all cases, either criminal or civil, addressing the possibility that the examinee is feigning symptoms (psychiatric, cognitive, or physical) must be considered and such consideration should be addressed in the forensic report. Common forensic evaluations of criminal defendants where malingering should be considered include competency to stand trial, criminal responsibility, competency to be sentenced, competency to be executed, sexually violent predator commitments, mentally disordered offender commitments, and appropriateness for community placement. The assessment of malingering is also important in civil litigation such as personal injury claims, social security evaluations, worker's compensation evaluations, and disability evaluations. This chapter provides an overview of malingering, discusses methods for evaluating malingering, and suggests how to incorporate the results of this malingering assessment into a forensic report.

18.1 Overview

Malingering of psychiatric symptoms is not a rare event. The reported incidence of malingering varies depending on the population in question. In a study of malingered mental illness in a metropolitan emergency department, 13% of patients were strongly suspected or considered to be malingering. Reasons identified for malingering included seeking hospitalization for food and shelter, attempting to gain medication, attempting to avoid incarceration, and seeking financial gain (Yates et al. 1996). Rogers et al. (1993) estimated that approximately half of the individuals evaluated for personal injury claims were feigning all or part of their cognitive deficits. A group of forensic psychologists estimated that malingering occurred in almost 16% of forensic patients and more than 7% of non-forensic patients (Rogers et al. 1994). Additionally, almost 21% of defendants undergoing evaluations of criminal responsibility engaged in or were suspected of engaging in malingering (Rogers 1986). In contrast, Cornell and Hawk (1989) found the incidence of malingering in a sample of defendants referred for an evaluation of competence to stand trial and/or criminal responsibility to be 8%. Our data, presented at the American Academy of Psychiatry and the Law annual meeting (McDermott et al. 2009), indicate that 18.4% of patients found incompetent to stand trial were malingering their psychiatric symptoms on admission for restoration. Gold and Frueh (1999) found that either 14% or 22% of veterans referred for an evaluation for PTSD were classified as "extreme exaggerators" on the MMPI-2, depending on the criteria used. Clearly, the context of the evaluation bears greatly on the probability that malingering will occur.

Research has been divided on whether individuals with antisocial personality disorder are more likely to malinger, as suggested by the DSM-IV-TR. For example, Gacono and his colleagues (1995) found that individuals adjudicated "not guilty by reason of insanity" who subsequently admitted feigning mental illness were more likely to be diagnosed with antisocial personality disorder and to score higher on a measure of psychopathy (Hare Psychopathy Checklist – Revised [PCL-R]; Hare 1991) than individuals receiving the same verdict who were not suspected to be malingering (and consented to participate in research). In contrast, Poythress et al. (2001) found that prisoners scoring high on a measure of psychopathy (Psychopathic Personality Inventory; Lilienfeld & Andrews 1996) were no more likely than other prisoners to successfully malinger. Delain et al. (2003) found that defendants in criminal court with a diagnosis of antisocial personality disorder were more likely to malinger memory deficits, as measured by the Test of Memory Malingering (Tombaugh 1996), than defendants without this diagnosis. However, recently it has been suggested that such inconsistent research findings may be related to how *successful* the individual is in malingering and that the real question should be: Are individuals with antisocial personality disorder more likely to *attempt* to malinger? Kucharski et al. (2006) found that criminal defendants scoring in the high psychopathy range (PCL-R score greater than 29) were more likely to score in the malingering range on standardized assessments. The authors concluded that their study provided some support for the DSM-IV-TR recommendation of suspecting malingering in the presence of antisocial personality disorder. Moreover, the affective and interpersonal features of psychopathic persons (which include pathological lying) were best at discriminating malingerers from non-malingerers.

There are several DSM-IV disorders from which malingering must be differentiated. Diagnostic confusion between malingering and other mental disorders, particularly factitious disorder, can be traced to Asher's (1951) original description of Munchausen syndrome. He attributed several possible motives to Munchausen syndrome, including "a desire to escape from the police" and "a desire to get free board and lodgings for the night" (p. 339), motives that would now clearly classify such feigned illness behavior as malingering. The tendency to include malingering within the factitious disorder spectrum was further reinforced by Spiro (1968), who recommended that in individuals with Munchausen syndrome, "malingering should only be diagnosed in the absence of psychiatric illness and the presence of behavior appropriately adaptive to a clear-cut long-term goal" (p. 569). As such, any individual with a psychiatric illness could not be considered a malingerer. There are, however, many examples of patients with factitious disorder who also malinger (Feldman 1995). Eisendrath (1996) described three such individuals, all of whom entered into civil litigation as a result of their feigned physical illnesses. In each case, it appeared that the feigned illness was intended to assume the sick role and only later was used to pursue financial incentives.

Other disorders to consider in the differential diagnosis of malingering include conversion disorder and/or other somatoform disorders. Although all of these diagnoses may involve physical symptoms, none involve the production of symptoms for external incentives. Individuals with conversion disorder or another somatoform disorder experience symptoms that cannot be fully explained by a medical condition and are often connected to psychological reasons, of which the person often is unaware. Somatoform disorders that may be confused with malingering include the following: Conversion Disorder, Hypochondriasis Disorder, Pain Disorder, and Somatization Disorder. Persons with Conversion Disorder present with one or more symptoms that affect voluntary motor or sensory function suggestive of a neurological or other medical condition. In contrast to malingering, the symptom is not intentionally produced and is judged to be a result of psychological factors associated with a preceding stressor (McDermott & Feldman 2007). Cases of Pain Disorder involve persistent complaints of pain that are not accounted for by tissue damage. Somatization Disorder cases involve chronic, unpleasant symptoms (often including pain) that appear to implicate multiple organ symptoms. In both Pain Disorder and Somatization Disorder, it is presumed that the patient actually experiences the pain they are reporting. The pain complaints may covary with psychological stressors. Unlike malingering, the pain reported in these disorders is not under conscious control, nor is it motivated by external incentives.

However, there are no reliable methods for affirmatively establishing that pain and other complaints are unconscious and involuntarily produced. When opining that pain and/or physical complaints are *voluntarily* produced, evaluators should explain how this determination was made. Such determinations usually involve objective evidence that symptoms have been feigned as well as clear-cut secondary gain (McDermott & Feldman 2007). Hypochondriasis is diagnosed in patients who unconsciously interpret physical sensations as indicative of serious disease. The patient may present with minor pains that they fear indicate some unrecognized, potentially life-threatening illness. When hypochondriac patients do simulate or self-induce illness, these deceptions often reflect a desire to convince physicians to perform further tests (Hamilton & Feldman 2001). These patients are eager to undergo diagnostic evaluations of all kinds. In contrast, the malingerer is often uncooperative with the diagnostic process and, unlike those with hypochondriasis, is unlikely to show any relief or pleasure in response to negative test results (McDermott & Feldman 2007).

Patients may have an underlying psychiatric illness that accounts for the feigning of symptoms. Consider the example provided by Drob et al. (2009) of a schizophrenic patient who has the delusional belief that the psychiatrist is actually an FBI agent sent by the government to interrogate him. In order to avoid questioning by this perceived persecutor, this patient fakes amnesia, which is detected on both the clinical interview and psychological testing. In this instance, the malingering of memory deficits is not the most relevant factor for treatment. The same issue is cogent in the feigning of physical illness. The examiner should assess whether or not those patients who present with unexplained somatic complaints actually have an illness that is not detected during an initial evaluation or with subsequent testing. Physicians and other providers may be inclined to presume that the patient is malingering physical symptoms, but should use caution in making this assumption. Finally, individuals who confabulate should be distinguished from malingerers because they are unintentionally filling in information that they believed to have happened, when, in fact, it did not happen at all (Newmark et al. 1999; Resnick 2000).

18.2 Informed consent and the malingering assessment

What the examinee should be told prior to the initiation of the evaluation is of critical importance. As part of the disclosure process, evaluators should disclose their name, the purpose of the evaluation, limits of confidentiality, the purpose for which the information will be used, the absence of current or future treatment relationship, and a warning that once the information is released to a third party, evaluators do not have control over the information (Gold & Shuman 2009, p. 6). Opinions vary regarding whether or not an examinee should be specifically warned that the evaluation will also assess possible malingering. Such warnings are generally not recommended *immediately* prior to giving a test of malingering due to the risk of decreasing the effectiveness of the assessment (Gervais et al. 2001; Iverson 2006). Are such warnings ever appropriate at *any* point in the examination? Youngjohn (1995) suggested that cautioning examinees of special techniques to detect malingering will likely reduce the sensitivity of these techniques. In contrast, Slick and Iverson (2003) recommend that it is ethically appropriate to provide a general warning *at the beginning* of the evaluation that malingering may be detected. These divergent opinions were also reflected in a survey of 29 "expert" neuropsychologists who were asked the following question: "Prior to commencing testing, do you give litigants any type of warning regarding the fact that psychological tests may be sensitive to poor effort, exaggeration or faking of deficits?" Fifty-four percent answered that they "never" provided such a warning, 8.3% reported that they "sometimes" gave this warning, and 37.5% responded that they "always" gave this type of warning (Slick et al. 2004). If the examiner elects to provide a caution regarding the assessment of malingering, written statements to be included in the informed consent section of the report might read:

- I informed the examinee at the beginning of the interview that methods of detecting exaggeration and poor effort were part of the evaluation process; or
- I informed the examinee at the beginning of the interview that I was evaluating his/her diagnosis and it was important for him/her to answer my questions as accurately as possible.

Generally speaking, option two is preferred to avoid "priming" the examinee and thus diminishing the chance of accurately detecting malingering. In addition, the second warning may actually enhance the evaluators' ability to detect malingering. It hardly can be argued that examinees should *not* be warned to answer as honestly as they can. Finally, the second option is appropriate whether or not the referral question specifically requests an evaluation of malingering in addition to general assessment of a psychiatric disorder.

18.3 Assessment methods

The assessment of malingering generally involves a clinical interview, a review of relevant collateral information, and psychological testing when indicated. Comparing the examinee's report of symptoms to any prior reports and collateral records is particularly important. In fact, in a study surveying 105 board-certified orthopedic surgeons and neurosurgeons from six states, factors that surgeons most strongly considered in making their estimates of malingering were not in fact related to external incentive, but were more closely associated with inconsistencies in the medical examination (Leavitt & Sweet 1986). The two inconsistencies most frequently cited as suggestive of malingering were weakness in the exam not seen in other activities, and disablement disproportionate to the objective findings. This suggests that one of the hallmarks of malingering is inconsistency between reports and observations, or inconsistencies between various methods of assessment. The various data should converge in order to best explain the relationship of malingering to the presentation of particular symptoms.

Unless examinees confess that symptoms have been fabricated for some type of external gain, the assessment of malingering will require collateral information from a variety of potential sources. The examiner must incorporate multiple sources of information to support or refute malingering. An evaluator should carefully record any inconsistencies that are noted during the course of the forensic evaluation. Seven types of inconsistencies that may indicate malingering and can be described in the forensic report are as follows (McDermott et al. 2008):

1. The individual presents an inconsistency during his or her own report of an alleged symptom. For example, a person may report being currently unable to talk while speaking eloquently throughout the interview.
2. The evaluator observes that the malingerer's exhibited behavior differs significantly from the symptoms reported. The person who describes active, continuous, disturbing hallucinations during the interview but shows no evidence of distraction illustrates this type of inconsistency.

3. Malingerers behave in a dramatically different way depending on who he or she believes is observing them. This disparity in presentation is illustrated by a person who acts in a confused, disoriented manner in the clinician's office and shortly after leaving is observed to be chatting casually with ward staff.
4. Malingerers often report symptoms that are inconsistent with how genuine symptoms normally manifest.
5. The person's actual level of functioning is inconsistent with the severity of the reported symptoms.
6. The examinee's report of prior history significantly contradicts records and other collateral information.
7. Psychological testing data are inconsistent with the history and symptom presentation provided by the examinee.

Psychological testing may be helpful in assessing the validity of the individual's reported mental health and/or cognitive symptoms in both civil and criminal litigation. The specific test or tests selected for the evaluation will likely vary depending on the individual case specifics and type of symptoms reported. For further discussion of structured assessments useful in the detection of malingering, please refer to Chapter 15. These assessments should always be used as an adjunct to the clinical assessment of malingering.

18.4   Malingering assessment of specific disorders

Although it is beyond the scope of this chapter to summarize the literature regarding the assessment of malingering of various symptoms and diagnoses, key factors to evaluate malingering in psychotic disorders, Posttraumatic Stress Disorder (PTSD), and depression are reviewed below. When evaluating malingering, the evaluator should begin by asking open-ended questions about the reported symptoms. This initial approach allows the examinee an opportunity to describe symptoms without specific prompts. Such general questions might include the following:

- Describe to me any symptoms you are experiencing.
- Is there anything else you can tell me about this to help me understand your situation more?
- When did your symptom first start?
- Had you ever had any of these symptoms before?
- Have you noticed any change in your symptoms over time?
- Is there anything that you have learned helps decrease (or tends to worsen) your symptoms?

Because information regarding psychiatric symptoms is readily available through a variety of sources about diagnoses, the examiner may also wish to ask:

- Do you know anyone else who has similar symptoms (or disorder)?
- Have you read or learned about this symptom (or disorder) from any source? If so, what?

18.4.1 Malingered psychosis

Individuals who present as potentially psychotic should be carefully observed to evaluate whether their behavior and interactions are consistent with the type and severity of reported symptoms. Resnick (1997a) has suggested a clinical decision model for the assessment of

Table 18.1 Clinical decision model for the assessment of malingered psychosis*

A. Understandable motive to malinger

B. Marked variability of presentation as observed in at least one of the following:

    1. Marked discrepancies in interview and non-interview behavior

    2. Gross inconsistencies in reported psychotic symptoms

    3. Blatant contradictions between reported prior episodes and documented psychiatric history

C. Improbable psychiatric symptoms as evidenced by one or more of the following:

    1. Reporting elaborate psychotic symptoms that lack common paranoid, grandiose, or religious themes

    2. Sudden emergence of purported psychotic symptoms to explain antisocial behavior

    3. Atypical hallucinations or delusions

D. Confirmation of malingered psychosis by either:

    1. Admission of malingering following confrontation

    2. Presence of strong corroboration information, such as psychometric data or history of malingering

* From Resnick, P. J. (1997a). Malingered psychosis. In *Clinical Assessment of Malingering and Deception*, 2nd edn., ed. R. Rogers. New York, NY: Guilford, pp. 47–67.

---

malingered psychosis, outlined in Table 18.1, that can be useful when organizing the malingering opinion in a forensic report.

In regard to specific psychotic symptoms, Resnick (1997a) has noted malingered hallucinations should be suspected if any combination of the following is observed:

- Continuous rather than intermittent hallucinations.
- Vague or inaudible hallucinations.
- Hallucinations not associated with delusions.
- Inability to state strategies to diminish voices.
- Self-report that all command hallucinations were obeyed.
- Visual hallucinations in black and white.

Some of the above symptoms are rarely reported (such as visual hallucinations in black and white) and therefore may not always serve as a useful indicator of malingering. However, when such atypical symptoms are described, the likelihood of malingering is increased and should prompt further investigation.

Resnick (1997a) has also noted that malingered delusions should be considered if a combination of the following factors is present:

- Abrupt onset or termination of delusion.
- Eagerness to call attention to delusions.
- Conduct markedly inconsistent with delusions.
- Bizarre content without disordered thinking.

18.4.2 Malingered PTSD

Posttraumatic stress disorder may be especially easy to malinger as the diagnosis is primarily made on the person's self-report. Information about PTSD criteria is readily available as

Table 18.2 Factors suggesting malingered PTSD*

When the examinee demonstrates the following, malingered PTSD should be suspected:

- Calls attention to symptoms early and frequently during the interview
- Reports flashbacks where only visual images are experienced without additional components such as auditory, olfactory, or tactile sensations
- Describes frequent nightmares that are always the same and occur every time the person sleeps or dreams
- Reports no problems prior to the alleged incident (in a way suggesting the absolute absence of even common problems)
- Seeks treatment only in the context of litigation
- Claims complete amnesia where no actions are recalled
- Describes sleep difficulties not confirmed by partner
- Exaggerates severity of symptoms with textbook rehearsed-sounding answers
- Enjoys recreational activities and justifies such activities as therapeutic
- Reports chronic nonfluctuating symptoms that do not improve to any extent with time or treatment
- No reported survivor guilt in situations where others were present and/or harmed
- History of multiple lawsuits and unstable work history

* Reproduced with permission from Hall, C. W. and Hall, C. W. (2006). Malingering of PTSD and diagnostic considerations, characteristics of malingerers and clinical presentations. *General Hospital Psychiatry*, 28, 525–535.

more than 2 million citations describing PTSD were noted in a recent Google search (Hall & Hall 2006).

In conducting the clinical assessment of PTSD, Resnick (1995) recommends that the evaluator take a detailed history of the traumatic event, the claimant's psychiatric symptoms, and treatment efforts. When taking the history, the examiner should be careful not to provide clues about how genuine PTSD presents and collateral informants should be interviewed separately from the examinee. To be effective, it is important that the evaluator have a good general knowledge of genuine PTSD symptom presentation in coming to an understanding of the relationship of reported PTSD symptoms to the alleged stressor in a particular case. Hall and Hall (2006) have suggested that malingered PTSD should be suspected under a number of circumstances, as listed in Table 18.2.

18.4.3 Malingered depression

As with PTSD symptoms, a diagnosis of depression relies significantly on an individual's self-report. An interview of several hours' duration provides an opportunity to assess whether the person's observed symptoms and behavior are consistent with his or her report of depressive symptoms. The possibility of malingered depression should be considered if the examinee demonstrates one or more of the following:

- Excellent concentration during a lengthy interview despite claims of being unable to concentrate or focus.
- Sense of humor (joking and laughing) in contrast to a depressed mood or restricted affect.
- A normal range of motor movements without evidence of psychomotor agitation or retardation.

- No loss or gain of weight noted in actual records in contrast to reported change in appetite or weight.
- Active exercise or physical activity in contrast to reports of extreme fatigue.
- Enjoyment of vacations or other social activities in contrast to reports of social isolation.

18.5 Forensic report writing

Examinees may interact with the examiner and respond to psychological test questions in a variety of ways that indicate their responses are not consistent with the objective evidence. Such presentations are often referred to as the person's *response style*. The forensic examiner should be familiar with definitions of these various response styles and appropriately incorporate them in the forensic report. Malingering represents only one of many possible response styles. Other terms used to describe interview behavior or responses on psychological testing include faking, simulating, dissimulating, magnifying, amplifying, and exaggerating. Numerous terms have been used to describe a person's *effort level* on psychological tests or neuropsychological testing. Such terms include non-optimal effort, submaximal effort, incomplete effort, negative response bias, suboptimal effort, and poor effort (Iverson 2006). Iverson (2006) recommends that the term *poor effort* be used when a person underperforms on neuropsychological tests and the term *exaggerating* used to describe symptom reporting during an interview, during psychological testing, or through behavioral observations. In contrast to these recommendations, Rogers and Payne (2006) caution against the use of terms such as suboptimal or poor effort because a person's ideal effort cannot be reliably measured.

In the forensic report, the forensic expert should carefully delineate all sources of information reviewed as part of the evaluation process, particularly in reference to malingering. Appropriate sources of information to review and list in the report may include the following: psychiatric and/or medical records; undercover video- or audiotapes; occupational records; criminal rap sheet and jail and/or prison records; deposition testimony; witness statements, collateral interviews, administered psychological testing, and other forensic mental health evaluations. Each interview should include information regarding those individuals who participated and the interview length of time. Documents reviewed should be appropriately identified to include the title, author, and date of the document.

Forensic vignette #1 provides an example of how inconsistencies can be summarized in a written format when malingering should be obvious. Forensic vignette #2 illustrates the difficulty an evaluator may have when the examinee's presentation of potentially malingered symptoms is more subtle and complex.

18.5.1 Forensic vignette #1: data

Mr. Grove is a 49-year-old man charged with stalking and making terrorist threats against his ex-wife after she filed a restraining order against him following an incident of domestic violence. During his court-appointed evaluation for trial competency, Mr. Grove appeared very withdrawn and told the examiner that he was "hearing voices" and was "confused about his charges." Mr. Grove was found trial incompetent with a diagnosis of Major Depressive Disorder with Psychotic Features and subsequently transferred to a state hospital for competency restoration. Early during the first week of his hospitalization, he was noted to have an excellent appetite and to sleep eight hours a day without difficulty. He was observed to joke with staff and other patients and was quickly elected ward president where he assertively used the patients' rights advocate to assist himself and other patients in meeting their demands. In rehabilitation therapy groups, he was observed to excel at games involving complex cognitive strategies. Mr. Grove was also an active participant in competency to stand trial restoration groups and sometimes served as the substitute leader of the groups when a staff member was late or could not attend. However, whenever Mr. Grove was formally tested for trial competency by the unit psychologist, he suddenly acted very depressed, would cry, and told the psychologist that he just "didn't have the energy" to help his attorney. Mr. Grove also informed the evaluating psychologist that he was so depressed that he could not remember important aspects of his charges. He added that his "depression" interfered with his short-term memory, yet then recalled six specific examples of poor memory recall from that same day. A review of Mr. Grove's treatment chart revealed that as soon as he left his competency evaluation, he quickly engaged with peers and staff and was very animated. Four hours after his competency evaluation (where he had reported a severe lack of energy), Mr. Grove won the hospital dance contest. Mr. Grove also filed a civil lawsuit against the hospital for not providing him a stimulant medication which he claimed helped his "attention" and improved his ability to answer trial competency questions. His ex-wife forwarded to the hospital a series of letters that Mr. Grove wrote indicating his detailed knowledge of the legal system, his plan to fake trial incompetency and then insanity, and his desire to eventually be released from the hospital so that he could kill his ex-wife.

18.5.2 Forensic vignette #1: writing sample

Although Mr. Grove's presentation of depressive symptoms may leap out as an obvious case of malingering, it is nevertheless critical that the forensic report outline the specific evidence that supports a malingering finding. When considering the possibility of malingering in the written report, the evaluator should outline key inconsistencies in the patient's presentation. A brief outline of how these inconsistencies from the above vignette might be summarized reads:

> I carefully considered the possibility that Mr. Grove was suffering from a Major Depressive Episode with Psychosis that renders him incompetent to stand trial as noted by the prior court examiner. However, the available evidence indicates that Mr. Grove is presently malingering his depressive symptoms in accordance with his stated purpose to avoid criminal punishment so that he can eventually be released and kill his wife. Mr. Grove has numerous inconsistencies in his presentation that are characteristic of individuals who are malingering. Examples of such inconsistencies include the following:

> 1. Mr. Grove's verbal report that he has a markedly impaired short-term memory is inconsistent with his actual excellent short-term memory. For example, he told the evaluating psychologist that he "couldn't remember anything" about activities in which he was involved on the morning of his evaluation but then later cited an example when a staff member was precisely ten minutes late for a group therapy meeting that same day. During the psychological examination, he accurately pointed out all questions that had previously been asked during the evaluation.
> 2. Mr. Grove's report that he is clinically depressed is inconsistent with others' observations of him. Although Mr. Grove describes to competency evaluators that he is so depressed that he cannot concentrate on his legal trial or cooperate with his attorney, on the same day he makes these reports, he is observed to laugh and joke with others, to efficiently advocate for patients as ward president, and to win memory recall games in rehabilitation therapy.

3. Mr. Grove's behavior changes dramatically depending on who is observing him. For example, he suddenly becomes quiet with markedly slowed motor movements whenever the evaluating psychologist walks by him. As soon as this evaluator leaves the room, he resumes his outgoing interactions with others and is noted to smile and laugh.
4. Mr. Grove's reported depressive symptoms are inconsistent with how depressive symptoms typically present. His sudden onset and termination of depression is not consistent with the more slowly developing and resolving nature of genuine depression.
5. Mr. Grove's assertion that he is so depressed that he cannot concentrate on his trial or assist his attorney is inconsistent with his actual level of functioning. He has been actively engaged in filing civil lawsuits from the hospital and demonstrates excellent concentration in preparing his legal complaints and studying law books in the library.

18.5.3 Forensic vignette #2: data

Mr. Jones is a 24-year-old man who was hit by a car making an illegal turn when he was riding his motorcycle to work. Mr. Jones sustained significant physical injuries as a result of this accident, including a fractured pelvis and a broken left arm. Mr. Jones is suing the driver's insurance company claiming that he has severe emotional distress as a result of the accident.

During the evaluation, Mr. Jones reported that at the time of the accident he thought he was going to die and felt afraid and helpless. He stated that he continues to have nightmares of the accident that vary when compared with the actual accident. He described experiencing flashbacks of the accident. He added that he does not like riding in any motor vehicle, particularly as a passenger because he feels more loss of control if he is not the driver. Mr. Jones noted that he avoids conversations or thoughts about the accident and will not drive on the road where the accident occurred. Mr. Jones also reports, however, that he drives a car several hours a day because he must take his sister to college and do shopping errands for his aunt. He did not describe feelings of being detached from others or an inability to have loving feelings. He reported difficulty concentrating, hypervigilance, an increased startle response, and impaired sleeping as a result of his physical pain. He also reported that he has impaired concentration and short-term memory. In addition, Mr. Jones answered affirmatively to a series of symptoms extremely atypical for PTSD, including having the compulsion to look at a picture of his mother, going on sudden unexplained shopping sprees, and an impulse to check light switches.

During the mental status examination, Mr. Jones was very quiet and became tearful when talking about the accident. He was able to concentrate and focus throughout the six-hour examination without evidence of cognitive impairment. Mr. Jones stated that he has not sought mental health treatment because he has no insurance coverage or money to pay a mental health provider. A review of his past history indicates a chaotic family environment with significant depression in high school. As a teenager, he attempted to hang himself though the rope he tied broke. No family member was aware that he tried to commit suicide despite his having a brief period of unconsciousness. He has never had any type of mental health treatment and there are no collateral mental health records for review. He reported a significant history of alcohol dependence prior to the accident that consisted of numerous blackouts. His school transcripts prior to the accident repeatedly comment on his problems with concentration and significant academic difficulties.

Mr. Jones was administered three tests to assess possible malingering: the Miller-Forensic Assessment of Symptoms Test (M-FAST), the Structured Inventory of Malingered Symptomatology (SIMS), and the Test of Memory Malingering (TOMM). On the M-FAST, he scored a 12, which is significantly above the cut off score of six or greater that indicates malingering. On the SIMS, he scored a 33, which is significantly elevated above the cutoff score of 15 or higher that indicates malingering. On the TOMM, he scored 49 out of 50 on the first learning trial and 50 out of 50 on the second learning trial, indicating that he was not malingering memory deficits on this test.

18.5.4 Forensic vignette #2: writing sample

The vignette described above provides mixed information regarding Mr. Jones' presentation and the assessment of malingering. By self-report alone, he would likely meet the diagnostic criteria for PTSD. However, he also over-endorses symptoms that are atypical for PTSD. In addition, he scores relatively high on two tests of malingered psychiatric symptomatology but does not present as malingering on a test to assess his short-term memory complaint. The forensic report must address this disparity in information. One possible abbreviated opinion for this vignette is provided below.

> It is my opinion, with reasonable medical certainty, that if Mr. Jones is honestly reporting his mental health symptoms, then he meets criteria for Posttraumatic Stress Disorder as a result of the motorcycle accident. Mr. Jones was noted to be tearful when describing the accident and although he endorsed three atypical symptoms of PTSD, he did not over-endorse all genuine symptoms of PTSD. In contrast to his clinical interview presentation, Mr. Jones scored in the malingering range on two psychological tests designed to assess faking or exaggeration of symptoms. His responses on these assessments raise a legitimate concern that he may be feigning or exaggerating his reported mental health symptoms.
>
> Mr. Jones has also reported some difficulty concentrating and remembering. I did not find evidence during my six-hour evaluation that he had concentration and/or memory impairments. In fact, Mr. Jones had an excellent detailed recall for various aspects of his life. Mr. Jones has prior risk factors for impaired cognitive functioning, including heavy alcohol use and the hanging attempt with a loss of consciousness that he reported. In addition, a review of his school records notes marked academic impairment that predates his accident. Mr. Jones also told me that he had difficulty in school because of problems with remembering information.
>
> In summary, Mr. Jones described the onset of PTSD symptoms such as dreaming of the accident, avoidance of cues that remind him of the accident, and hypervigilance when driving or when around cars. Because he scored in the malingering range on two psychological tests assessing psychiatric symptoms, the accuracy of his reported psychiatric symptoms is very difficult to assess based on his self-report alone.

18.6 Summary

The guidelines outlined above are tools that can assist the expert in assessing and writing a forensic report that involves the consideration of malingering. To summarize, the evaluator should focus on how malingered symptomatology presents during the interview, acquire as many relevant collateral records as possible, interview as many relevant collateral contacts as feasible, and conduct psychological testing appropriate to evaluate the reported symptoms. The expert should utilize these multiple sources of information in the written report to examine potential inconsistencies and atypical aspects of presented psychiatric symptoms. Malingering assessments can be extremely challenging as malingering itself involves two opposite ends of the forensic spectrum: it is so easy to suspect, yet so difficult to prove.

References

American Heritage Dictionary of the English Language, 4th edn., s.v. "malingering." Retrieved July 6, 2009, from Dictionary.com website: http://dictionary.reference.com/browse/malingering

American Psychiatric Association (2000) Diagnostic and Statistical Manual of Mental Disorders, Fourth Edition, Text Revision. Washington, DC: American Psychiatric Association.

Asher, R. (1951) Munchausen's syndrome. Lancet 1: 339–341.

Cornell, D. G. & Hawk, G. L. (1989) Clinical presentation of malingerers diagnosed by experienced forensic psychologists. Law and Human Behavior 13: 375–383.

Delain, S. L., Stafford, K. P., & Ben-Porath, Y. S. (2003) Use of the TOMM in a criminal court forensic assessment setting. Assessment 10: 370–381.

Drob, S. L., Meehan, K. B., & Waxman, S. E. (2009) Clinical and conceptual problems in the attribution of malingering in forensic evaluations. Journal of the American Academy of Psychiatry and the Law 37: 98–106.

Eisendrath, S. J. (1996) When Munchausen becomes malingering: factitious disorders that penetrate the legal system. Bulletin of the American Academy of Psychiatry and the Law 24: 471–481.

Feldman, M. D. (1995) Illness or illusion? Distinguishing malingering and factitious disorder. Primary Psychiatry 2: 39–41.

Gacono, C. B., Meloy, J. R., Sheppard, K., & Speth, E. (1995) A clinical investigation of malingering and psychopathy in hospitalized insanity acquittees. Bulletin of the American Academy of Psychiatry and the Law 23: 387–397.

Gervais, R. O., Green, P. Allen, L. M., & Iverson, G. L. (2001) Effects of coaching on symptom validity testing in chronic pain patients presenting for disability assessments. Journal of Forensic Neuropsychology 2: 1–20.

Gold, P. B. & Frueh, B. C. (1999) Compensation-seeking and extreme exaggeration of psychopathology among combat veterans evaluated for posttraumatic stress disorder. Journal of Nervous and Mental Disease 187: 680–684.

Gold, L. H. & Shuman, D. W. (2009) Taking the high road: ethics and practice in disability and disability-related evaluations. In Evaluating Mental Health Disability in the Workplace, ed. L. H. Gould & D. W. Shuman. New York: Springer, pp. 1–24.

Hall, C. W. & Hall, C. W. (2006) Malingering of PTSD and diagnostic considerations, characteristics of malingerers and clinical presentations. General Hospital Psychiatry 28: 525–535.

Hamilton, J. C. & Feldman, M. D. (2001) "Chest pain" in patients who are malingering. In Chest Pain, ed. J. W. Hurst & D. C. Morris. Armonk, NY: Futura Publishing Co., Inc., pp. 443–456.

Hare, R. D. (1991) The Hare Psychopathy Checklist – Revised Manual. Toronto, ON, Canada: Multi-Health Systems.

Iverson, G. L. (2006) Ethical issues associated with the assessment of exaggeration, poor effort, and malingering. Applied Neuropsychology 13: 77–90.

Kucharski, L. T., Duncan, S., Egan, S. S., & Falkenbach, D. M. (2006) Psychopathy and malingering of psychiatric disorder in criminal defendants. Behavioral Sciences and the Law 24: 633–644.

Leavitt, F. & Sweet, J. J. (1986) Characteristics and frequency of malingering among patients with low back pain. Pain 25: 357–364.

Lilienfeld, S. O. & Andrews, B. P. (1996) Development and preliminary validation of a self-report measure of psychopathic personality traits in noncriminal populations. Journal of Personality Assessment 66: 488–524.

McDermott, B. E. & Feldman, M. D. (2007) Malingering in the medical setting. Psychiatric Clinics of North America 30: 645–662.

McDermott, B. E., Leamon, M. H., Feldman, M. D., & Scott, C. L. (2008) Factitious disorder and malingering. In The American Psychiatric Publishing Textbook of Psychiatry, 5th edn., ed. R. E. Hales, S. C. Yudofsky & G. O. Gabbard.

Washington, DC: American Psychiatric Publishing, Inc., pp. 643–664.

McDermott, B. E., Rabin, A., Scott, C. L., & Warburton, K. (2009) *Triaging the IST Patient: A Brief Screen to Reduce LOS.* American Academy of Psychiatry and the Law Annual Meeting.

Newmark, N. & Adityanjee, K. J. (1999) Pseudologia fantastica and factitious disorder: review of the literature and a case report. *Comprehensive Psychiatry* 40: 89–95.

Poythress, N. G., Edens, J. F., & Watkins, M. M. (2001) The relationship between psychopathic personality features and malingering symptoms of major mental illness. *Law and Human Behavior* 25: 567–582.

Resnick, P. J. (1995) Guidelines for the evaluation of malingering in posttraumatic stress disorder. In *Posttraumatic Stress Disorder in Litigation: Guidelines for Forensic Assessment*, ed. R. Simon. Washington DC: American Psychiatric Association.

Resnick P. J. (1997a) Malingered psychosis. In *Clinical Assessment of Malingering and Deception*, 2nd edn., ed. R. Rogers. New York: Guilford, pp. 47–67.

Resnick, P. J. (1997b). Malingering of posttraumatic disorders. In *Clinical Assessment of Malingering and Deception*, 2nd edn., ed. R. Rogers. New York: Guilford, pp. 130–152.

Resnick, P. J. (2000) The clinical assessment of malingered mental illness. In *Annual Board Review Course Syllabus*. Bloomfield, CT: American Academy of Psychiatry and the Law, pp. 842–866.

Rogers, R. (1986) *Conducting Insanity Evaluations.* New York: Van Nostrand Reinhold.

Rogers, R. & Payne, J. W. (2006) Damages and rewards: assessment of malingered disorders in compensation cases. *Behavioral Sciences and the Law* 24: 645–658.

Rogers, R., Harrell, E. H., & Liff, C. D. (1993) Feigning neuropsychological impairment: a critical review of methodological and clinical considerations. *Clinical Psychology Review* 13: 255–274.

Rogers, R., Sewell, K. W., & Goldstein, A. M. (1994) Explanatory models of malingering: a prototypical analysis. *Law and Human Behavior* 18: 543–552.

Slick, D. J. & Iverson, G. L. (2003) Ethical issues arising in forensic neuropsychological assessment. In *Handbook of Psychological Injuries*, ed. I. Z. Schultz & D. O. Brady. Chicago, IL: American Bar Association, pp. 2014–2034.

Slick, D. J., Tan, J. E., Strauss, E. H., & Hultsch, D. F. (2004) Detecting malingering: a survey of experts' practices. *Archives of Clinical Neuropsychology* 19: 465–473.

Spiro, H. R. (1968) Chronic factitious illness: Munchausen's syndrome. *Archives of General Psychiatry* 18: 569–579.

Tombaugh, T. N. (1996) *Test of Memory Malingering (TOMM).* New York: Multi-Health Systems.

Wiley, S. (1998) Deception and detection in psychiatric diagnosis. *Psychiatric Clinics of North America* 21: 869–893.

Yates, B. D., Nordquist, C. R., & Schultz-Ross, R. A. (1996) Feigned psychiatric symptoms in the emergency room. *Psychiatric Services* 47: 998–1000.

Youngjohn, J. R. (1995) Confirmed attorney coaching prior to a neuropsychology evaluation. *Assessment* 2: 279–283.

19

Psychiatry and ethics in UK criminal sentencing

John O'Grady

19.1 Introduction

This chapter describes an ethical journey undertaken by forensic psychiatrists in the UK. Until recently, general medical ethics had been assumed to be sufficient to guide the work of psychiatrists in court. Changes in legislation and, in particular, new, indeterminate, sentencing provision have forced the profession to review its ethical framework.

That ethical framework has to recognize the conflicting obligations facing psychiatrists when the psychiatrist's opinion can contribute to an outcome, for instance a longer sentence, which the person being assessed sees as contrary to their interests. Related conflicts can also occur at the pre-trial stage, however, when examining competency to stand trial. Nor are such conflicts confined to psychiatrists' encounters with the criminal law. A physician providing a report on their patient to an insurance company can reach a medical opinion that results in refusal of insurance. Civil commitment of psychiatric patients can result in commitment not necessarily for the patient's welfare but justified by protection of others. Public health physicians, occupational health physicians, and military doctors all routinely operate as dual agents in their clinical practice. Medical ethical frameworks have to be capable of addressing dual agency conflicts. Otherwise, many physicians will find themselves practicing outside of accepted ethical frameworks.

It is important to note also that laws permitting preventative detention are not exclusive to the UK. In Germany, life imprisonment can be imposed on offenders regarded as dangerous, potentially without parole (Van Zyl Smit 2006). Australian state statutes allow for indeterminate sentences based on future risk (McSherry et al. 2006). American states use a medical model of sexual deviance to justify the post-sentence detention of "dangerous" sexual offenders. Australian legislation uses a judicial rather than a medical model to achieve similar ends (McSherry et al. 2006). In all of these cases, however, psychiatric evidence on disorder and risk is central to legal decision-making.

19.2 Sentencing changes in the UK

In the UK, prior to 2003, case law governed the role of psychiatric evidence in cases where the court could impose an indeterminate sentence (for a summary and case references see O'Grady 2002, 2009). The judgments suggest that courts considered mental instability (not otherwise defined but usually interpreted to include both mental illness and abnormal personality traits) to be associated with risk to the public, especially where the disorder

---

The Psychiatric Report, ed. Alec Buchanan and Michael A. Norko. Published by Cambridge University Press. © Cambridge University Press 2011.

was thought likely to be long term. In cases where the court was concerned about mental instability and risk, psychiatric evidence was sought, not to address the welfare of a defendant, but to determine if there was evidence which would justify an indeterminate or longer than normal sentence. Where there was evidence of mental disorder and a hospital bed was available, however, courts usually chose hospital treatment over imprisonment.

With the passing of the Criminal Justice Act 2003 English criminal law was subjected to a radical overhaul. Defendants convicted of certain specified violent or sexual offenses can now receive an Indeterminate Sentence for Public Protection. Such a sentence comprises two elements:

- A fixed term of imprisonment representing the minimum to be served for punishment/retribution purposes.
- An indeterminate (i.e., life) sentence where release is dependent on a judgment that the offender no longer represents a significant risk to the public.

The court is obliged, by law, in passing such sentences to take account of the type of offense, antecedents of the offender, and patterns of social functioning and emotional life of the defendant. The court is guided by probation and medical reports. Psychiatric practitioners provide evidence to support or undermine the reasonableness of the risk assessment and presumption of dangerousness. Psychiatric reports are expected to address the issue of serious harm, risk, and dangerousness for the "guidance of the sentencing judge."

19.3 The background to the sentencing changes

Feeley and Simon (1992, 1994) would regard the Criminal Justice Act 2003 as an exemplar of what they have termed Actuarial Justice, or New Penology. In their terms Old Penology is based on "just desserts," that is, the appropriate punishment for a crime. Old Penology is based on the individual's guilt, responsibility, and obligations to society. Crime is seen as a deviant activity and the individual as being held responsible for deviant actions.

Actuarial Justice or New Penology is, by contrast, concerned with the containment of suspect populations based on actuarial assessment of the likelihood of offending. The emphasis is on profiling, preventative detention, and incapacitation. Feeley and Simon (1992, 1994) regard this change as rooted in societal attitudes which have been identified by Garland (2001) as:

- High crime rates are regarded as normal.
- Emotional investment in crime is widespread with fascination, fear, and resentment about offenders.
- Crime is highly politicized.
- Concern about victims and public safety dominates public discourse around offending.
- The criminal justice system (and by implication psychiatric community care) is seen as ineffective and suspect.
- Professionals are viewed as distanced from crime with attempts to understand difficult people rooted in their own elitism and lack of personal contact with crime.
- Reintegration of offenders is seen as unwelcome and unrealistic.
- Society exhibits a general willingness to bear the costs of rising penal numbers.

The aim is to identify high-risk offenders and manage those offenders by incapacitation, thus attempting to reduce the crime rate. The punishment is not based on "just desserts" but on a sentence that reflects an assessment of the offender's future potential for reoffending.

Hudson (2001) comments that offenders are then assessed as risk posing on the basis that they display "whatever characteristic the specialist responsible for the definition of preventative policy have constituted as risk factors." Offenders then become correctly incapacitated if risk factors have been correctly identified; not whether the individual will or will not reoffend. This gets around the problem of false positives as there is no need to verify predictions at an individual level when the policy objective is to correctly identify the right population to be incapacitated. The burden of proof is shifted to the offender, who has to prove that he or she no longer "dangerous" in order to firstly avoid the sentence and then to justify release.

As justice systems increasingly embrace actuarial justice, assessment of risk becomes the central issue and incapacitation of risk groups the policy objective. The forensic psychiatrist plays a central role in evidence to the court on mental disorder and risk. Mullen and Ogloff (2009), correctly in my view, justify risk assessment on the basis that "risk assessment finds its ultimate justification in risk management." In clinical practice, the risk assessment can be continuously re-evaluated as interventions for risk factors are implemented. However, in court, though the risk assessment will be presented in terms of probabilities, the court has to make an all or none dichotomous decision such as imposing an indeterminate rather than a determinate sentence. Especially when there is a low base rate for the behavior under consideration, which is usually the case for violence to others, false positives will be high.

Another way of putting this is that the confidence interval for any one risk evaluation is very wide (Hart et al. 2007). For example, in a group deemed to be at 50% risk of future violence, individuals within that group could vary from 25% risk to 75% risk. There is thus no way of accurately distinguishing the true risk of any one member of such a group, accuracy being possible only at the group level. All actuarial risk instruments are designed round a trade-off between high specificity and sensitivity. This leads Mullen (2007) to argue that "the margins of error in every actual or conceivable risk assessment instrument are so wide at the individual level that their use in sentencing, or any form of detention, is unethical."

Whilst the court may recognize the limitations of risk assessment and attendant ethical concern, nevertheless the court can legitimately argue that evaluation of risk for the mentally disordered falls outside the "common knowledge" of judge and jury (see below) and conclude that the psychiatrist is the only witness with the necessary expertise to inform them on questions of risk and mental disorder. In practice, this is the approach in the UK. Case law has determined that where a defendant is thought to have a mental disorder and the court is considering a sentence under the 2003 Criminal Justice Act, that court should hear psychiatric evidence. Australian law goes further, requiring psychiatric evidence when considering any defendant for an indeterminate sentence (McSherry et al. 2006). Whilst courts may be sophisticated enough to recognize the limitations of psychiatric evidence on risk, there is nevertheless a danger that preventative detention laws lead to an unhealthy alliance between psychiatrists and social forces that construe certain classes of criminal (i.e., the dangerous mentally disordered offender) as needing special forms of containment.

19.4 The ethical challenge posed by the changes

Stone (1984, 1994, 2008) questioned the moral underpinning of forensic psychiatry. He identified several hazards:

1. That psychiatrists might not have "true" answers to the legal and moral questions posed by law.
2. That psychiatrists might go too far and twist the rules of fairness and justice to help the patient.
3. That psychiatrists might deceive the patient in order to serve justice and fairness.
4. That psychiatrists might be seduced by the adversarial system and prostitute the profession.

Stone was concerned that psychiatrists lacked clear guidelines as to what was proper and ethical in forensic practice, guidelines that might help them to avoid these hazards.

Stone used the term "dual role" to describe the psychiatrist's role in a legal context. In Stone's view the roles of the physician and medical examiner for court were irreconcilable. Stone was troubled particularly that the defendant might be unable to distinguish the role of court expert from that of personal physician and that medical skills would then be being used, in effect, to seduce a patient into an inadvertent disclosure. The psychiatrist's therapeutic and empathic medical skills, which in a simpler doctor/patient encounter are designed to help the patient, would contribute to an outcome contrary to the patient's interests. Stone (1994) argued that once the encounter becomes in any way "therapeutic" doctors should excuse themselves from providing a report to the court.

Appelbaum's (1997, 2008) response to Stone's concerns emphasized the differences between the roles of clinician and evaluator. He suggested a more formal distinction, with a different set of ethical guidelines to assist the "forensicist." Mental health law in the UK, however, seems to make a dual role inevitable in three respects. First, courts can impose treatment in hospital as a sentence following a finding of guilt. Once the defendant is sentenced to hospital, the criminal justice system ceases to have any power over them and the patient's subsequent management is governed by health legislation and process. UK forensic psychiatrists effectively act as gatekeepers to health service facilities throughout the criminal justice pathway from the courtroom to prison.

Second, courts have available other sentences including indeterminate life sentences. Where there is mental disorder but no offer of a welfare disposal, the court can use the psychiatric evidence as part of the justification for the imposition of a longer than normal or indeterminate sentence. Before evaluation, the psychiatrist has no "a priori" means of determining whether the evidence will have a welfare benefit to the defendant or be used by the court to justify an indeterminate sentence. Third, as discussed in the previous section, psychiatrists in court may find themselves using their clinical skills, skills that involve monitoring with a view to therapeutic intervention, to make static predictions of questionable validity.

19.5 Response to the ethical challenge

19.5.1 A doctor is always a doctor

In assessing the proper response to the new law, the Royal College of Psychiatrists' (2005) starting point was that "psychiatry is a medical discipline and psychiatrists are first and foremost doctors, both in their technical training and in the ethical core within which they work." Pellegrino (1998) stated "medical ethics derives from the universal predicament of human illness, from the vulnerability, dependence and exploitability of those the physician attends. The aims of medicine are healing, helping, comforting and curing." Norko (2008) argues that compassion is similarly central to the practice of forensic psychiatry. It is difficult to see how a doctor can be other than a doctor when examining a defendant. A defendant, at least within UK culture, is likely at some level to consider that the doctor before them will consider their individual welfare. As already argued, the UK forensic psychiatrist's role in any case involves both legal and welfare evaluation.

19.5.2 Doctors have wider duties

The Royal College of Psychiatrists (2005) considered also the nature of the state's claim on psychiatrists. Human rights not only provide for the rights of individuals but also a right to be protected from harm that may arise from the action of others, including the mentally disordered. Psychiatrists may therefore legitimately argue that they have a duty to participate in procedures to provide that human right to be protected from harm from others. If it is accepted that the state has a legitimate right to scientific knowledge beyond the experience and knowledge of judge and jury, in an adversarial judicial system it is surely unjust for only one side to have access to evidence that is relevant. That argument would seem to preclude a solution to act only where there is a likelihood of welfare benefit to the offender (or only for the defense), one possible answer to the dual agent dilemma.

The Royal College report offered a public health argument to the participation of psychiatrists in indeterminate sentencing proceedings and put the argument thus:

> The core purpose of medicine is the identification and treatment, or at least amelioration, of human pain, disease and distress. For many medical conditions, it is convenient to consider the pathology as existing within the individual and to treat accordingly. However, for mental disorders, that disorder exists in the context of relationships, family, workplace and society. There is a known association (ignoring for the purposes of this argument any issues of causation) between mental disorder and violence. A violent act carried out in the context of mental disorder will have effects, not only on that individual, but upon their family, the victim, the victim's family and wider society. (Royal College of Psychiatrists 2005, p. 74)

The European Convention of Human Rights acknowledges this in recognizing that there is a human right to be protected from known risk from others. The Royal College report continues, "Is it therefore part of the core purpose of the medical specialty of psychiatry to identify, treat or, at least, ameliorate the effect of and consequences of violence associated with mental disorder? Some would argue that this approach would extend to the point of there being a public health perspective on the prevention of violence within populations of people who are mentally disordered." This is very close to the justification put forward for actuarial/preventative sentencing.

19.5.3 Limits to "wider duties"

To work ethically within this framework presupposes a just state. To deprive offenders of their liberty based on future assessment of risk to the public requires good quality evidence for its moral coherence which, in the case of mentally disordered offenders, can only come from high quality evidence from psychiatrists. Expert evidence to court in the UK is governed by a "common knowledge" rule which states that "an expert opinion is admissible to furnish the courts with scientific information which is likely to be outside the experience and knowledge of a judge or jury" (*R* v. *Turner*; also see O'Grady 2009). That same judgment went on to say, "Jurors do not need psychiatrists to tell them how ordinary folk who are not suffering from any mental illness are likely to react to the stresses and strains of life." Diagnosis, treatability, and risk assessments of offenders with mental disorder can be expected to fall outside the, "experience and knowledge of a judge or jury." Psychiatric evidence on offenders without mental disorder usually will not.

19.5.4 Contrast with developments in the United States

Any evaluation for treatment recommendations requires the examining psychiatrist to engage therapeutically with the offender/patient. From a UK perspective, the ethical debate in the United States seems focused on "pure" medical ethics and to pay insufficient attention to the wider perspective of the clinician's duties to the court and society. Furthermore it ignores the powerful influence of culture, social meaning, and politics. Forensic practitioners must understand their role within a cultural framework or narrative that recognizes the cultural factors relevant to the defendant's disorder, psychological state, belief systems, and in some cases experience of belonging to a non-dominant group in society (Griffith 1997, 2008). Zedner (2009) similarly says of expert testimony, particularly the technological application of risk assessment in the legal context, "While technology itself is neutral, it is shot through with social meaning, it is politicised and filtered through the cultural lens of those applying it in ways that technological determinism accounts belie."

19.6 Unresolved questions

Stone's (2008) most basic objection to the role of the psychiatrist in court is that the psychiatrist does not have true answers to the legal and moral questions posed by the law. This is by no means an issue just for medical experts. Courts recognize this issue and have sought to define the limits and usefulness of expert testimony more generally (for a detailed account see Hodgkinson & James 2007). Judgments in the English courts have identified three limbs for the admissibility of expert testimony in court:

- First, whether the expert evidence is beyond the "common knowledge" of judge and jury.
- Second, whether the expert's evidence "forms part of a body of knowledge which is sufficiently organised or recognised to be accepted as a reliable body of knowledge" and thereby of assistance to the court on matters beyond their common knowledge.
- Third, whether the witness has acquired by study or experience knowledge of the subject to render their opinion of value to the court.

Psychiatric evidence would seem to fulfill these three criteria but, as the courts themselves recognize, there are formidable problems with applying this reasoned and pragmatic approach to expert testimony. Thus, as one UK judge put it, astrologers possess a body of knowledge recognized by their fellow practitioners and have appropriate training and accreditation for their work. Nevertheless it is unlikely that a court would allow evidence that a particular constellation of the stars at the time of the offense robbed the offender of responsibility for their actions. How then is the court to decide whether the expert has scientific knowledge which the court can accept?

In the United States, the landmark case of *Daubert* v. *Merrell Dow Pharmaceuticals* established criteria that included that the body of knowledge can be tested, has been subjected to peer review and publication, has a known rate of error, is subject to maintenance of standards and controls, and is generally accepted by the scientific community. It is by no means clear how courts can undertake this task and UK courts have steered clear so far from a *Daubert*-type test. Instead, they have taken the approach that psychiatry is part of medicine and properly trained and informed psychiatrists do have a body of knowledge of assistance to the court. Nevertheless courts will have difficulty distinguishing between evidence that is properly informed by a recognized and accepted body of knowledge and evidence that is based on novel or controversial theory.

Stone sees psychiatric evidence as evidence that pertains to moral questions of responsibility and punishment. I agree with Grubin (2008) that this is a misunderstanding of the expert's role. Psychiatrists inform the courts of an individual's mental disorder and how that disorder may affect the thinking and behavior of the defendant. It is then for the jury to determine, with the judge's assistance, the moral implications of the findings. Psychiatrists should confine their evidence to their area of expertise, namely that of diagnosis, risk, treatability, etc. There is of course a real danger that a distinguished witness's aura of profound knowledge and arcane wisdom may overly influence the jury but that is a problem, however great it is, for the court and does not mean the psychiatrist has nothing true to say. There is a real danger too of bias when expert witnesses identify themselves with one or other party to the legal process.

I believe the moral issue here is not one of a basic boundary issue but one of professional governance. The task for psychiatry is to ensure that psychiatric experts are properly trained, and understand their role and the limitations of psychiatric evidence. Governing bodies and professional organisations should, through professional development, appraisal and revalidation, ensure that experts maintain throughout their career a high standard of practice. Courts in most jurisdictions use regulatory rules to this end. However helpful such court rules might be, the most powerful means of ensuring good quality evidence in court is through professional self-regulation. At a personal level this must mean a willingness to submit one's work to peer scrutiny and a willingness to tackle poor practice in one's colleagues, however distinguished the practitioner might be, through the regulatory bodies for the profession (in the UK, the Royal College of Psychiatrists and the General Medical Council).

19.7 Conclusion

One trainee in forensic psychiatry commented to me that, "life is a moral adventure and forensic psychiatry is for the particularly adventurous." One task for those writing in the fields of forensic practice and ethics should be to make the adventure less dangerous. In the UK context O'Grady (2002) proposed that forensic practice should be guided by principles drawn both from medicine (beneficence and non-malfeasance) and criminal justice (truthfulness, respect for autonomy, and balancing the distribution of benefits and risks for the patient and society).

How then is the ethical dual agent to proceed? I suggest:

1. Be aware that a doctor is always a doctor, but also of the different roles a doctor can adopt.
2. Act within a wide ethical framework that encompasses medical and justice ethics, recognizing that there will be conflict between these differing perspectives.
3. Consider whether one has a public health duty to consider managing the risk to others arising from mental disorder.
4. Understand the legal framework within which one practices including relevant court rules.
5. Act regularly for both defense and prosecution, ensuring that one provides the same opinion regardless of whether it is defense, prosecution, or court who commissions it.

At the same time be aware of inevitable subtle bias that will arise through interaction with the commissioning agent.

6. Act only within one's competence including ensuring that one has the necessary scientific knowledge and training to answer the court's questions.

7. Submit reports regularly to peer review and comply with the professional standards for continuing professional development (including, in the UK, relicensing of clinicians).

The forensic practitioner is first and foremost a member of society and then a member of a profession. Medicine is practiced within a social context. Individuals, and that includes doctors, are embedded within a complex social network of individuals, families, and communities with distinct cultural and historical backgrounds. Society, correctly in my view, expects medical knowledge to be utilized towards the advance of the general health of society (Pellegrino & Thomasma 2004; Pellegrino 2005). In this context Pellegrino and Thomasma (2004) state: "A truly dynamic philosophy of society recognises the necessity for continuously negotiating a struggle to balance individual and common good." Translated to forensic practice, there is a need to continuously negotiate a struggle between the welfare of the individual defendant, the legitimate needs of the court for expert testimony, and the public health argument that psychiatry has a duty to address the risk to others posed by individuals with mental disorder.

Criminal law is concerned with justice, fact-finding, and the attribution of guilt whilst psychiatry concerns itself with the welfare of the individual, their mental disorder, and its treatment. If one accepts the principle that courts have a legitimate right to psychiatric expertise on matters outside the "common knowledge" of judge and jury, then notwithstanding the formidable hurdles to ethical practice outlined by Stone (1994, 2008), psychiatrists have in my view a duty to participate in society's legal system. The dual agency dilemma is but one of a set of dilemmas that doctors face in their interaction with society. Whilst physicians must consider their patients' good, the same physicians are also bound to consider societal good and both have to be "sensed simultaneously" (Pellegrino & Thomasma 2004).

Do the arguments in this paper lead one full circle back to Stone's contention that forensic psychiatry is without an adequate ethical foundation? I do not think so. In other spheres of life, many situations are in conflict where one clear overarching ethical theory or framework is inadequate. Modern perspectives on ethics (for a particularly clear account, see Blackburn 2001) reject categorical ethical frameworks as inadequate to address the subtleties of moral decisions facing human beings. The approach by Beauchamp and Childress (2009), which expands medical principles of beneficence and non-malfeasance to include justice and respect for autonomy, is a good starting point. Such an ethical framework suggests practitioners should understand their dilemmas in the context of a set of interrelated ethical principles which at times will be in conflict with one another and where one principle does not override others.

I have found the approach termed narrative ethics (Martinez & Candilis 2005) to be particularly helpful as it offers an alternative framework, one in which professionalism and "disciplined subjectivity" do justice to the diversity of personal, societal, cultural, and professional perspectives which shape the forensic practitioner's ethical outlook. If there is a universal ethical principle that should guide our work then perhaps Norko's (2008) contention that compassion should be at the heart of our practice could fulfill that role. If embedded within the wider ethical framework offered by the cultural perspective of Griffith and the narrative ethics of Martinez and Candilis (2005), then Appelbaum's ethical principles of respect for others and truth-telling (1997) can become a central plank of an adequate ethical framework but as argued in this paper cannot by themselves adequately tackle the dual agency dilemma.

References

Appelbaum, P. S. (1997) A theory of ethics for forensic psychiatry *Journal of the American Academy of Psychiatry and the Law* **25**: 233–247.

Appelbaum, P. S. (2008) Ethics and forensic psychiatry: translating principles into practice. *Journal of the American Academy of Psychiatry and the Law* **36**: 195–200.

Beauchamp, T. L. & Childress, J. F. (2009) *Principles of Bioethics*, 6th edn. New York: Oxford University Press.

Blackburn, S. (2001) *Ethics: A Very Short Introduction*. Oxford: Oxford University Press.

Daubert v. *Merrell Dow Pharmaceuticals Inc.*, 509 US 575 (1993).

Feeley, M. & Simon, J. (1992) The new penology: notes on an emerging strategy of corrections and its implications. *Criminology* **30**: 449–474.

Feeley, M. & Simon, J. (1994) "Actuarial justice": the emerging new criminal law. In *The Futures of Criminology*, ed. D. Nelden. London: Sage.

Garland, E. (2001) Crime Complex: the Culture of High Crime Societies. In *The Culture of Control: Crime and Social Order in Contemporary Society*. Oxford: Oxford University Press, pp. 139–165.

Griffith, E. E. H. (1997) Ethics in forensic psychiatry: a cultural response to Stone and Appelbaum. *Journal of the American Academy of Psychiatry and the Law* **26**: 171–184.

Griffith, E. E. H. (2008) Stone's views of 25 years ago have now shifted incrementally. *Journal of the American Academy of Psychiatry and the Law* **36**: 201–205.

Grubin, D. (2008) Commentary: Mapping a changing landscape in the ethics of forensic psychiatry. *Journal of the American Academy of Psychiatry and the Law* **36**: 185–190.

Hart, S. D., Michie, C., & Cooke, D. J. (2007) Precision of actuarial risk assessment instruments. Evaluating the margins of error of group versus individual predictions of violence. *British Journal of Psychiatry* **190** (Supp 49): s60–s65.

Hodgkinson, T. & James, M. (2007) *Expert Evidence: Law and Practice*, 2nd edn. London: Sweet and Maxwell.

Hudson, B. (2001) Punishment, rights and difference: defending justice in the risk society. In *Crime Risk and Justice: The Politics of Crime Control and Liberal Democracies*, ed. K. Stenson and R. R. Sullivan. Cullompton, UK: Willan Publishing.

McSherry, B., Keyzer, P., & Freidberg, A. (2006) Preventative Detention of "Dangerous" offenders in Australia: a Critical Analysis and Proposals for Policy Development. Assessed at http://www.criminologyresearchcouncil.gov.au/reports/200405-03.pdf

Martinez, R. & Candilis, P. J. (2005) Commentary: Toward a unified theory of personal and professional ethics. *Journal of the American Academy of Psychiatry and the Law* **33**: 382–385.

Mullen, P. E. (2007) Dangerous and severe personality disorder and in need of treatment. *British Journal of Psychiatry* **190**: s3–s7.

Mullen, P. E. & Ogloff, J. R. (2009) Assessing and managing the risks of violence towards others. In *New Oxford Textbook of Psychiatry*, 2nd edn., ed. M. Gelder, N. C. Andreason, J. J. Lopez-Ibor Jr., & J. R. Geddes. Oxford: Oxford University Press, pp. 1991–2002.

Norko, M. A. (2008) Commentary: Compassion at the core of forensic psychiatry. *Journal of the American Academy of Psychiatry and the Law* **33**: 386–389.

O'Grady, J. C. (2002) Editorial: Psychiatric evidence and sentencing: ethical dilemmas. *Criminal Behaviour and Mental Health* **12**: 179–184.

O'Grady, J. C. (2009) The expert witness in the Criminal Court: assessment, reports and testimony. In *New Oxford Textbook of Psychiatry*, 2nd edn., ed. M. Gelder, N. C. Andreason, J. J. Lopez-Ibor Jr., & J. R.

Geddes. Oxford: Oxford University Press, pp. 2003–2008.

Pellegrino, E. D. (1998) Forum: Psychiatrists and the death penalty: some ethical dilemmas, Comment. *Current Opinion in Psychiatry* **11**: 5.

Pellegrino, E. (2005) The "telos" of medicine and the good of society. In *Clinical Bioethics, a Search for the Foundations*, ed. C Viafora. Dordrecht, Netherlands: Springer.

Pellegrino, E. D. & Thomasma, D. C. (2004) The good of patients and the good of society: striking a moral balance. In *Public Policy and Ethics*, ed. M. Boylan. Dordrecht, Netherlands: Kluwer Academic Publications, pp. 17–37.

R v. *Turner* [1975] QB 834 and 841.

Royal College of Psychiatrists (2005) The psychiatrist, courts and sentencing: the impact of expended sentencing on the ethical framework of forensic psychiatry. Council Report CR129. *Psychiatric Bulletin* **29**: 73–77.

Available at http://pb.rcpsych.org/cgi/content/full/29/2/73-a. Accessed June 9, 2010.

Stone, A. A. (1984) The ethical boundaries of forensic psychiatry: a view from the ivory tower. *Bulletin of the American Academy of Psychiatry and the Law* **12**(3): 209–219.

Stone, A. A. (1994) Revisiting the parable. Trust without consequences. *International Journal of Law and Psychiatry* **17**(1): 79–97.

Stone, A. A. (2008) The ethical boundaries of forensic psychiatry: a view from the ivory tower. *Journal of the American Academy of Psychiatry and the Law* **36**: 177–174.

Van Zyl Smit, D. (2006) Life imprisonment: recent issues in national and international law. *International Journal of Law and Psychiatry* **29**(5): 405–421.

Zedner, L. (2009) Fixing the future? The pre-emptive turn in criminal justice. In *Regulating Deviance*, ed. B. McSherry & S. Bronitt. Portland, OR: Hart Publishing.

Conclusion

Alec Buchanan and Michael A. Norko

Introduction

The psychiatric report serves as a focal point for many of the skills of forensic practice. Good report writing requires the ability to assemble and organize relevant material (see Chapter 2), conduct a psychiatric evaluation, understand the clinical condition of the subject of that evaluation, and relate clinical findings to the questions being asked. It requires an awareness of the needs of an audience and an ability to convey one's conclusions in language that a non-medical reader can understand. It also requires an understanding of the particular ethical tensions that emerge when employing clinical skills to non-clinical ends. For these reasons, the examination of the skills of forensic writing contained in this volume offers a perspective on forensic skills more generally. What themes have emerged? In particular, in which areas do the concerns of the authors collected here suggest avenues for future research in forensic psychiatry?

Narrative

All of the contributors to this volume have adopted a sequential structure to the psychiatric report, one that starts with scene-setting, continues with a narrative account of the material under discussion and ends with a conclusion. As Chapter 7 indicated, some others include a "preview" of their conclusions at the beginning of the report, but the preview is usually brief and the conclusion proper appears only after the background material has been presented. Griffith et al. (Chapter 5) suggest that even within this sequence there is room for substantial variation. In particular, their espousal of a series of different narratives, each true to the viewpoint of one or more actors but not necessarily consistent one with another, is an original departure that seems to require a response (see Appelbaum 2010).

First, it challenges those who adopt the traditional model to show that the process by which a single narrative is generated from a series of sometimes inconsistent reports can be a valid one, and is not inevitably distorted by the cultural and personal characteristics of the person writing the report. Second, by allowing each voice in the story to express not just their observations of what happened but their interpretations and moral judgments as well, the proposal would allow more information into the report, both factual and interpretative. It remains for proponents of the traditional model to show that this information is unlikely to be valuable or, at least, that its inclusion will be unlikely to improve the overall quality of the report.

Griffith et al.'s proposal also suggests avenues for its own further development. It raises the question of at what point the various disagreements between sources will be addressed, and how this will be done. The problem already arises in respect of factual disagreements. It would presumably become a much more common one if the value judgments of witnesses in criminal cases, for instance, are to be included in a report's narrative account.

The Psychiatric Report, ed. Alec Buchanan and Michael A. Norko. Published by Cambridge University Press. © Cambridge University Press 2011.

The conclusion of a criminal responsibility report, for instance, may make it clear that the authors do not share the view of a witness who noted that the act was cold and deliberate. Where is the disagreement to be discussed? And to what extent is it to be explained? Defendants' denials of events that obviously happened are often quoted without further comment, but doing justice to all of the voices in a report seems to require more than this.

Respect for persons

The obligation on the report writer to respect properly the subject has been a recurring theme of this volume. It is central also to US forensic psychiatry's response to the challenge that psychiatrists in court lack an ethical compass (see the Foreword; also Appelbaum 1990, 1997; Stone 1980, 1994). Ensuring respect for the subject is critical in other areas also. It requires a forensic reporter to take appropriate steps to protect a subject's confidentiality. It determines the content of the warning given to the subject at the start of a forensic evaluation, and the way in which that warning is presented. It is a central consideration when deciding whether or not to obtain the subject's permission before obtaining collateral information when the law does not require this. This is particularly the case when the source of that information is someone known to the subject. Finally, respect is a key consideration when deciding how much information, and of what kind, to include in the "Background" section of any report.

The centrality of respecting people to the work described here raises several, related, questions. One of the most intriguing is its relation to the subject's consent. Consent presumably permits many things to be done respectfully that would otherwise be disrespectful. But not everything. Even if the subject has given permission for the assessor to contact family members and include what they say in a report, for example, there is no reason to include embarrassing and irrelevant material (see Chapters 4 and 8). Just as the victim's consent is not automatically a defense to a charge of assault (see Shipley 2009; Chiesa 2011; *Laskey, Jaggard and Brown* v. *United Kingdom*), so a subject's consent does not seem always to be a defense to an allegation that the subject has been treated disrespectfully. Then there is the question of when consent is valid, and who should be able to give it when the subject's mental state prevents him or her from being able to give it. Those who lack decision-making capacity presumably deserve the same respect as other people, but their agreement seems to be a less reliable safeguard against their being treated disrespectfully.

There is also the question of timing. People change their minds, sometimes quickly. When consent has been sought and given, does a telephone call withdrawing that consent, received after an evaluation has been completed but before any report is submitted, change matters? Finally, there has been little discussion in the literature of what amounts to an adequate explanation for the purposes of obtaining consent. When risk is an issue and consent is sought to speak to a subject's family, it seems clear that the assessor should mention the possibility that they will describe past behavior that may count against the subject. But what of cases where risk is not initially an issue, but becomes one as a result of what a family member says? In US states where clinicians are obliged to breach confidentiality when they obtain details of child abuse, providing details of the relevant statutes to sex offenders in sentencing evaluations is common practice. But it is not common practice in other evaluations, where the same issues can arise (Kapoor & Zonana 2010). Should it be?

Integration and separation

Many of the preceding contributions emphasize the value of integrating the data presented in the report not just in, but before, the Opinion section. It quickly becomes apparent that this imposes a limit on the degree of structure that can be prescribed for the report. Thus a history of head trauma demands more attention to premorbid intellectual functioning and more detail in describing present cognitive function, both in the evaluation and in the report. Additional sub-headings may help the reader. Integrating information in this way can make obvious the assessor's diagnostic impression, thus previewing the Opinion section of the report. It is not clear that this is always a problem, and it may leave more space, literally and metaphorically, for the Opinion to address the legal issues. On the other hand, adopting this course requires some assumptions regarding the likely focus of legal interest and all assumptions involve a degree of risk. In some instances, assuming a diagnosis in the Background section of the report will be clearly inappropriate. Where a diagnosis is central, for instance, as with posttraumatic stress disorder in cases of alleged psychological damage, the evidence for and against will usually have to be gone through in detail in the Opinion section.

Ethics

Martinez and Candilis reflect that there can be no ethical report without ethical practice (Chapter 4). Which ethical questions has this volume suggested require further elucidation? The complicated role of consent as a guarantor of respect for persons has been discussed above. A related concern is the coercive environment in which consent to psychiatric evaluation is often provided. The criminal justice system provides the most graphic examples. Undergoing a psychiatric evaluation may be the only way of mounting a successful defense or of avoiding imprisonment. But plaintiffs in civil actions have little option but to participate in an assessment if they wish to pursue a claim that includes reference to psychological damage. And for suspended employees in fitness for duty cases a psychiatric evaluation may be their only way back to work.

Do these pressures require that particular safeguards be put in place to protect the subject, particularly the vulnerable subject? If so, is it the job of the person or authority requesting the evaluation to guarantee these safeguards, or does it fall to the forensic evaluator? If the answer to the latter question is "Both," are there situations in which the view of the authority requesting the report and that of the evaluator are likely to differ, and what is to be done then?

One setting in which these questions arise is the assessment of prisoners for sexually violent predator (SVP) commitment, as described by Pinals et al. (Chapter 10). The situation there is made more complicated by the fact that many of the statutes are relatively recent and commitment can be for life. The long-term implications for a prisoner of refusing to be evaluated cannot yet be clear, although it is likely that sufficient cases have now been adjudicated for most attorneys to feel able to advise their subjects. In practice, the refusal can apply only to certain aspects of the evaluation, such as the release of records and submitting to a psychiatric examination. Where an evaluator feels able to proceed, a limited assessment can be carried out without the subject's cooperation. Is this ethical? The question has to be answered with one eye on the possibility that if a majority of clinicians pull out the evaluations may simply be conducted by those with fewest ethical scruples. This seems less than satisfactory.

It is also the case that safeguards, if they make psychiatric evaluations less likely to happen, may be counterproductive. Ethical safeguards designed to protect prisoners may have reduced the amount of clinical research in prisons. Whether this has been to the benefit of prisoners seems debatable. Presumably some of that research would have looked at which treatments work best in a prison setting and the quality of prison health care in general, and prison psychiatric care in particular, would have risen. If ethical safeguards to prevent vulnerable potential subjects from consenting to evaluations that would not help them are appropriate, they should presumably be tailored to ensure that the same prisoners are not prevented from participating in evaluations from which they might derive benefit.

Underlying these questions is a more fundamental one. This asks whether traditional medical ethical principles are sufficiently broad and flexible to be applied to the practices of writing and testifying to someone's clinical condition in the variety of settings described in this book. A national, perhaps even a cultural, divide seems to emerge from the contributions contained here. Most of the arguments suggesting that the nature of forensic psychiatric practice makes traditional ethical principles insufficient come from the United States. Most of those that suggest the opposite, and advocate an ethical framework for forensic work that derives from the same principles that are evident elsewhere in medical practice, derive from other parts of the English-speaking world. The coming years will reveal whether this split widens or is resolved.

The role of professional organizations: clinical guidelines and peer review

One way in which medical ethics can affect forensic practice is through the activities of regulatory bodies and professional organizations. O'Grady (Chapter 19) argues that many concerns over inappropriate and low quality courtroom evidence can be addressed by professional organizations. Those organizations, after all, can choose who will become a member. They are in a position to ensure that anyone who does so has been properly trained. They can also contribute, with regulatory bodies, to ensuring that their members take appropriate steps to maintain their skills, and most have very significant roles in determining what form continuing education will take. Many in the United States, including the American Medical Association, the American Psychiatric Association, and the American Academy of Psychiatry and the Law, issue ethical and practice guidelines as well as participating in professional development.

In many ways, professional organizations are in a better position than the courts to achieve an object, the reliable production of ethical testimony, that both share. Professional organizations have a wider and deeper expertise than courts. They have available to them a wider array of sanctions: courts can do little beyond exclude testimony. They are in a position to help impaired physicians through re-training and mentorship. Finally, they can offer more general assistance through their contributions to improving clinical practice, for instance by providing the opportunity for expert testimony to be reviewed by peers. The involvement of professional organizations in ensuring standards of forensic practice also presents challenges, however. Concern has been expressed that the interests of the profession may be put before those of the courts or the public, for instance by restricting the types of evidence against fellow practitioners that will be deemed "ethical" in malpractice cases (see Appelbaum 2002).

Empirical research

Many aspects of psychiatric report writing can benefit from improved training and from the application of theories and principles, for instance in relation to ethics. Some aspects of that writing, however, seem able to benefit from empirical research also. Malingering is one example, where improvements in the resolution and availability of advanced neuroimaging techniques may allow the consequences of brain injuries, for instance, to be mapped with less reliance on the victim's description of symptoms. It may also be that interview-based empirical research will improve our understanding of the reasons that people give accounts of their symptoms that are inconsistent with the observations of others. Malingering can coexist with "real" symptoms (see Chapter 18). Presumably it can interact with them also.

Descriptive research may also be able to help refine the problematic concept of "reasonable medical certainty." Given the lack of clarity surrounding the definition of the term, it seems unlikely that all courts mean the same thing when they use it. As Chapter 16 points out, attempts to anchor a definition in clinical practice, or perhaps in evidence-based medicine, are unlikely to work for the simple reason that the term is not used there. It remains to be seen whether anything can be done to derive a consistent definition from the numerous conflicting suggestions. One way forward may be for professional organizations to develop guidelines addressing the level of confidence to be sought in evaluations for the courts, and the best way of articulating that level of confidence.

Conclusion

Just as the psychiatric report reflects the practices that generated it, so the questions raised by report writing reflect broader questions that derive from and affect forensic practice as a whole. Finding answers to these questions is partly a task for academic writing, empirical research, and books like this one. But it is also a task for practitioners and for the professional bodies that represent them. The answers to those questions will derive in part from the practice of psychiatry, but in part also from related professional disciplines and from academic fields outside medicine. Writing a psychiatric report is an exercise in synthesis. So is the task of improving the quality of report writing.

References

Appelbaum, K. (2010) Commentary: the art of forensic report writing. *Journal of the American Academy of Psychiatry and the Law* **38**: 43–45.

Appelbaum, P. (1990) The parable of the forensic psychiatrist: ethics and the problem of doing harm. *International Journal of Law and Psychiatry* **13**: 249–259.

Appelbaum, P. (1997) A theory of ethics for forensic psychiatry. *Journal of the American Academy of Psychiatry and the Law* **25**: 233–247.

Appelbaum, P. (2002) Policing expert testimony: the role of professional organizations. *Psychiatric Services* **53**: 389–390, 399.

Chiesa, L. (2011) Consent is not a defense to battery: a reply to Professor Bergelson. *Ohio State Journal of Criminal Law* 9(1), available at ssrn.com/abstract=1636537.

Kapoor, R. & Zonana, H. (2010) Forensic evaluations and mandated reporting of child abuse. *Journal of the American Academy of Psychiatry and the Law* **38**: 49–56.

Laskey, Jaggard and Brown v. United Kingdom (1997) 24 EHRR 39.

Shipley, J. (2009) Consent as defense to charge of criminal assault and battery. *American Law Reports* **58**: 662–665.

Stone, A. (1980) Presidential address: conceptual ambiguity and morality in modern psychiatry. *American Journal of Psychiatry* **137**: 887–891.

Stone, A. (1994) Revisiting the parable: truth without consequences. *International Journal of Law and Psychiatry* **17**: 79–97.

Index

Note: page numbers in *italics* refer to figures and tables

Printed in the United States
by Baker & Taylor Publisher Services